Social Media and Mobile Technologies for Healthcare

Mowafa Househ
College of Public Health and Health Informatics, King Saud Bin Abdulaziz University for Health Sciences, Saudi Arabia

Elizabeth Borycki
University of Victoria, Canada

Andre Kushniruk
University of Victoria, Canada

A volume in the Advances in Healthcare
Information Systems and Administration (AHISA)
Book Series

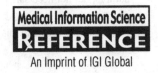

Managing Director: Lindsay Johnston
Production Editor: Jennifer Yoder
Development Editor: Austin DeMarco
Acquisitions Editor: Kayla Wolfe
Typesetter: Kaitlyn Kulp
Cover Design: Jason Mull

Published in the United States of America by
        Medical Information Science Reference (an imprint of IGI Global)
        701 E. Chocolate Avenue
        Hershey PA, USA 17033
        Tel: 717-533-8845
        Fax: 717-533-8661
        E-mail: cust@igi-global.com
        Web site: http://www.igi-global.com

                        Library of Congress Cataloging-in-Publication Data

Social media and mobile technologies for healthcare / Mowafa Househ, Elizabeth Borycki, and Andre Kushniruk, editors.
        p. ; cm.
  Includes bibliographical references and index.
  Summary: "This book provides insight on the tools that are integral to understanding and implementing emerging technolo-
gies in health-related fields"--Provided by publisher.
  ISBN 978-1-4666-6150-9 (hardcover) -- ISBN 978-1-4666-6151-6 (ebook) -- ISBN 978-1-4666-6153-0 (print & perpetual
access)
  I. Househ, Mowafa, 1977- editor. II. Borycki, Elizabeth, 1968- editor. III. Kushniruk, Andre W., 1958- editor.
  [DNLM: 1. Medical Informatics--trends. 2. Mobile Applications--trends. 3. Social Media--trends. W 26.5]
  R858.A2
  610.285--dc23
                        2014013792

This book is published in the IGI Global book series Advances in Healthcare Information Systems and Administration
(AHISA) (ISSN: 2328-1243; eISSN: 2328-126X)

British Cataloguing in Publication Data
A Cataloguing in Publication record for this book is available from the British Library.

For electronic access to this publication, please contact: eresources@igi-global.com.

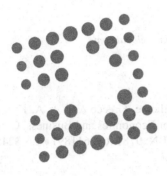

Advances in Healthcare Information Systems and Administration (AHISA) Book Series

Anastasius Moumtzoglou
Hellenic Society for Quality & Safety in Healthcare and P. & A. Kyriakou Children's Hospital, Greece
Anastasia N. Kastania
Athens University of Economics and Business, Greece

ISSN: 2328-1243
EISSN: 2328-126X

MISSION

The **Advances in Healthcare Information Systems and Administration (AHISA) Book Series** aims to provide a channel for international researchers to progress the field of study on technology and its implications on healthcare and health information systems. With the growing focus on healthcare and the importance of enhancing this industry to tend to the expanding population, the book series seeks to accelerate the awareness of technological advancements of health information systems and expand awareness and implementation.

Driven by advancing technologies and their clinical applications, the emerging field of health information systems and informatics is still searching for coherent directing frameworks to advance health care and clinical practices and research. Conducting research in these areas is both promising and challenging due to a host of factors, including rapidly evolving technologies and their application complexity. At the same time, organizational issues, including technology adoption, diffusion and acceptance as well as cost benefits and cost effectiveness of advancing health information systems and informatics applications as innovative forms of investment in healthcare are gaining attention as well. **AHISA** addresses these concepts and critical issues.

COVERAGE

- Role of Informatics Specialists
- Clinical Decision Support Design, Development and Implementation
- IT Applications in Physical Therapeutic Treatments
- E-Health and M-Health
- Telemedicine
- Medical Informatics
- Nursing Expert Systems
- IS in Healthcare
- Decision support systems
- IT Security and Privacy Issues

IGI Global is currently accepting manuscripts for publication within this series. To submit a proposal for a volume in this series, please contact our Acquisition Editors at Acquisitions@igi-global.com or visit: http://www.igi-global.com/publish/.

Titles in this Series

For a list of additional titles in this series, please visit: www.igi-global.com

Cloud Computing Applications for Quality Health Care Delivery
Anastasius Moumtzoglou (Hellenic Society for Quality and Safety in Healthcare, Greece & P. & A. Kyriakou Children's Hospital, Greece) and Anastasia N. Kastania (Athens University of Economics and Business, Greece)
Medical Information Science Reference • copyright 2014 • 342pp • H/C (ISBN: 9781466661189) • US $245.00 (our price)

Achieving Effective Integrated E-Care Beyond the Silos
Ingo Meyer (empirica, Germany) Sonja Müller (empirica, Germany) and Lutz Kubitschke (empirica, Germany)
Medical Information Science Reference • copyright 2014 • 332pp • H/C (ISBN: 9781466661387) • US $245.00 (our price)

Advancing Medical Practice through Technology Applications for Healthcare Delivery, Management, and Quality
Joel J.P.C. Rodrigues (Instituto de Telecomunicações, University of Beira Interior, Portugal)
Medical Information Science Reference • copyright 2014 • 361pp • H/C (ISBN: 9781466646193) • US $245.00 (our price)

Handbook of Research on Patient Safety and Quality Care through Health Informatics
Vaughan Michell (University of Reading, UK) Deborah J. Rosenorn-Lanng (Royal Berkshire Hospital Foundation Trust Reading, UK) Stephen R. Gulliver (University of Reading, UK) and Wendy Currie (Audencia, Ecole de Management, Nantes, France)
Medical Information Science Reference • copyright 2014 • 486pp • H/C (ISBN: 9781466645462) • US $365.00 (our price)

Research Perspectives on the Role of Informatics in Health Policy and Management
Christo El Morr (York University, Canada)
Medical Information Science Reference • copyright 2014 • 323pp • H/C (ISBN: 9781466643215) • US $245.00 (our price)

Cross-Cultural Training and Teamwork in Healthcare
Simona Vasilache (Bucharest University of Economic Studies, Romania)
Medical Information Science Reference • copyright 2014 • 326pp • H/C (ISBN: 9781466643253) • US $245.00 (our price)

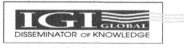

www.igi-global.com

701 E. Chocolate Ave., Hershey, PA 17033
Order online at www.igi-global.com or call 717-533-8845 x100
To place a standing order for titles released in this series, contact: cust@igi-global.com
Mon-Fri 8:00 am - 5:00 pm (est) or fax 24 hours a day 717-533-8661

Table of Contents

Section 1
Conceptual Frameworks and Models

Section 2
Overview of the Field

Section 3
Real Life Implementations and Cases

Detailed Table of Contents

Section 1
Conceptual Frameworks and Models

This section provides an overview of various conceptual frameworks and models used in the research and application of social media and mobile technologies in healthcare.

Chapter 1
    Eh Eh Tin, University of Tasmania, Australia
    Elizabeth Cummings, University of Tasmania, Australia
    Elizabeth Borycki, University of Victoria, Canada

Cummings, Borycki, and Roehrer (2013) developed a Consumer Perspectives Framework that identified a range of consumer-related issues and concerns that should be considered when downloading and using healthcare applications for mobile phones. The framework identifies data-related issues with mobile applications, such as ownership, location, completeness, corporate use, storage, and privacy. This chapter documents research undertaken in confirming the Consumer Perspectives Framework. Finally, the authors propose a method by which the Consumer Perspectives Framework can be implemented for use by consumers prior to downloading healthcare applications.

Chapter 2
    Haitham Alali, Ministry of Health, Jordan
    Juhana Salim, Universiti Kebangsaan Malaysia, Malaysia

The existing studies on online Communities of Practice (CoPs) in healthcare organizations have not adequately focused on the factors affecting KM initiative success and acceptance. Thus, establishing an evaluation framework has become essential for the advancement of research and practice in this area. In online communities of practice, the process of measuring and developing an evaluation framework has become quite complicated and challenging due to the intangible nature of the knowledge. Moreover, the lack of standards and studies, related to online CoPs measurements and evaluation frameworks, respectively, triggers the need for intensive studies in this area. In this context, this chapter reviews online CoPs success factors and identifies the gaps in our understanding. The authors classify the existing studies based on the area of evaluation, such as health and non-health domains. The chapter concludes by proposing a conceptual framework to measure the success of online CoPs in the healthcare sector.

Chapter 3

The use of mobile devices in healthcare is increasing in prevalence and poses different constraints for use than traditional desktop computing. This chapter introduces several usability testing methods that are appropriate for use when designing and developing mobile technologies. Approaching the development of mobile technologies through a user-centered approach is critical to improve the interaction and use of the hardware and software that is implemented on a mobile platform in healthcare. User-centered design adds value by getting feedback about functionality, design, and constraints that need to be built into the system prior to its completion. Future work in this domain will require further tailoring and use of novel usability methods to evaluate and improve the design of mobile healthcare technologies.

Chapter 4

Hand-held and mobile technology is steadily expanding in popularity throughout the world. Mobile technologies (e.g. mobile phones, tablets, and smart phones) are increasingly being used in Emergency Departments (ED) around the world. As part of this international trend towards introducing mobile technologies into the ED, health professionals (e.g. physicians, nurses) are now being afforded opportunities to access patient information and decision supports anywhere and anytime in the ED. In this chapter, the authors present a model that describes the current state of the research involving mobile device use in the ED, and they identify key future directions where mobile technology use is concerned.

Section 2
Overview of the Field

The focus of this section is on providing a high-level overview of the field of social media and mobile technologies in healthcare.

Chapter 5

This chapter presents the current state and outlines future directions in the possibilities of applying and exploiting social media in supporting healthcare processes. Starting from the abstracts of the Medicine 2.0 conference in 2012, the authors identify categories of application purposes for social media-based healthcare applications. The applications of social media tools and data are categorized into five groups:

1) supporting the treatment process, 2) for information gathering and prevention, 3) for networking and information exchange, 4) for knowledge management, and 5) for research and monitoring. Use of social media for information gathering and disease prevention is most prevalent. Existing applications mainly concentrate on supporting treatment of chronic and mental diseases. Technology is ready for supporting such applications. To go further in that direction, organizational and legal issues need to be addressed, including developing concepts for integrating with clinical information settings, establishing financing models, and ensuring security and trust.

Chapter 6

This chapter examines how the rapid diffusion of social media and Mobile Web is impacting personal healthcare management amongst those living with chronic disease. Despite a recent increase in research in this area (Moorhead, et al., 2013), evaluating the "social" still poses challenges to conventional notions of the "Internet empowered" patient and the best ways to support the management of chronic disease (Østbye, et al., 2005). The chapter argues that there is a need for advancing conceptual thinking on how health and IT are now interacting at the level of individual patients/citizens and how this is continuing to transform health professional-patient interactions (Glasgow, et al., 2008). By drawing on examples of e-health research, the chapter illustrates how notions of the "social" and "technology" have evolved over time from medically centred e-health through to patient-centred e-health. The chapter considers how this evolution may lead to a future focus on community-centred personal healthcare of chronic disease supported by "social" e-health tools, applications, and services that continue to blur the more conventional boundaries between health professionals, patients, and their social networks.

Unfortunately, many users are unaware of the risks and limits that arise from the use of health-related and medical apps in a medical context. Often, problems arise from insufficient, misleading, or false information, but they also arise from errors within the app or inappropriate hardware that is running on the app. Provided information is often inadequate to enable users to assess whether a medical or health app is reliable and safe. Laws and regulations that are meant to provide consumer safety (for patients and medical professionals alike) only apply to a limited number of apps with a specific medical purpose. For non-regulated apps used in a health context, there are various projects and initiatives, for example relating to app certification, but not all of these provide the information they collect about an app in a comprehensible and verifiable manner. The app synopsis presented in this chapter aims at alleviating the situation. The authors propose that manufacturers and developers use its clear structure for providing users with information about an app, ideally in a place where they commonly look (e.g. the app stores).

    Sharazade Balouchi, Sewanee: The University of the South, USA
    Karim Keshavjee, InfoClin Inc, Canada & University of Victoria, Canada
    Ahmad Zbib, Heart and Stroke Foundation, Canada
    Karim Vassanji, InfoClin Inc, Canada
    Jastinder Toor, InfoClin Inc, Canada

Consumer electronic healthcare applications and tools, both Web-based and mobile apps, are increasingly available and used by citizens around the world. "eTools" denote the full range of electronic applications that consumers may use to assess, track, or treat their disease(s), including communicating with their healthcare provider. Consumer eTool use is prone to plateauing of use because it is one-sided (i.e., consumers use them without the assistance or advice of a healthcare provider). Patient eTools that allow patients to communicate with their healthcare providers, exchange data, and receive support and guidance between visits is a promising approach that could lead to more effective, sustained, and sustainable use of eTools. The key elements of a supportive environment for eTool use include 2-way data integration from patient home monitoring equipment to providers and from provider electronic medical records systems to patient eTools, mechanisms to support provider-patient communication between visits, the ability for providers to easily monitor incoming data from multiple patients, and for provider systems to leverage the team environment and delegate tasks to appropriate providers for education and follow-up. This is explored in this chapter.

Section 3
Real Life Implementations and Cases

This section includes real implementation examples from the field of social media and mobile technologies in healthcare.

    Mary Schmeida, Kent State University, USA
    Ramona McNeal, University of Northern Iowa, USA

Increasingly, the healthcare burden of an aging population in the United States is being "relieved" through family members caring for aging and ill loved ones at home. Today, families are turning to mobile technology to lessen their burden and to cope with the stress of caring for loved ones through activities ranging from healthcare information searches to social interactions with online health communities. The purpose of this chapter is to analyze factors predicting the characteristics and context of the U.S. home caregiver population. In addition, this chapter explores how mobile technologies are helping to mitigate some of the weight placed on the family caregiver. The authors explore these questions using multivariate regression analysis and individual level data from the Internet and American Life Project. The findings suggest that interaction with others in online support groups may be more important for the e-caregiver than other online activities.

Continuing professional development is mandatory for all healthcare professionals in Australia. This chapter explores how the expectations of the regulatory and professional organisations of nursing and midwifery can be integrated within the profession by enrolled and registered nurses and midwives to meet the requirements and maintain their registrations. Using actual case studies as a basis, the chapter demonstrates how continuing professional development can be delivered as mobile or m-learning using social media or mobile technologies within this health profession. This chapter focuses on case studies from the Australian healthcare sector; however, it appears that similar issues arise in other countries and so the challenges and solutions described in the case studies can inform practice in other countries. It concludes by discussing the potential for continuing professional development m-learning into the future.

An anticipated research activity in healthcare is the involvement of populations and social media to identify health problems, including environmental ones. In this chapter, the authors propose an Android mobile-based system for collection and targeted distribution of the latest alerts and real-time environmental factors to the Malaysian population. This mobile system is designed to facilitate and encourage research into environmental health quality issues by providing a comprehensive tracking and monitoring tool correlated to social media networks. This system is embedded with Google Maps and Geocoding services to visualize the location and environmental health reports from the aggregated social media news feeds; the output is also shared across the social media networks.

Chapter 12

Prompt and efficient access to patient records is vital in providing optimal patient care. The Cancer Agency Information System (CAIS) is the primary patient record repository for the British Columbia Cancer Agency (BCCA) but is only accessible on traditional computer workstations. The BCCA clinics have significant space limitations resulting in multiple healthcare professionals sharing each workstation. Furthermore, workstations are not available in examination rooms. A novel and cost-efficient solution is necessary to improve clinician access to CAIS. This prompted the BCCA and the Provincial Health Services Authority (PHSA) Information Management Information Technology Services (IMITS) team to embark on an innovative provincial collaboration to introduce and evaluate the impact of a mobile device to improve access to CAIS. The project consisted of 2 phases with over 90 participants from multiple clinical disciplines across BCCA sites and other PHSA facilities. Phase I evaluated the adoptability, effectiveness, and costs associated with providing access to CAIS using desktop virtualization via Citrix. Citrix is a server solution that provides remote access to clients via the Web or to dummy terminals in a network. Phase II incorporated the feedback and findings from Phase I to develop a customized mobile application. Phase II also addressed privacy and security requirements and included additional users and workflows. This is explored in this chapter.

Chapter 13

This chapter outlines the recent advances in self-tracking technology both for wellness and healthcare purposes. It addresses one of the key challenges in mobile health: how to link the data from self-tracking devices with data in clinical data systems, such as Personal Health Records and Electronic Health Records systems. This chapter also discusses advances in visualisation and analysis for personally controlled data from self-tracking and PHR systems.

Chapter 14

The aim of this chapter is to highlight the current issues and the challenging process of the adoption of social media by Italian local health authorities (ASL). After a literature review of the role of social media for health organizations, the authors focus their attention on how social network sites are modifying health communication and relations with citizens in Italy. They conduct an exploratory study articulated in three stages: after mapping the presence of local health authorities on the most popular social media platforms (Facebook, Twitter, YouTube), they carry out a content analysis to describe the prevalent kinds of messages published in the official Facebook timelines; in the third phase, using several interviews with healthcare directors and communications managers, the authors investigate implementation issues, managerial implications, and constraints that influence proper use of these participative platforms by Italian public health organizations. Limitations and further steps of the research are discussed.

This chapter explores the effects of social media in influencing the behavior of young people in relation to HIV/AIDS. The platform used for the project is an online discussion forum. The study is a One Group Pretest and Posttest inquiry. Formative evaluation is performed at the beginning of the study to establish participants behaviour, the intervention is introduced, then a summative evaluation is done to find out whether the intervention had any effect on the behaviour of the participants. The findings of the study indicate that there is a significant change in the behaviour of participants in relation to HIV/AIDS due to the use of the online forum. The study recommends that more efforts need to be directed to the use of various technologies that young people have at their disposal in the fight against HIV/AIDS as this can be very economical and effective.

Section 4
Challenges and Issues

This section focuses on the various challenges and issues facing the use of social media and mobile technologies in healthcare.

Consumers' access to their health records is increasing, and one of the ways they can gain access and potentially contribute to their records is by using a mobile Personal Health Record (mPHR). mPHRs emerged as a combination of mHealth and Personal Health Records (PHRs). Despite the current shortage of evidence supporting mPHR use, these systems are already being deployed, and examples of currently available mPHRs are provided. mPHRs have an array of potential uses and different target user groups, but there are also several challenges impeding their success. The physical constraints of mobile devices, health literacy, and usability all create obstacles for mPHRs. However, mPHRs create opportunities due to the affordances of mobile devices and the potential to integrate consumer mHealth applications. The challenges and opportunities of these nascent systems are outlined in this chapter, as they inform research topics with respect to mPHRs.

Chapter 17

Tridib Bandyopadhyay, Kennesaw State University, USA
Bahman Zadeh, Kennesaw State University, USA

ICT technologies like the Internet, mobile telephony, and other enabled handheld gadgets have penetrated our lives in an unprecedentedly disruptive fashion. Explosive computing and communicating power with ever-decreasing price of service over the passage of time have been the hallmark of this success. The success of these technologies has been effectively appropriated in many business processes and systems including the banking sector and the social media applications. However, in spite of having stupendous potential in the healthcare sector, especially in providing access to service for patients in rural and difficult-to-reach areas, very limited ICT appropriation has been witnessed. The authors explain the current extent of ICT penetration and seek reasons for such lackluster inclusion of ICT and mobile technology in the healthcare sector. They use the TAM model to identify the critical factors of technology adoption, and use such understandings to help readers understand the barriers of adoption of ICT and mobile technologies in the healthcare sector. The authors also provide indicative guidelines about how such barriers may be overcome, and widespread adoption and deployment of these technologies can be made possible in the healthcare sector, yielding benefits to large sections of population in the US.

Foreword

Within the first decade-and-a-half of the 21st century, we have lived through little short of a revolution in the ways in which many people, in many parts of the world, obtain information and interact with each other (whether they be on opposite sides of the world or within the same room). Not only has the reality of such interactions changed rapidly, but so have people's expectations, such that individuals from all age groups (not just Generation Y and their successors) have an expectation of "always on" Internet access, instant responses, and being able to find any information at the push of a button or swipe of a touchscreen – to such an extent that many exhibit signs akin to drug withdrawal symptoms if they are unable to do these things for even a short period.

However, while the increasing ubiquity of smart portable devices (such as smartphones, tablets, and similar devices that increasingly bridge the divide), of fast and "always on" Internet access, and social media applications have altered the ways in which many of us perform many common activities, from booking flights, holidays, hotels and restaurants, accessing news, consuming films and other "broadcast" media, they have had less impact on the ways in which most people access health services. It is only as people's expectations have changed (if I can almost instantly book a hotel on the far side of the world online, they ask, then why can't I book my doctor on the next street?) that we have seen the health services in many countries slowly begin to realise the potential and provide such services. Health services have long been seen by many as slow adopters of new technologies – and they seem, so far, to have been little different in terms of adopting, and adapting to, the challenges afforded by people's expectations of their uses of social media and new technologies. Using new technologies to do things in different ways is, though, only one aspect of the ways in which social media, and the "always connected" potential of mobile devices, is changing people's modes of communication and interaction. Crowdsourcing of opinion, for example through popular restaurant and hotel review sites, is used by many to choose where to eat and stay, and similar sites are being used, albeit slowly at present, to review people's experiences of healthcare provision.

Much of the literature to date and many conference presentations on the use of social media and mobile technologies, however, have been and tend to remain at the level of opinion and even "hype," and there exists a lack of demonstrated evidence from scientific work on the real benefits and impact of using new tools and technologies. Perhaps it is, to some degree, not surprising that we lack a substantive scientific literature at present. After all, many of the popular social networking tools are less than 10 years old, and more specialised variants for specific health purposes are even more recent. LinkedIn was launched in 2003, Facebook in 2004, and Twitter in 2006, while among the iconic mobile devices, the iPhone was launched in 2007 and the iPad in 2010. Given the typical timeline from conception to publication of rigorous funded and peer-reviewed scientific studies, we are only now beginning to see published results from health professionals and researchers who have explored the reality of using such new tools.

This volume begins to fill the gap, and hopefully will be an early example of a new era of research-based evidence for whether we can actually see significant benefit, behaviour change, or health impacts from the use of social media and mobile technologies in healthcare. As the editors note in their Preface, four main themes are addressed, each in itself important, but taken together help to introduce examples of the work that increasingly needs to be undertaken: 1) conceptual frameworks and models; 2) overview of the field; 3) real life implementations and cases; and 4) challenges and issues in social media and mobile technologies in healthcare. In addition to being useful for students, the 16 chapters will also provide food for thought for educators and researchers, and hopefully stimulate more exploration of the current status and issues surrounding the use of social media and mobile technologies in healthcare.

We are still in the early days of what we recognise as social media. One thing that we can be sure of is that the landscape will change increasingly rapidly. We will see the emergence of new social media applications – some may be designed specifically for health use, especially with the growing impact of citizens and patients driving both healthcare and health promotion, but more often we are likely to see the adaptation of more generic tools to health-related uses. We cannot be sure that some of the behemoths of the modern social media landscape will still be with us in 10-15 years, unless they adapt to the new and innovative uses to which they will undoubtedly be put; if they do not adapt, then others will rapidly fill the void. We will also likely see the emergence of new approaches to research into their use, perhaps based in more collaborative models of care and research, and almost certainly driven by the focus of citizens and patients, rather than the often-esoteric interests of traditional healthcare researchers. New research approaches will certainly need to be more agile, producing meaningful findings far more quickly than traditional methods.

It is also increasingly likely that the non-traditional and unexpected technology actors and providers will have an impact on the future, at least in respect of some areas of health and wellbeing promotion and provision; some of these may also impact traditional providers and be adopted by hospitals and other providers of institutional healthcare. At the time of writing this, the first glimpses and rumours are emerging of Apple's new HealthBook App – will it be a game-changer, as so many Apple products have been, or will it be consigned to the dustbin of history along with Google Health? Only time will tell, but we can be certain that we will be living in very interesting times.

Might the combination of social media tools and approaches, together with mobile technologies, provide us, sometime in the near future, with the wherewithal to make a genuine contribution towards helping people achieve the goal of health as a state of complete physical, mental, and social well-being and not merely the absence of disease or infirmity, as defined by the World Health Organization? On their own, no technologies can achieve this, but if they can provide better ways of supporting access to and sharing knowledge, then social media and mobile technologies may speed the achievement of these goals. The examples of real use that are explored in this volume provide a valuable starting point from which to change health and healthcare for the better, for the benefit of all.

Peter J. Murray
International Medical Informatics Association (IMIA), Germany

Peter J. Murray *is currently CEO of the International Medical Informatics Association (IMIA), an international not-for-profit association that acts as a bridging organisation, bringing together constituent health and medical informatics societies and their members. He worked in the health services (NHS) in the United Kingdom as a coronary/cardiac care nurse before moving into nurse education, where he worked in several Schools of Nursing, and for The Open University in the UK, where he developed distance and online educational materials for nurses and other health professionals. He is a Fellow and Chartered Information Technology Professional of the British Computer Society.*

Preface

Social Media and Mobile Technologies in healthcare is an evolving topic area within both the healthcare and information technology domains. Thousands of mobile health (mHealth) applications exist on the market today targeting a variety of health consumer/patients, clinicians, and academics. MHealth applications exist for health education, self-management, monitoring, health promotion, and other uses. For years, there has been a disconnect in the literature between the field of mHealth and social networking for healthcare. Much of the literature on mHealth has focused on interventions at the individual level without considering the influence of group social interactions and their impact on behavioral change. Recently, there has been an increase in mHealth applications that incorporate social networking elements to promote healthy group behavior. Nevertheless, the field remains in its infancy, with few frameworks, models, or definitions for the integration of social networking into mHealth applications. The use of social networking in mHealth applications will shift the focus from the individual's attempts to modify or monitor their health to group support of the individual through social networking via mHealth software and hardware. Consequently, individuals will receive differing levels of support from groups of people, which may result in improved health. The impetus behind this book is to promote the use of social networking within mHealth applications, which is a field referred to as Mobile Social Networking in Healthcare (MSNET-Health).

Due to the book being grounded in current research, it can be used for graduate courses in health informatics, healthcare policy, health management, medicine, and other health professional courses. The book will play a role in helping students to understand the various frameworks, models, challenges, and real life applications of social media and mobile technologies in healthcare.

The book is organized into 17 chapters that address the topic of social media and mobile technologies in healthcare. The book addresses innovative concepts and critical issues from various parts of the world including the United States of America, Canada, Australia, Germany, Italy, Malaysia, Jordan, and Botswana. This represents the international character of the book, which is an indication of growth in the topic and its importance globally.

The 17 chapters are organized into 4 overall themes: 1) conceptual frameworks and models; 2) overview of the field; 3) real life implementations and cases; and 4) challenges and issues in social media and mobile technologies in healthcare. Four chapters discuss the first theme of conceptual frameworks and models. Chapter 1, "Review of the Consumer Perspective Framework for Healthcare Applications," discusses a range of issues and concerns that should be considered when downloading mHealth applications. Chapter 2, "Success Dimensions of the Online Healthcare Communities of Practice: Towards an Evaluation Framework," provides an overview of the use of social media technologies by health communities of practice. Chapter 3, "Incorporating Usability Testing into the Development of Healthcare

Technologies," concentrates on providing a model for understanding of how use-centered design processes can be incorporated into the design and development of mobile applications. Chapter 4, "Mobile Technologies in the Emergency Department: Towards a Model for Guiding Future Research," presents a model that describes the current state of research in using mHealth technologies in the emergency department.

The second theme of the book focuses on various review papers that represent a high-level view of social media and mobile technologies in healthcare. Chapter 5, "Use Cases and Application Purposes of Social Media in Healthcare," examines the role of social media in healthcare and the various possibilities it presents. Chapter 6, "The Past, the Present, and the Future: Examining the Role of the 'Social' in Transforming Personal Healthcare Management of Chronic Disease," argues for the need to advance conceptual thinking on how health and IT are now interacting at the level of patients and citizens. Chapter 7, "Synopsis for Health Apps: Transparency for Trust and Decision Making," centers on developing a case for the formation of a clear structure for the providing credible and trustworthy information on the use of mHealth applications. Chapter 8, "Creating a Supportive Environment for Self-Management in Healthcare via Patient Electronic Tools," reviews "eTools" for the assessment, tracking, and treatment of diseases.

The third theme focuses on real cases where social media and mobile technologies have been implemented in healthcare. Chapter 9, "Online Health Information: Home Caregiver Population Driving Cyberspace Searchers in the United States," examines the use of social media and mobile technologies in healthcare in relation to aging. Chapter 10, "Nurses Using Social Media and Mobile Technology for Continuing Professional Development: Case Studies from Australia," looks at the use of social media and mobile technologies for continuing professional education in Australia. Chapter 11, "An Android Mobile-Based Environmental Health Information Source for Malaysian Context," provides an overview of a mHealth application that is used to visualize location and environmental health reports from aggregated social media feeds in Malaysia. Chapter 12, "The Introduction and Evaluation of Mobile Devices to Improve Access to Patient Records: A Catalyst for Innovation and Collaboration," discusses the authors' work in providing access to the British Columbia Cancer Agency Information System through mobile devices. Chapter 13, "Analysis and Linkage of Data from Patient-Controlled Self-Monitoring Devices and Personal Health Records," discusses the current landscape of self-tracking devices and examines how the data collected from such devices could be integrated into the clinical health record of the patient or consumer, thereby making the data more useful for management of chronic conditions and maintaining good health. Chapter 14, "Social Media for Health Communication: Implementation Issues and Challenges for Italian Public Health Authorities," analyses the official communication of healthcare organizations within Italy. Chapter 15, "Social Media in Promoting HIV/AIDS Prevention Behavior among Young People in Botswana," explores the impact of social media on influencing the behavior of young people in relation to HIV/AIDS.

The fourth and final theme of the book focuses on the upcoming challenges for mHealth and social media technologies. Chapter 16, "Personal Health in my Pocket: Challenges, Opportunities, and Future Research Directions in Mobile Personal Health Records," discusses the various challenges and opportunities and future research for the development, implementation, and use of mobile personal health records. The final chapter, Chapter 17, "Mobile Health Technology in the US: Current Status and Unrealized Scope," reviews the challenges associated with implementing mobile technologies in healthcare institutions in the United States of America.

Mowafa Househ
College of Public Health and Health Informatics, King Saud bin Abdulaziz University for Health
Sciences, Saudi Arabia

Elizabeth Borycki
University of Victoria, Canada

Andre Kushniruk
University of Victoria, Canada

Acknowledgment

This work could not have been carried out without the dedication of the authors who have spent hours reviewing, updating, and writing their book chapters for this important text that will hopefully be the first of its kind in exploring the role of social media and mobile technologies in healthcare. We appreciate the originality, comprehensiveness, and professionalism of their work. We also acknowledge the work of the reviewers and appreciate all of their effort.

In addition, we would like to thank the College of Public Health and Health Informatics at King Saud Bin Abdulaziz University for Health Sciences and the School of Health Information Science, University of Victoria for their support of this work.

Mowafa Househ
College of Public Health and Health Informatics, King Saud bin Abdulaziz University for Health
   Sciences, Saudi Arabia

Elizabeth Borycki
University of Victoria, Canada

Andre Kushniruk
University of Victoria, Canada

Section 1
Conceptual Frameworks and Models

This section provides an overview of various conceptual frameworks and models used in the research and application of social media and mobile technologies in healthcare.

Chapter 1
Review of the Consumer Perspective Framework for Healthcare Applications

Eh Eh Tin
University of Tasmania, Australia

Elizabeth Cummings
University of Tasmania, Australia

Elizabeth Borycki
University of Victoria, Canada

ABSTRACT

Cummings, Borycki, and Roehrer (2013) developed a Consumer Perspectives Framework that identified a range of consumer-related issues and concerns that should be considered when downloading and using healthcare applications for mobile phones. The framework identifies data-related issues with mobile applications, such as ownership, location, completeness, corporate use, storage, and privacy. This chapter documents research undertaken in confirming the Consumer Perspectives Framework. Finally, the authors propose a method by which the Consumer Perspectives Framework can be implemented for use by consumers prior to downloading healthcare applications.

INTRODUCTION

The ubiquity of mobile phone accessibility around the world is increasing. Worldwide the number of mobile phones in use grew from fewer than 1 billion in 2000 to around 6 billion in 2012. Recent estimates conclude that over 75% of the world's population have access to a mobile phone (World Bank, 2012). Globally, there has been a rapid rise

in the use of smart phones by consumers with over 1 billion Smart Phones subscribers (Approximately 30% of smartphone users are likely to use wellness apps by 2015, (Bjornland, Goh, Haanæs, Kainu, & Kennedy, 2012) with more than 30 billion mobile applications being downloaded in 2011 (World Bank, 2012).

Along with this increase in penetration, there has been a significant increase in the development

DOI: 10.4018/978-1-4666-6150-9.ch001

and deployment of mobile software applications across multiple computing platforms (e.g. smart phones, tablets and laptops). The most popular of these include Apple's iOS and Google's Android software. Both were designed for use with touch screen mobile devices such as iPhones. Today, there are a plethora of differing types of software applications that have been made available for use with the iOS and Android platforms. Software applications written for mobile or smart phones serve a range of purposes and uses, including; business, financial, educational, entertainment, gaming, lifestyle, health and fitness, news, music, photography, productivity, reference, graphics and design, developer tool, medical and health care consumer applications.

More recently, there has emerged significant interest in health care applications written for mobile phones. Mobile phone software applications are of particular interest because of their ability (in some cases) to improve lifestyle habits in well individuals and improve health outcomes in the chronically ill (Katz, Mesfin, & Barr, 2012).

In conjunction with this there has emerged a significant growth in the number of consumers that are downloading these health specific software applications for self-use (Kay, Santos, & Takane, 2011). Research suggests that mobile phone users use differing types of software applications in conjunction with their smart phones and their use of specific software applications may be role dependent. For example, research has found that physicians and other health care professionals tend to use mobile health applications that differ from those used by patients or members of the general public. Physicians and health professionals are more likely to use mobile software applications that provide them with access to references to health care information (e.g. guidelines, information found in journal articles). These applications provide information to health professionals (i.e. they allow health professionals to review evidence-based research) that can be used in their clinical decision making. Unlike

health care consumers that input data into mobile health applications, health professionals are less likely to employ mobile applications in the process of collecting data about patients. This may be because health professionals may perceive there to be privacy and security issues associated with collecting, transmitting and storing patient data via a mobile device (Jones, Hook, Park, & Scott, 2011). As well, mobile phone applications present a potential risk for public health as some software applications have been questioned in regards to their clinical efficacy and other such software applications have been noted to induce technology-induced errors. Technology induced errors are errors made by software/hardware users that "arise from the: design and development of a technology; implementation and customisation of a technology; and interactions between the operation of a new technology and the new work processes that arise from the technology's use" (Borycki & Kushniruk, 2008).

Therefore, even as some software applications have been shown to improve consumer health and wellness, there have emerged concerns about the quality of these applications, the privacy and confidentiality of the information captured by these software applications (Spiekermann & Lorrie, 2009) and the ability of the technology to introduce technology-induced errors (Borycki & Kushniruk, 2008). This has led to calls by some researchers to achieve a balance between patient safety and innovation in mobile application development with the intent that no harm should occur to the general public (Barton, 2012) and for a deep integration of consumers' perspectives into the development of applications. More user centric applications for Smart Phones are needed (Jones et al., 2011).

This has led some researchers to develop frameworks that can aid consumers and health professionals to better understand and make decisions regarding the use of the technology. For example, researchers such as Cummings, Borycki and Roehrer (2013) have identified a number of issues that should be considered by consumers and health professionals when considering using these applications. In their work they developed a consumer perspective framework that identifies the relation between the use of health related consumer software applications and privacy, confidentiality and safety of the applications. The framework describes a method that can be used by consumers to evaluate health related applications before purchasing the software for use with a mobile or smart phone. The framework can be used by consumers as an aid to selecting the right health related software applications for their own personal use. Therefore, in order to better understand how these mobile software applications are being used as well as some of the issues that have arisen in recent years, the authors have conducted a review of the literature and a review of a range of free iOS applications in relation to the Consumer Perspective Framework.

CONSUMER PERSPECTIVES FRAMEWORK

The potential benefits of mobile software applications in assisting consumers in obtaining, managing and maintaining healthy lifestyles is evident. For example, the ability to incorporate Global Positioning Systems (GPS) and location tracking into a mobile software application provides additional opportunities for health and lifestyle maintenance as well as community-based data collection that can be used in public health surveillance (Aanensen, Huntley, Feil, al-Own, & Spratt, 2009). However, there continue to be a number of risks associated with the use of these technologies – they include issues in and around confidentiality of citizen information and security risks associated with using the technology.

Many of these mobile software applications are easy to purchase on the WWW so consumers can easily buy this technology for use. Therefore, the burden of assessing where the technology is appropriate rests with the individual consumer. To date there have been few published frameworks that can help consumers evaluate software for issues and risks associated with its use. One such framework that can be used by consumers and health professionals to assess their mobile device software is the *Consumer Perspectives Framework* by Cummings et al. (2013).

Cummings et al.'s (2013) *Consumer Perspectives Framework* allows the consumer or health professional to consider (for their personal use) mobile health care applications and helps the consumer to determine if the mobile health care application is appropriate for them. The framework emphasises some key aspects of mobile application use that should be considered by consumers in relation to health and lifestyle prior to purchase (see Table 1). In the framework mobile phones and their associated applications are reviewed in context of data and software issues. Data issues include storage and privacy, ownership, corporate use, location, and completeness. Software issues include accessibility, clinical effectiveness, credibility, information quality, and consumer usage.

In relation to the category of data issues, storage and privacy refer to ensuring the privacy of data is not violated and that it is stored in a secure manner. Ownership refers to who claims or maintains ownership of the data that is collected and stored through use of the software application. Corporate use is related to ownership but refers to the use of data by the application developer for their own purposes that are not necessarily evident at the time of collection or storage. Location relates to the actual location at which data is stored, which can be an issue if data crosses national borders. Completeness relates to the completeness of the data that is collected.

Software issues are the other main category described in the consumer perspectives framework. This includes such things as accessibility which refers to the ability to easily identify and access reliable applications. Clinical effectiveness refers to whether there is evidence of the effectiveness of

Table 1. Consumer Perspectives Framework

Data Issues	Software Issues
Storage and Privacy	Accessibility
Ownership	Clinical Effectiveness
Corporate Use	Credibility
Location	Information Quality
Completeness	Consumer Usage

Source: (Cummings et al., 2013)

the app. Information quality relates to the quality and accuracy of information and advice provided through the software and consumer usage refers to the motivation behind a consumer's use of the application. Each of these issues needs to be considered by consumers when purchasing mobile health care applications.

METHOD

During January 2013, a broad literature search was conducted using ProQuest and Web of Knowledge using the following key words; Storage and Privacy, Ownership, Corporate Use, Location, and Completeness, Accessibility, Clinical Effectiveness, Credibility, Information quality, Consumer Usage, and mobile app*. We chose to focus our search on consumer medical, health and fitness applications used on mobile phones as this is the focus of the *Consumer Perspectives Framework*. Following this, the abstracts of articles focusing on the above outlined key areas that were published after 2006 were reviewed by two individuals trained in health informatics. Articles post 2006 were used as this is the timeframe for the rise in the use of mobile phones and subsequent increase in the development of mobile applications. Articles

that met the following criteria were reviewed more fully for their quality and within the context of Cummings and colleagues' framework:

- Articles that described the use of mobile phone applications in relation to consumers in the community;
- Articles outlined the issues with mobile phone applications in relation to consumers in the community; and
- Articles where mobile phone application use was not prescribed by a medical practitioner.

Grey literature, including web based publications, were sourced from a Google search to supplement the original search and ensure completeness.

RESULTS

Forty articles were returned. Eighteen articles met our criteria and were read. As each article was read the researchers developed a table (see Table 2) that describes the articles more fully (i.e. author name, year of publication, sample, setting, methods and key findings). From our review of the literature using the lens of the Cummings et

Figure 1. Literature search method

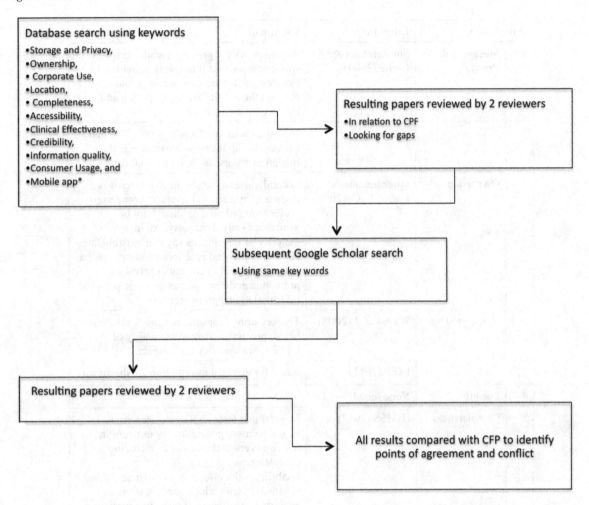

al. framework we identified several themes that emerged and are in keeping with the Consumers Perspectives Framework (see Table 2).

In our review of the literature we found that few researchers fully address the elements of the Consumer Perspectives Framework. This may indicate that few consumers are aware that mobile software applications have issues associated with their use or that consumers may have little interest in understanding the technology. More research is needed to understand the underlying reasons for this phenomenon. However, there were also some concerns noted in the literature that were outside the expectations of the framework. A broader dis-

cussion in relation to the literature highlights and a number of considerations will be discussed in the next section. The authors begin by discussing those aspects of the literature review that validate the framework.

Storage and Privacy

Computing activities such as data collection, storage and processing may lead to an invasion of privacy and may raise privacy concerns among consumers (Spiekermann & Lorrie, 2009). Most mobile applications require interaction with internal or external systems to produce expected results.

Table 2. Consumer Perspective Framework related literature example

Data Issues		Literature	Comment
1	Storage and Privacy	Spiekermann & Lorrie (2009)	A framework for privacy friendly systems was discussed: the framework provides the two designs for systems development through the use of Privacy by policy and Privacy by architecture.
		Croll A. (2011)	How data is used affects its value. The main concern for application consumers is the inappropriate use of their personal data.
2	Ownership	Spiekermann, S., & Lorrie, F. C. (2009)	Secondly use of data by third parties was discussed by various literature: Some users prefer their online data should not be available to any third party. An increasing majority of US citizens say that existing laws and organizational practices do not provide a reasonable level of consumer privacy protection and that companies share personal information inappropriately.
3	Corporate Use	Whitaker, J (2008)	The key things consumers want from their health privacy include trust, quality of service, transparency and respect.
		IAPP (2011)	Cases for misused information are discussed.
4	Location	None found	
5	Completeness	HIMSS (2012)	Suggest that instead of completeness, it would be more general to say as *usability* which covers usability issues including completeness. Usability is the effectiveness, efficiency and satisfaction with which specific users can achieve a specific set of tasks in a particular environment.
Software Issues		**Literature**	**Comment**
6	Accessibility	Luxton, McCann, Bush, Mishkind, & Reger (2011)	More research is needed to provide data on the usability and clinical effectiveness of Smart Phone technology in the behavioural health field.
7	Clinical Effectiveness	(Gustafson et al. (2011)	It is too early to generalize about the usefulness applications especially for non-evaluated applications.
		Gerdes, A., & Øhrstrøm. P (2011)	Although methods exist to evaluate software credibility there is still a need for more measurements and evaluation.e.g. further refinement as well as empirical support informing us about issues of system credibility.

A recent study found that integrated personal health records (PHRs) can have a huge impact upon patient care, leading to transformational changes in health care delivery as well as self-care by patients (Detmer, Bloomrosen, Raymond, & Tang, 2008). Electronic exchange of personal health information is a major concern for the public. Survey research suggests that consumer concerns about confidentiality and security issues still remain where technology is concerned (Detmer et al., 2008). With the rise in popularity of Smart Phone applications (with varying functions) among medical practitioners, clinicians, medical students and patients, there has also arisen an increased concern about patient privacy (Mosa, Yoo, & Sheets, 2012). This indicates that high use of mobile applications by those working in the health sector and by the general public will also lead to increased awareness of sharing patient and personal information via mobile applications.

Privacy has become a major concern for individuals. Survey research suggests that people are very concerned about privacy especially in the U.S where the majority of people say there is no reasonable level of consumer privacy protection and this allows companies to share personal information inappropriately (IAPP, 2011; Spiekermann & Lorrie, 2009; Whitaker, 2008). The key things consumers want from their health privacy include trust, quality of service, transparency and respect (Whitaker, 2008). The consumer perspective framework suggests there are data issues relevant to storage and privacy of a consumer's data stored on their Smart Phones or remotely on servers. Location based software applications may even collect consumers' data to identify a customer's location for accuracy. However, some businesses or application developers fail to notify users of how sensitive data are stored. There are two main approaches towards ensuring the privacy of consumers' data. They are privacy by policy and

privacy by architecture (Spiekermann & Lorrie, 2009). In the future application developers will need guidance, where the design and development of mobile applications, is concerned.

Ownership of the Data

Acquiring ownership of data in the digital age is quite a challenge as there is no physical possession of collected data to establish a boundary of ownership. Data storage and processing are required as part of many smartphone applications (Barton, 2012; Detmer et al., 2008; Laakko, Leppanen, Lahteenmaki, & Nummiaho, 2008; Mosa et al., 2012; Ng, Sim, & Tan, 2006; Perrig, Stankovic, & Wagner, 2004; Shi & Perrig, 2004; Spiekermann & Lorrie, 2009). However, Smart Phones have limited capabilities for storing and processing data so they may require external storage and processing power (Laakko et al., 2008). Data that flows out of users' devices may be accessible by third parties in various ways and may be used for many purposes. Consumers need to understand how secure the security mechanism build is in the type of Smart Phone they are using as well as the level of security being considered in application development. Nowadays many software applications utilise centralised storage for easy access to data and interoperability between different Smart Phone platforms.

The privacy-by-policy approach focuses on the implementation of the notice and choice principles of fair information practices, while the privacy-by-architecture approach minimises the collection of identifiable personal data and emphasises anonymisation and client-side data storage and processing (Spiekermann & Lorrie, 2009). A number of studies have investigated individuals' privacy concerns (Brown & Muchira, 2004) and there are seven areas of activity that cause concerns (Smith, Milberg, & Burke, 1996):

collection and storage of extensive amounts of personal data, unauthorised secondary use by the collecting organisation, unauthorised secondary use by an external organisation with whom personal data has been shared, unauthorised access to personal data, e.g., identity theft or snooping into records, errors in personal data, whether deliberately or accidentally created, poor judgment through decisions made automatically based on incorrect or partial personal data, and a combination of personal data from separate databases to create a combined and thus more comprehensive profile for a person.

Corporate Use

According to Cummings et al. (2013), corporate use and access to data collected by and entered into a mobile software application should be considered an important issue by consumers and health professionals who are reviewing mobile software applications and making decisions about using them. Here, the researchers identified that some mobile software applications developed by some corporations were collecting data about the users and it was unclear how the data was being used. In the research literature few publications described this potential consumer/health professional concern. In addition, there was little research that described how such data were used by corporations (if it was collected). Instead, much of the dialogue in the literature focused on the importance of maintaining the privacy of consumer data (see earlier section above). There were a few case studies that were published in the literature and described the misuse of information collected by mobile devices (IAPP, 2011). More research is needed in this area to determine if health care consumers and health professionals are concerned about health data being collected by corporations and to what extent the corporate analysis of that data (e.g. for marketing purposes) is a concern for consumers.

Location

Cummings and colleagues (2013) suggested that location based information collected by mobile devices and their software should be a concern for health care consumers and health professionals. Here, the researchers suggested that some consumers or health professionals do not want their location to be tracked on a daily or ongoing basis. In reviewing the literature focusing on the ability of mobile devices to continually provide information about the location of an individual, there was little literature that specifically identified location as an important type of data that health care consumers were concerned about reporting to an organisation or to other individuals.

It is interesting and worthy to note, that new mobile software applications are being developed that allow health care consumers to provide information about their location and the type of activity they are engaging in. In the case of these applications, such software not only report on the location of the individual, but on other individuals that they are tracking or others who may be in the same area or region of a park, city block etc. Such software applications allow individuals to track each other's locations. Such tracking may provide some individuals with incentives to continue engaging in an activity or to find other individuals who are engaging in a similar activity at the same time. For example, a jogger may wish to know if his or her friends are also jogging and where they are located so they can jog to that persons location and then jog as a group rather than an individual. The ability to track the location of individuals can turn a solitary physical activity into a group-based one and this may motivate some individuals to exercise more often. More research is needed to determine if disclosure of location is a concern for those who use these types of applications and if such disclosure of location in conjunction with a physical activity can lead to greater physical activity by those using such applications.

Completeness

Completeness of the mobile software application is another aspect of the Cummings framework that needs to be considered. Completeness can be defined as having all the necessary or appropriate parts (Oxford University Press, 2013). In the research literature, completeness is linked to the usability of mobile software. Here, researchers such as Kushniruk et al. (2005) have suggested that all software needs to be efficient, effective, enjoyable, safe and learnable in order for it to be usable. Tied to this is the ability of the mobile software to collect all information that is needed to provide feedback to the user, but at the same time to be usable. Research is needed to identify those mobile phone interface designs that balance the need to collect sufficient information for the software application to act as a true aid to the health care consumer while at the same time be easy to use or usable so the software application's design is not a barrier to its full use. More research will be needed to understand the nature of this balance between clinical effectiveness, completeness and usability.

Accessibility

Accessibility is degree to which an application is available to as many people as possible. There are two aspects to this: firstly, it is related to how easy it is to access and download applications, and secondly, it relates to the ability to be accessed and used by all people irrespective of ability or disability. Currently there is a lack of interoperability between mobile application platforms and so applications need to be developed for specific platforms (Cummings et al., 2013; Qiang, Yamamichi, Hausman, & Altman, 2011). To maximise the benefits and potential power of health and wellbeing applications as tools for assisting consumers take control it is necessary to create an open-source platform that can be used across operating systems (Qiang et al., 2011)

Clinical Effectiveness

Clinical Effectiveness or the ability of the mobile software application to improve a patient's clinical outcomes is an important area of research. In the framework, Cummings and colleagues (2013), identify that it is important for all mobile software applications to be reviewed in terms of their clinical effectiveness. Here, a consumer or health professional should ask the question; will the mobile phone software improve my health outcomes? (e.g. help me reduce my weight if I am obese, help me control my blood glucose levels if I have diabetes). In recent years there have been a number of studies have attempted to determine if such mobile software can lead to improvements in health outcomes. Some researchers have found that some mobile software, when targeted to a specific aspect of a disease and when designed to be usable and easy to integrate into an individual's life, can effectively improve health outcomes in that individual. Yet, this is not the case for all software. Here, consumers and health professionals need to be cognisant that some software does not provide clinically effective interventions that could improve a person's health outcomes. As well, poorly designed software that is neither usable nor easily used in the context of one's lifestyle may not be clinically effective. There is a need to for future research to fully describe how mobile phone software can be clinically effective and what consumers should look for to determine if the software they are purchasing leads to better health outcomes.

Credibility

Cummings and colleagues (2013) identify that mobile software credibility should be considered from a consumer perspective. Credibility can be defined as the quality of being trusted and believed in (Oxford University Press, 2013). Over the past several years, there have been numerous research publications that have documented the importance of obtaining information from a credible source when looking for information on the world wide web. Internationally, the credibility of health information remains a significant concern that many countries and individuals continue to struggle with when assessing information found on websites. Many government and health care organisations provide credible information for consumers to review and use in their health care journeys. For example, the government of the United States provides information on the National Institutes of Health website for health professionals and consumers. The information is developed by individuals who have a health care background and specialist expertise in varying health care conditions and diseases. Health care organisations such as the Canadian Lung Association also provide information to health care consumers about specific lung disease to help them not only learn about the disease but to identify health care resources in their community. As well, there are several tools that can be used by consumers to assess the quality of information published on a website and there are organisations that certify the quality of information on a given health care website.

There is a range of organisations that offer health care consumers the ability to purchase health care software. Many of these organisations guarantee the quality of the software itself, but may not guarantee the credibility of the corporation that developed the software. Some health care consumers may find this confusing. Future research may involve developing and testing tools that can help health care consumers evaluate the credibility of mobile phone software.

Information Quality

Information quality and credibility are linked together in some of the mobile software literature. Interestingly, information quality remains a concern even when considered in the context of mobile applications. There is concern about the clinical effectiveness of mobile software applications, the credibility of the organisations who produce these technologies and also the quality of the information provided or produced by these devices. In the research literature a key theme has emerged where information quality is considered in the context of mobile software applications. The key theme in this area is the need for education for consumers about the importance of information quality and how information quality should be assessed by consumers when considering using such applications (AHIMA, 2007). As some researchers suggest, it is possible to gather large quantities of low quality data as easily as high quality data and care is required for consumers to understand the difference (Chhablani et al., 2012; Luxton et al., 2011; Palmier-Claus et al., 2012). If consumers understand this issue they will give careful consideration to quality of the information presented and gathered by mobile software applications. Future research will need to attend to the need to develop tools that will help consumers assess the quality of the information provided by software applications as well as the quality of the information gathered by these applications to ensure consumers are fully supported in their health care related decision making.

CONCLUSION

In summary research has shown that mobile software applications can help health care consumers to self-manage their health and wellness (Barton, 2012). There has been some demonstration that mobile applications can lower costs and improve the quality of health care. It is also believed that mobile applications can change behaviour to increase the prevention of diseases and combined these can improve long term health outcomes (Qiang et al., 2011).

There is however a paucity of data on the actual impact of m-health services and this has led to challenges for policymakers and governments in regulating the industry. Qiang et al. (2011) suggest that strategies for regulation of the industry should focus on the health care system's most urgent needs.

Katz et al. (2012) find that in relation to chronic disease management there are certain challenges that mobile applications may be successful in addressing, namely improving patient skills and self-management techniques. However, there is a need for improved quality assurance in relation to mobile health applications. Currently approximately 95% of all health related applications are consumer only products and many are not based upon rigorous research and so the outcome from their use is not well researched.

FUTURE RESEARCH DIRECTIONS

Although the research in the area of mobile phone software has advanced considerably, there remain a number of gaps. For example, there is a need to understand how consumers view continuous connectivity. Some health care consumers do not want to be continuously connected to their health care software, preferring to turn it on and off when needed and only in times where they need their health related decision making supported. Other consumers may wish to be continually monitored by their mobile phone application. In addition to this researchers have identified that it is challenging for mobile phone technologies to continuously monitor health and physiologic status as there may be a need for continuous connectivity. Issues such as limited battery life and variability in mobile signalling continue to affect continuous monitoring. As well, many mobile health applications will not function without continuous data exchange with an external server via the Internet. Maintaining such a continuous connection may be challenging due to limited wireless connectivity in some locations and due to the cost of maintain such as connection.

More recently, the safety of mobile software applications has emerged as an issue. Many software applications used in medical diagnosis or treatment have had their safety called into question. Researchers have identified that some software features and functions may introduce new types of errors (i.e. technology-induced errors). In the upcoming years, governments will be introducing new regulations and safety standards to prevent harm arising from technologies used by health care consumers and health care providers in treating patients. Research is needed to better understand how the safe and unsafe features and functions of the technology.

In keeping with our previous work, we found that security was identified by researchers as being important to consider when purchasing mobile health applications (Jones et al., 2011). However, we noted that utilising wireless sensor networks along with health care applications brings a new dimension to mobile phone use – a dimension that requires a well-design security mechanism (Ng et al., 2006). This includes fast authentication for sensor nodes and efficient key distribution in a large network (Ng et al., 2006). Resource constraints sometimes bring challenges as they may be difficult to embed in a multi-layer security solution (Ng et al., 2006) to protect against data leaks. There are many key aspects to ensuring digital traffic flows within mobile health care applications. Many mobile phone software applications that utilise sensor networks are vulnerable to security breaches. Therefore, a secure sensor network that maintains data aggregation, secure group management, secure routing, resilience to node compromise, availability, integrity and authentication, confidentiality and privacy, and key establishment and trust set-up is key to ensuring the security of mobile software applications (Perrig et al., 2004; Shi & Perrig, 2004).

Currently mobile applications are developed for single operating systems and need to then be redeveloped if there is a requirement to use on another operating system. This can lead to issues with interoperability. Additionally, medical, and health and fitness applications are more regularly incorporating external devices for data collection. These devices need to be interoperable with the mobile operating systems. Research will be needed in this area. Some of this work will need to include standards. There are variety of international standards that provide specifications for services, products and best practices. The standards can be accessed by category from the International Standards Organisation (ISO) website and there is a variety of standards available for software developers. Mobile applications development is an emerging area of software developer practice where the ISO has not fully developed standards covering mobile application development. As mobile devices and their applications are becoming more and more consumers focused, application developers are forced to overcome issues through the use of appropriate practices. Research on standards involving mobile devices and mobile health care software will need to be undertaken. Choosing the right health care application requires certain knowledge that encompasses the development of Smart Phones applications. Not all application developers consider notifying the applications consumers of how data entered into the applications will be processed. The consumer perspective framework is a starting point that would guide consumers to better decide and choose the application with limited security risks.

REFERENCES

Aanensen, D., Huntley, D., Feil, E., Al-Own, F., & Spratt, B. (2009). EpiCollect: Linking smartphones to web applications for epidemiology, ecology and community data collection. *PLoS ONE*, *4*(9), e6968. doi:10.1371/journal.pone.0006968 PMID:19756138

AHIMA. (2007). *Statement on Quality Healthcare Data and Information*. Retrieved 10 Jan 2013, from http://library.ahima.org/xpedio/groups/public/documents/ahima/bok1_047492.pdf

Barton, A. J. (2012). The regulation of mobile health applications. *BMC Medicine*, *10*(46). PMID:22569114

Bjornland, D., Goh, E., Haanæs, K., Kainu, T., & Kennedy, S. (2012). *The Socio-Economic Impact of Mobile Health*. The Boston Consulting Group.

Borycki, E. M., & Kushniruk, A. W. (2008). Where do Technology-Induced Errors Come From? Towards a Model for Conceptualizing and Diagnosing Errors Caused by Technology. In A. W. Kushniruk, & E. M. Borycki (Eds.), *Human, Social, and Organizational Aspects of Health Information Systems* (pp. 148–166). Hershey, PA: IGI Global. doi:10.4018/978-1-59904-792-8.ch009

Brown, M., & Muchira, R. (2004). Investigating the Relationship between Internet Privacy Concerns and Online Purchase Behavior. *Journal of Electronic Commerce Research*, *5*(1), 62–70.

Chhablani, J., Kaja, S., & Shah, V. (2012). Smartphones in ophthalmology. *Indian Journal of Ophthalmology*, *60*(2), 127–131. doi:10.4103/0301-4738.94054 PMID:22446908

Croll, A. (2011). *Who Owns Your Data?* Retrieved 17 December, 2012, from http://mashable.com/2011/01/12/data-ownership/

Cummings, E., Borycki, E. M., & Roehrer, E. (2013). Issues and considerations for healthcare consumers using mobile applications. *Studies in Health Technology and Informatics*, *183*, 227–231. PMID:23388288

Detmer, D., Bloomrosen, M., Raymond, B., & Tang, P. (2008). Integrated Personal Health Records: Transformative Tools for Consumer-Centric Care. *BMC Medical Informatics and Decision Making, 8*(45). PMID:18837999

Gerdes, A., & Øhrstrøm, P. (2011). The role of credibility in the design of mobile solutions to enhance the social skill-set of teenagers diagnosed with autism. *Journal of Information. Communication and Ethics in Society, 9*(4), 253–264. doi:10.1108/14779961111191057

Gustafson, D., Boyle, M., Shaw, B., Isham, A., McTavish, F., & Richards, S. et al. (2011). An E-Health Solution for People with Alcohol Problems. *Alcohol Research & Health, 33*(4), 327–337. PMID:23293549

HIMSS. (2012). *Selecting a Mobile App: Evaluating the Useability of Medical Applications.* Retrieved 17 December, 2012, from http://www.yumpu.com/en/document/view/10378687/himssguidetoappusabilityv1mhimss

IAPP. (2011). *US Privacy Enforcement Case Studies Guide.* Retrieved 17 December, 2012, from https://www.privacyassociation.org/media/pdf/certification/CIPP_Case_Studies_0211.pdf

Jones, J., Hook, S., Park, S., & Scott, L. (2011). *Privacy, security and interoperability of mobile health applications.* Paper presented at the 6th International Conference on Universal Access in Human-Computer Interaction. New York, NY.

Katz, R., Mesfin, T., & Barr, K. (2012). Lessons from a community-based mHealth diabetes self-management program: It's not just about the cell phone. *Journal of Health Communication, 17*(1), 67–72. doi:10.1080/10810730.2012.650613 PMID:22548601

Kay, M., Santos, J., & Takane, M. (2011). mHealth: New horizons for health through mobile technologies. Geneva, Switerland: World Health Organization.

Kushniruk, A., Triola, B., Borycki, E., Stein, B., & Kannry, J. (2005). Technology Induced Error and Usability: The Relationship Between Usability Problems and Prescription Errors When Using a Handheld Application. *International Journal of Medical Informatics, 74*(7-8), 519–526. doi:10.1016/j.ijmedinf.2005.01.003 PMID:16043081

Laakko, T., Leppanen, J., Lahteenmaki, J., & Nummiaho, A. (2008). Mobile Health and Wellness Application Framework. *Methods of Information in Medicine, 47*(3), 217–222. PMID:18473087

Luxton, D., McCann, R., Bush, N., Mishkind, M., & Reger, G. (2011). mHealth for mental health: Integrating smartphone technology in behavioral healthcare. *Professional Psychology, Research and Practice, 42*(6), 505–512. doi:10.1037/a0024485

Mosa, A. S. M., Yoo, I., & Sheets, L. (2012). A Systematic Review of Healthcare Applications for Smartphones. *BMC Medical Informatics and Decision Making, 12*(67). PMID:22781312

Ng, H. S., Sim, M. L., & Tan, C. M. (2006). Security issues of wireless sensor networks in healthcare applications. *BT Technology Journal, 24*(2), 138–144. doi:10.1007/s10550-006-0051-8

Ozdalga, E., Ozdalga, A., & Ahuja, N. (2012). The Smartphone in Medicine: A Review of Current and Potential Use Among Physicians and Students. *Journal of Medical Internet Research, 14*(5), e128. doi:10.2196/jmir.1994 PMID:23017375

Palmier-Claus, J., Ainsworth, J., Machin, M., Barrowclough, C., Dunn, G., & Barkus, E. et al. (2012). The feasibility and validity of ambulatory self-report of psychotic symptoms using a smartphone software application. *BMC Psychiatry, 12*, 72. doi:10.1186/1471-244X-12-172 PMID:22759565

Perrig, A., Stankovic, J., & Wagner, D. (2004). Security in wireless sensor networks. *Communications of the ACM, 47*(6), 53–57. doi:10.1145/990680.990707

Qiang, C. Z., Yamamichi, M., Hausman, V., & Altman, D. (2011). *Mobile Applications for the Health Sector*. Washington, DC: ICT Sector Unit, World Bank.

Savitz, E. (2012). 5 Ways Mobile Apps Will Transform Healthcare. *CIO Network: Insights and Ideas for Technology Leaders*. Retrieved 10 Jan 2013, from http://www.forbes.com/sites/ciocentral/2012/06/04/5-ways-mobile-apps-will-transform-healthcare/

Shi, E., & Perrig, A. (2004). Designing secure sensor networks. *IEEE Wireless Communications, 11*(6), 38–43. doi:10.1109/MWC.2004.1368895

Smith, J., Milberg, S., & Burke, S. (1996). Information Privacy: Measuring Individuals' Concerns about Organizational Practices. *Management Information Systems Quarterly, 20*(2), 167–196. doi:10.2307/249477

Spiekermann, S., & Lorrie, F. C. (2009). Engineering privacy. *IEEE Transactions on Software Engineering, 35*(1), 67–82. doi:10.1109/TSE.2008.88

Whitaker, J. (2008). *Health Privacy: What Consumers Want*. Retrieved 17 December 2012, from http://www.privacy.org.au/Papers/HealthInfoPrivacy-081110.pdf

World Bank. (2012). *Information and Communications for Development 2012: Maximizing Mobile*. Washington, DC: World Bank.

ADDITIONAL READING

Bjornland, D., Goh, E., Haanæs, K., Kainu, T., & Kennedy, S. (2012). The Socio-Economic Impact of Mobile Health: The Boston Consulting Group

Katz, R., Mesfin, T., & Barr, K. (2012). Lessons from a community-based mHealth diabetes self-management program: It's not just about the cell phone. *Journal of Health Communication, 17*(1), 67–72. doi:10.1080/10810730.2012.650613 PMID:22548601

Kay, M., Santos, J., & Takane, M. (2011). mHealth: New horizons for health through mobile technologies. Geneva, Switerland: World Health Organization

Qiang, C. Z., Yamamichi, M., Hausman, V., & Altman, D. (2011). *Mobile Applications for the Health Sector*. Washington, DC: ICT Sector Unit, World Bank.

KEY TERMS AND DEFINITIONS

Accessibility: The ability to easily identify and access reliable applications.

Clinical Effectiveness: The presence/absence of evidence of the effectiveness of an application.

Completeness: The completeness of the data that is collected.

Consumer Perspective Framework: A simple framework that assists mobile app consumers to determine if a specific mobile health care application is appropriate for their needs.

Consumer Usage: The motivation behind a consumer's use of the application.

Corporate Use: Refers to the use of data by the application developer for their own purposes that are not necessarily evident at the time of collection or storage.

Credibility: The quality of being trusted and believed in.

Health Apps: Software that claim to provide health related information or services via mobile devices.

Information Quality: The quality and accuracy of information and advice provided through the software.

Location: The actual location at which data is stored.

Mobile Applications (Apps): Software designed for use on mobile or handheld devices.

Ownership: Who claims or maintains ownership of the data that is collected and stored during use of an application.

Chapter 2
Success Dimensions of the Online Healthcare Communities of Practice:
Towards an Evaluation Framework

Haitham Alali
Ministry of Health, Jordan

Juhana Salim
Universiti Kebangsaan Malaysia, Malaysia

ABSTRACT

The existing studies on online Communities of Practice (CoPs) in healthcare organizations have not adequately focused on the factors affecting KM initiative success and acceptance. Thus, establishing an evaluation framework has become essential for the advancement of research and practice in this area. In online communities of practice, the process of measuring and developing an evaluation framework has become quite complicated and challenging due to the intangible nature of the knowledge. Moreover, the lack of standards and studies, related to online CoPs measurements and evaluation frameworks, respectively, triggers the need for intensive studies in this area. In this context, this chapter reviews online CoPs success factors and identifies the gaps in our understanding. The authors classify the existing studies based on the area of evaluation, such as health and non-health domains. The chapter concludes by proposing a conceptual framework to measure the success of online CoPs in the healthcare sector.

INTRODUCTION

This book chapter provides an overview of the pertinent literature of the online communities of practice (CoPs), where the development, main characteristics and dimensions of online CoPs measurement, which are considered in the online CoPs literature have been examined. Moreover, this book chapter has reviewed past empirical studies related to online CoPs success and acceptance that have highlighted the major themes and criteria of online CoPs measurement; in addition

DOI: 10.4018/978-1-4666-6150-9.ch002

to the earlier online CoPs success and acceptance models have also been reviewed. The output of this review has identified the most critical dimensions that constitute towards the success and acceptance of online CoPs.

Online CoPs have emerged as a new robust interactive channel using available social media, by supporting all characteristics used as part of the knowledge management system (KMS) (Tseng & Kuo, 2014). According to Wenger, McDermott, and Snyder (2002), online CoPs help knowledge management by capturing and sharing the expertise of members and by imparting skills, ideas, problems, innovations, talents, and experiences. Members of online CoPs are held together by a common purpose and require information on what others know (Wenger et al., 2002). However, the importance of measuring the effectiveness of online CoPs has been recognized by practitioners and researchers in the knowledge management (KM) field as supportive of knowledge sharing (Alali & Salim, 2013; Kankanhalli & Tan, 2005; Tseng & Kuo, 2014). Measuring the success of online CoPs includes the process of assessing their value in managing knowledge by identifying success and acceptance factors (Alali & Salim, 2013; Nistor, Schworm, & Werner, 2012).

Success measures of online CoPs support organizations in different ways, such as suggesting approaches to improve usage and operation of online CoPs. Furthermore, success measures of online CoPs can enhance decision-making related to online CoPs and KM projects investments (Ho et al., 2010; Wenger et al., 2002), as well as instruments to be used as benchmarks for future measurement and enhancement of online CoPs. Fundamentally, literature review helps researchers to determine the missing gap that can be compensated in the future (Fernandez, Gonzalez, & Sabherwal, 2004; Kankanhalli & Tan, 2005). From the theoretical perspective, the wide implementation of online CoPs in various industries with high levels of success had been reported by Wenger and other scholars, in con-

trast to the limited studies that evaluated online CoPs in the healthcare sector. In addition, these existing limited studies are descriptive, and hence have motivated this book chapter to review and to compare the literature pertaining to healthcare online CoPs and that of various industries. Ultimately, this book chapter aims to identify the main dimensions that determine the success of online CoPs. We have analysed and synthesized successful literature of online CoPs to identify the main taxonomy related to their success.

Theoretical Background

Evaluating online CoPs is a vital aspect, especially for measuring the effectiveness of CoPs. The evaluation might ensure the accomplishments of CoPs, particularly in supporting healthcare practitioners in their knowledge sharing activities (Alali & Salim, 2013; Kankanhalli & Tan, 2005). Online CoPs evaluation refers to the process of assessing their value in managing knowledge by defining determinants of success and acceptance. Success measures of online CoPs should support healthcare organizations in various ways, such as providing suggestions to improve the design, implementation, usage, and operation of online CoPs, by addressing and understanding the main factors that affect their success and acceptance (Alali & Salim, 2013). Furthermore, success measures of online CoPs can enhance their investment decisions and KM initiatives, as well as aid in the development of instruments to be used as benchmarks for future evaluation and comparison. In addition, online CoPs evaluation provides researchers the opportunity to determine and address missing gaps that can improve online CoPs in the future (Fernandez et al., 2004; Kankanhalli & Tan, 2005; Tseng & Kuo, 2014).

In evaluating online CoPs, researchers and practitioners must consider information technology, which is a component of online CoPs (Nistor, Schworm, & Werner, 2012; Alali & Salim, 2013). According to Wasko and Faraj (2005), online CoPs are self-organizing groups of practitioners that facilitate the process of knowledge sharing specific practices. The users can handle computer-mediated collaborative activities and various types of social media (Wasko & Faraj, 2005), such as bulletin boards, online forums, and e-mail, to build the social space (Fang & Chiu, 2010; Nistor, Schworm, & Werner, 2012). The social space is where users, who experience the same problems, challenges, occupational practice, and interests, will help and collaborate with each other (Wasko, Teigland, & Faraj, 2009; Tseng & Kuo, 2014). Furthermore, Wenger (2004) has stated that, generally CoPs consist of three main elements, namely, domain, community, and practice. The domain refers to the area of knowledge that brings the community together, provides its identity, and defines key issues that members must address. The community refers to the group of people for whom the domain is relevant, the quality of relationships among members, and the boundary that separates inside and outside societies. The practice refers to the body of knowledge, methods, tools, stories, cases, and documents that members share and develop together.

Healthcare organizations spend a large amount of money towards implementing KM initiatives in terms of the development of practitioners and expert resources (Davenport & Prusak 1998; WHO 2005). Executives subsequently question about the actual benefits and the value of investment in KM initiatives (Armstrong & Kendall, 2010; Kankanhalli & Tan, 2005; Wenger et al., 2002). On the other hand, Kankanhalli and Tan (2005a) and Wang et.al, (2011) recommended additional evaluation studies on online CoPs because of reported failures in KM initiatives and the lack of evaluation studies on online CoPs. However, evaluating the success and acceptance of online CoPs is challenging for both KM researchers and practitioners (Wang et al., 2012). In similar vein, Kankanhalli and Tan (2005a) reported that, most information systems (IS) studies, related to the success and acceptance of KMS have focused on

theoretical modelling of controls and measurement. A few earlier studies have been conducted on KMS usability and on KMS usage, specifically on online CoPs (Kankanhalli & Tan 2005a; Wang et al. 2012).

Previous Research on Evaluation of Online CoPs

To comprehensively review the literature pertaining to the success of online CoPs, we searched cited research from 1995 to 2011 in the fields of health informatics, information systems, and social science databases, including journal websites such as Pub Med, Science direct, Springer Link, Emerald, ProQuest, Wiley, Sage, EBSCO, Taylor, and ACM. Additional sources were obtained using Yahoo and Google Scholar search engines, locating references with key terms such as 'electronic', 'virtual', 'online', 'web-based', 'communities of practice', 'professional network', 'knowledge network', 'evaluation', 'assessment', 'success', 'effectiveness', and 'healthcare'. Search terms with the same meaning were combined using 'OR' and the terms had been paired with other terms using 'AND' and 'NOT' Boolean operators.

As shown in Figure 1, the selection process has a number of steps. Firstly, 634 relevant studies were identified after the initial screening of their titles and abstracts. Among these studies, 589 references were retained after removing duplicates, and another 240 articles were excluded based on their obvious irrelevance to the research aims. In cases of doubt about the exclusion, the full article was obtained for further assessment. After reading the full articles and excluding studies that were irrelevant that had not examined CoPs under a virtual setting, and were non-empirical, only 40 studies remained for the evaluation of online CoPs success. Four articles were added from tracing the bibliographical references of the articles. Research articles had been selected according to the following criteria: (i) the studies that have empirically evaluated online CoPs, (ii) the studies that have a

Figure 1. An overview of the study selection and the exclusion process

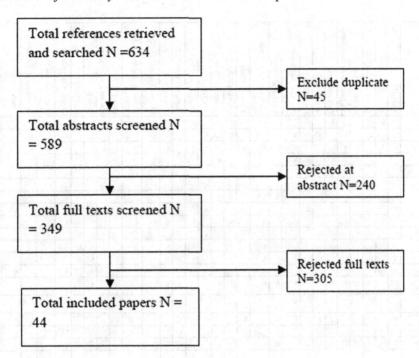

clear research methodology, and (iii) the studies that have presented complete research findings. Systematic review was conducted to extract and synthesize the main concepts and dimensions that measure online CoPs success in the literature. The 44 articles were categorized based on their relation to online CoPs in healthcare (11 articles) and to other domains (23 articles). However, the non-health studies have been included in the review, since the health studies did not cover all factors that influence the success and acceptance of online CoPs.

Success Dimensions

The main purposes of this book chapter are: (1) to identify the main dimensions and factors that determine online CoPs success, and (2) to determine the gaps between health and non-health literature in terms of studying online CoPs success. The comparisons are crucial for designers, research-

ers, policymakers, and adopters to be certain of the relative value of online CoPs in healthcare. Questions about relative differences in measuring online CoPs success are necessary, both during the early phases of development and as the field matures, to summarize main determinants and to suggest reliable methods to measure success, which will provide more credibility and direction. The last aim of this book chapter is to propose a conceptual framework in measuring the success of online CoPs in the healthcare sector

The data in Table 1 and Table 2 indicate the main dimensions and the related factors in literature. The social, human, semantic, and technical dimensions of online CoPs success and acceptance have been discussed in the succeeding section. Specific measures have been discussed for each dimension and each measure has been validated by a number of variables and indicators discussed in the literature. Main dimensions, related factors, and their association have also been explained.

Table 1. Online CoPs analyzed factors

Dimensions	Factors	Lin and Lee (2006)	Wang et al. (2011)	Fang and Chiu (2010)	Yu, Lu, and Liu (2010)	Lin, Hung, and Chen (2009)	Yang and Lai (2010)	Jin et al. (2009)	Lin (2008a)	Chiu, Hsu, and Wang (2006)	Wasko et al. (2009)	Chen, Chen, and Kinshuk (2009)	Lin et al. (2007)	Chen and Hung (2010)	Chang and Chuang (2011)	Lin (2008b)	Zhang et al. (2010)	Zhang and Watts (2003)	Kuo et al. (2003)	Hsu, Ju, Yen, and Chang (2007)	Vavasseur and MacGregor (2008)	Chen (2007)	Cheung and Lee (2009)	Choi, Kang, and Lee	Lin (2007)	Lin and Huang (2009)	Rosenbaum and Shachaf (2010)	Kankanhalli et al. (2005b)	Urbach, Smolnik, and Riempp (2010)	Dubé, Bourhis, and Jacob (2005)	Kankanhalli, Tan, and Wei (2005a)	Wasko and Faraj (2005)	Ackerman (1998)	Casaló et al. (2010)
Social	Reputation	X				X									X																X	X	X	
	Trust		X		X					X	X			X	X	X	X			X			X		X		X							
	Norms		X							X		X	X	X					X				X			X	X			X				X
	Shared Identity			X		X				X					X					X										X				X
	Commitment										X												X									X		
	Member Belonging								X						X												X							
	Social Ties									X	X	X			X								X		X									
Human	Member Satisfaction	X				X	X	X									X	X					X	X	X			X				X		
	Self-efficacy		X		X					X				X			X		X	X	X				X	X				X				
	Enjoyment in helping				X																				X							X	X	
	Attitude										X							X							X									X
	Intention	X	X					X			X							X	X				X		X	X								X
	Usage													X												X		X		X				
	Knowledge Sharing Behaviour		X	X			X			X	X	X		X	X				X	X					X							X		
	Human Related Expectation										X												X											
Semantic	Knowledge Quality	X					X	X						X		X	X						X				X	X						
	Information Consistency																X																	
	Knowledge Resources											X					X																	
	Relevancy of Contents				X																								X					
	Knowledge Quantity									X	X																							
	Information Retrieval																															X		
	Knowledge Usefulness			X																												X		
	Knowledge Format																																	
	Types of Knowledge																																	
Technical	System Quality	X							X					X			X						X	X						X				
	Service Quality	X																						X										
	Perceived Ease of Use		X							X																	X							X
	Perceived Usefulness		X		X					X										X							X						X	X

Social Dimension

Communities can meet face to face or virtually through ICT and social media, such as online forums, bulletin boards, and e-mail (Fang & Chiu, 2010). Knowledge is created and shared through social interaction, anchoring the essential information in a social context and for specific purposes (Tseng & Kuo, 2014; Wenger, 1998; Wenger et al., 2002) . Communities also collaborate with interdisciplinary curriculum development units (Vavasseur & MacGregor, 2008).

Basically, online CoPs consist of practitioners who interact, collaborate, learn together, and build relationships based on trust and mutual respect, motivating the intention to share best practices and experiences, identify common problems, and address existing challenges (Wenger et al., 2002). Practitioners in online CoPs can overcome difficult challenges that may negatively affect KMS by addressing knowledge overload using prioritization and filtering mechanisms. Moreover, they can reduce replication and can pool resources using new ICTs, such as teleconferences and web-based forums.

Previous studies recognized that people tend to select others as their favourite source of knowledge, and this personal contact is essential in enhancing the knowledge-seeking behaviour (Nistor, Schworm, & Werner, 2012; Parcell,

Table 2. Health online CoPs analyzed factors

Dimensions	Factors	Ho et al. (2010)	Brooks and Scott (2006a)	Bertulis and Cheeseborough (2008)	Brooks and Scott (2006b)	Beer et al. (2005)	Stergiou et al. (2009)	Docherty, Hoy, Topp, and Trinder (2005)	Booth, Sutton, and Falzon (2003)	Clarke, Lewis, Cole, and Ringrose (2005)	Armstrong and Kendall (2010)	Russell, Greenhalgh, Boynton, and Rigby (2004)
Social	Trust									X		
Social	Shared Identity	X										
Social	Social Ties										X	
Social	Member Satisfaction							X				
Human	Self-efficacy			X			X	X				
Human	Attitude			X								
Human	Knowledge/Information Quality					X						
Semantic	Availability of Knowledge Resources							X				
Semantic	Knowledge Quantity								X			
Semantic	Knowledge Format								X			
Semantic	Types of Knowledge											X
Semantic	System Quality									X		
Technical	Perceived Ease of Use	X	X					X			X	
Technical	Perceived Usefulness	X	X			X	X	X		X	X	

2005). Knowledge-based organizations, including the healthcare sector, are attentive and consider the knowledge, skills, and experiences of professionals as the most central asset (Lubon, 2005). Moreover, the knowledge domain and the community (practitioners) can be integrated to enhance patient safety, population health, and healthcare delivery, which correlates to the interaction of practitioners and the collaboration among peers. Geoffery (2008) stated that organizations should focus on understanding the social capital of CoPs. Consequently, communities might have a significant role in creating and sharing new ideas that can increase social capital through human relations.

The social dimension in online CoPs literature is exhibited by an individual's reputation/social image, trust, sharing norm, identification, commitment, sense of belongingness, and social interaction ties. Social action is simply achieved in online CoPs, in which ties are determined by a high level of intention, social bonds, and prospects of voluntary behaviour that are proposed to assist other participants. Trust is another characteristic of social ties in online CoPs, which is ordinarily linked to social action. To this end, the social dimension depends on the strength of the relationships and communication among members in online CoPs, which are determined by individual commitment, interpersonal trust, reputation, and norm of reciprocity (Nahapiet & Ghoshal, 1998; Wasko et al., 2009).

Over time, members will build a sense of common history, identity, belongingness, and mutual commitment from trusted relationships. Meanwhile, the traditional hierarchy and barriers between practitioners will decrease the involvement of individuals in the same area and interests to participate in online CoPs. According to Wasko et al. (2009) additional relational dimensions of network ties, including obligation to and identification with the community, commitment, affiliation, and organizational citizenship, are associated with social interaction.

Human Dimension

Knowledge is intrinsic in humans and is closely connected to the human senses and to previous experiences, thus, knowledge is unique to each individual. Knowledge is considered to be subjective and closely related to human action (Nonaka & Takeuchi 1995). Therefore, knowledge can be regarded as both the capacity and the results of human action (Nonaka & Takeuchi 1995). Individuals are crucial to knowledge management in online CoPs. Individuals perform KM functions using IT, and can create, manage, and use content to resolve problems and to achieve goals of online CoPs. Parcell (2005) stated that "to be connected to the people who have the knowledge is more important than capturing all the knowledge" (p. 68). Moreover, online CoPs do not require the formulation of high capability and ability criteria and are well-appreciated in fields such as medicine, management, and nursing.

Human capital has been considered as a key factor that impacts the success of online CoPs functions. In this context, Armstrong and Hegel (1996) mentioned, "a community full of half-empty rooms offers visitors a very unsatisfactory experience. The value of participating in a community lies in users' ability to access a broad range

of people and resources quickly and easily" (p.89). Thus, characteristics of individual, such as belief, attitude, personality, experience, motivation, and behaviour can lead to the success of online CoPs. Therefore, the human dimension of online CoPs success refers to the characteristics and senses of individuals who influence behaviour in online CoPs, consequently affecting knowledge sharing behaviour.

The literature has described different human factors that determine the human dimension of online CoPs. Majority of studies adopted user satisfaction, and many focused on human efficacy in using websites and on knowledge sharing self-efficacy. Online CoPs usage has been commonly studied based on general use and knowledge sharing behaviour (Tseng & Kuo, 2014).

Behavioural intention was studied by implementing two different methods that are presented in Table 1. The first method measures the intent of individuals to use online CoPs and the second method measures their intent to continue using online CoPs (Fang & Chiu 2010; Zhang et al. 2010). In addition, individual's attitude toward using online CoPs by knowledge seeking and contributing. Many studies adopted human factors as an output, such as use (Kankanhalli et al., 2005a; Kankanhalli, Tan, & Wei, 2005b; Lin, Fan, Wallace, & Zhang, 2007; Lin & Huang, 2008) and behavioural intention (Chen, 2007; Chen et al., 2009; Cheung & Lee, 2009; Fang & Chiu, 2010; Jin, Cheung, Lee, & Chen, 2009; Lin, 2007; Zhang, Fang, Wei, & Chen, 2010), to measure the effectiveness level of online CoPs (Lin, 2007; Zhang et al., 2010).

Semantic Dimension

Knowledge and information as an output or as the content of online CoPs can be measured at several levels. In IS research, DeLone and McLean (1992) adopted three levels of IS as suggested by Shannon and Weaver (1949), namely, technical, semantic, and effectiveness levels. The semantic level refers to the success of the information in expressing its intended meaning (DeLone & McLean, 1992; Shannon & Weaver, 1949).

Online CoPs is about knowledge management, in which members of the community must seek and contribute to the knowledge base. Furthermore, online CoPs are not purely a personal or social network. Members of CoPs must have initial knowledge to fulfil their needs (Alali & Salim, 2013). They actually adopt a specific knowledge domain. Regardless of time, they build their proficiencies in the knowledge domain, which refers to a set of key issues related to a specific knowledge area, which have to be addressed by members. The domain inspires members to participate and contribute, to create a community identity, to provide meaning to their actions, and to acquire guidance on their learning process (Wenger et al., 2002). For example, by examination of the G-I-N Emergency Care Community, their domain is emergency care practices, which is defined by the creation of clinical guidelines for clinicians (G-I-N, 2010).

Online CoPs provide an opportunity for their members to enhance interactions with their colleagues. Vavasseur and MacGregor (2008) emphasized that successful professional development stresses on the significance of focusing on the content rather than on the software and on the needs of professionals, as basis in grouping professionals by teams.

The semantic dimension refers to the success of the information in expressing its intended meaning and the user's expectations in terms of its usefulness and value. Chiu et al. (2006) measured the semantic level of online CoPs by qualitative and quantitative outcomes of knowledge sharing. The quality of knowledge can influence the members on the extent to which they interacts with others (Chen, 2007). Furthermore, Kulkarni et al. (2007) measured knowledge quality based on relevance,

accuracy, timeliness, applicability, comprehensibility, presentation formats, extent of insight, and availability of expertise and advice.

Several measurements of semantic level were adopted in online CoPs literature, such as availability of knowledge resources (Docherty et al., 2005; Wasko et al., 2009; Zhang & Watts, 2003), number of messages posted (Booth et al., 2003; Wasko et al., 2009), knowledge usefulness (Wasko & Faraj, 2005; Yu et al., 2010), information retrieval and access (Ackerman, 1998), relevance of content to members (Dubé et al., 2005; Yu et al., 2010), information consistency (Zhang & Watts, 2003), format (Booth et al., 2003), and types of knowledge exchanged (Russell et al., 2004). In sum, majority of research pertaining to online CoPs consider the semantic level by measuring shared knowledge/information quality.

Technical Dimension

Technology, especially the Internet, is a very significant aspect of knowledge sharing. The Internet obviously encompass a number of social functions, such as e-commerce, government, and private community interactions. The Internet facilitates online CoPs members to interact, contribute, and to increase professionalism among employees by social interaction, without highly spending for the learning process and the difficulty of transferring members. In addition, based on the perspective of human-computer interaction, scholars have indicated that, the quality of websites is a significant feature that can predict the tendency of members to use online CoPs (Preece, 2001).

At present, ICT supports online CoPs to expand their contacts using technologies, such as websites and electronic bulletin boards (Wasko & Faraj, 2005). Information technology (IT), particularly the social media, is an essential medium that facilitates knowledge storing, retrieving, and sharing by many users. The networking technology offers numerous opportunities for knowledge transfer across the world (Armstrong & Kendall, 2010). Consequently, the success of the technical dimension of online CoPs influences members on how they use information and communication-related technologies within their surroundings for KM activities.

Online CoPs employ the online social media to learn about the process of knowledge creation, capture, and use by healthcare practitioners (Brooks & Scott, 2006a). KM in online CoPs is carried out through its website (i.e., online forums). Many scholars have recognized the significance of website quality in knowledge seeking and contributing behaviour of members (Choi et al., 2008; Clarke et al., 2005; Lin et al., 2007; Lin, 2008a, 2008b; Lin & Lee, 2006; Urbach et al., 2010). Generally, websites support communication and interaction among members, enable interaction by removing geographical obstructions and allow knowledge sharing across online CoPs. A high-quality website can persuade its existing members to continuously utilize it (Alali & Salim, 2013; Chen, 2007).

Brooks and Scott (2006b) emphasized on the enabling role of technology that can help knowledge work, including the effective transfer of tacit knowledge. The success of online CoPs depends on the accumulation and enhancement of knowledge in the warehouse (Chen, 2007), which is obtained from discussion forums, newsletters, and recommended articles in the website of online CoPs. As shown in Table 1 and Table 2, the technical dimension in literature pertaining to online CoPs is mainly exhibited based on four constructs, namely, system quality, service quality, perceived usefulness, and perceived ease of use of online CoPs.

Discussion

In KM research, success refers to the improvement of organisational effectiveness that comes from reusing data by providing timely and accurate

knowledge (Jennex, 2008). Conversely, KMS success was defined as the effect of the successful employment of KMS components in encouraging the use of KMS. The successful implementation of KMS processes and their improved usage will be reflected in the management of knowledge (Jennex, 2008).

As mentioned previously, DeLone and McLean (1992) divided IS into three levels, namely, technical, semantic and effectiveness, based on the study by Shannon and Weaver (1949). The effectiveness level refers to the effect of the information to the receiver (DeLone & McLean, 1992; Shannon & Weaver, 1949). Many studies considered user satisfaction as an essential indicator in measuring the success of IS because of its ease of use and applicability as an indicator (Zviran & Erlich, 2003).

Many studies also associated user satisfaction with attitude and behaviour, while attempting to define it. For example, Baroudi et al. (1986) defined user satisfaction as the degree to which users believe that, IS has been available to them and it might help them to meet their information needs. User satisfaction has been frequently highlighted in literature as an attitude toward IS (DeLone & McLean, 2003) and recently has been widely accepted. According to Doll and Torkzadeh (1991), user satisfaction is a vital hypothetical feature due to its capability in establishing both upstream and downstream links in the value chain. As presented in Figure 2, upstream activities consist of factors that cause satisfaction, in which user satisfaction has been considered as a dependent variable. Downstream activities consist of behaviours affected by satisfaction, in which user satisfaction has been treated as an independent or antecedent factor. The relationship between user satisfaction and IS effectiveness is one of the inherent hypotheses made by researchers in employing user satisfaction measurements for the evaluation of IS effectiveness.

KMS success, for online CoPs, can be measured by various methods, including the achievement of objectives and learning enrichment (Tremblay,

Figure 2. System to value chain

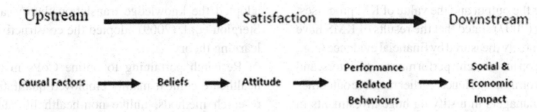

2007). Recently, scholars have begun shifting towards measuring intangible outcomes of KMS (Maier, 2007). In this context, Wenger et al. (2002) identified several advantages of CoPs to the organization in term of improve business outcomes, such as problem solving, obtaining quick answers to questions, minimised time and costs, enhanced quality of decisions, broadened perspectives on problems, coordination, consistency and collaboration among units, acquisition of resources for the application of strategies, and strengthened quality assurance. Several advantages also benefit community members in terms of enhanced professional experience, such as problem solving, access to expertise, increased ability to contribute to team-oriented activities, confidence in one's approach, fun with colleagues, more meaningful participation, and sense of belongingness. An additional benefit for the healthcare system is that

online CoPs can fill the existing gap in translating research findings and evidence-based practices into action (Know-Do gap) in daily healthcare practices.

As shown in Figure 3, with the intention to build a conceptual framework to measure the success of online CoPs, which is consistent with that by Jennex, Smolnik, and Croasdell (2008), the success of online CoPs has been determined by measuring two levels. The first level involves in measuring the success or effectiveness of knowledge creation, codification, sharing, and use processes. This level can be established by determining the factors that affect KM processes in the context of online CoPs. Based on the literature review, the present study argues that the success dimensions for KM processes are mutually associated with technical, social, semantic, and human dimensions. The second level involves

Figure 3. Conceptual framework of the success of online CoPs

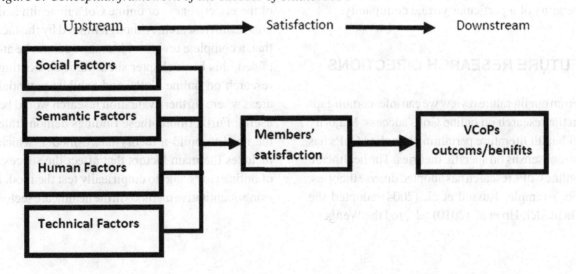

effectiveness evaluation of online CoPs by measuring the output and the value of KM processes. Maier (2007) stated that the results of KMS have been mostly measured by financial evidence (e.g., return on investment, performance indicators, and return on assets). Hence, earlier tangible outcomes help managers in justifying huge investments in KM initiatives (Wenger et al., 2002). However, investigating intangible outcomes of KMS (such as skills of practitioners, best practices, and intellectual property) has been considered as a complicated task. Many organisations, still consider that, intangible outcomes aid them in achieving a competitive advantage.

'Online CoPs outcomes' refer to the actual benefits that participants receive from using online CoPs, including intangible benefits that can address subsequent effects of the utilization. The intangible benefits of online CoPs can be classified into two categories. The first category comprises individual benefits, which primarily consist of knowledge sharing behaviour related to the use of online CoPs for knowledge sharing activities (such as information retrieval and publishing, communication, networking, collaboration, and completed work processes). The second category comprises community benefits that refer to the effect of a successful online CoPs to members, including their efforts to invite new members to join and to open discussions concerning the benefits of a particular virtual community.

FUTURE RESEARCH DIRECTIONS

From our literature review we can infer certain gaps in the research on online CoPs success. Majority of health literature pertaining to online CoPs has no consensus on specific theories. The healthcare online CoPs research has adopted diverse theories. For example, Russell et al. (2004) adopted the Ba model, Ho et al. (2010) adopted the Wenger's

CoPs framework, Armstrong and Kendall (2010) adopted the knowledge translation theory, and Stergiou et al. (2009) adopted the constructivist learning theory.

Research pertaining to online CoPs in the healthcare context mainly employed qualitative research methods, unlike non-health literature that employed quantitative research methods. In the literature review, majority of studies on online CoPs are apparently anecdotal in nature (Kankanhalli & Tan 2005), while those in the healthcare sector have a limited ability in evaluating the success and acceptance of online CoPs because of their use of the quantitative research approach. The qualitative research approach, specifically, the descriptive method has been often applied in online CoPs research (Armstrong & Kendall, 2010; Dubé et al., 2005), with their corresponding conceptual frameworks (Ho et al., 2010; Merrill & Hripcsak, 2008; Stergiou et al., 2009), or in anecdotal case studies (Brooks & Scott, 2006b; Russell et al., 2004).

The literature of online CoPs in the healthcare setting has focused on the learning process of staff members and professionals via the social environment and with the use of technology as enabler to increase the level of professionalism. The findings indicated that research on online CoPs should consider technical, social, semantic, and human dimensions that balance measurement of the effectiveness of online CoPs in health and non-health research. Although limited by the fact that, a complete review of literature cannot be attained, this book chapter sheds light on existing research on online CoPs, and exhibits potential areas where further evaluation research would be useful. Furthermore, these findings demonstrate the need to build a theory-based model, which includes the main factors that affect the success of online CoPs, and to empirically test the model using quantitative methods in the healthcare sector

REFERENCES

Ackerman, M. S. (1998). Augmenting organizational memory: A field study of answer garden. *ACM Transactions on Information Systems, 16*(3), 203–224. doi:10.1145/290159.290160

Alali, H., & Salim, J. (2013). Virtual Communities of Practice Success Model to Support Knowledge Sharing behaviour in Healthcare Sector. *Procedia Technology, 11*(0), 176–183. doi:10.1016/j.protcy.2013.12.178

Armstrong, A., & Hagel, I. J. (1996). The Real Value of ON-LINE Communities. *Harvard Business Review, 74*(3), 134–141.

Armstrong, K., & Kendall, E. (2010). Translating knowledge into practice and policy: The role of knowledge networks in primary health care. *The Health Information Management Journal, 39*(2), 9–17. PMID:20577019

Baroudi, J. J., Olson, M. H., & Ives, B. (1986). An empirical study of the impact of user involvement on system usage and information satisfaction. *Communications of the ACM, 29*(3), 232–238. doi:10.1145/5666.5669

Beer, M., Slack, F., & Armitt, G. (2005). Collaboration and teamwork: Immersion and presence in an online learning environment. *Information Systems Frontiers, 7*(1), 27–37. doi:10.1007/s10796-005-5336-9

Bertulis, R., & Cheeseborough, J. (2008). The Royal College of Nursing's information needs survey of nurses and health professionals. *Health Information and Libraries Journal, 25*(3), 186–197. doi:10.1111/j.1471-1842.2007.00755.x PMID:18796079

Booth, A., Sutton, A., & Falzon, L. (2003). Working together: Supporting projects through action learning. *Health Information and Libraries Journal, 20*(4), 225–231. doi:10.1111/j.1471-1842.2003.00461.x PMID:14641495

Brooks, F., & Scott, P. (2006a). Exploring knowledge work and leadership in online midwifery communication. *Journal of Advanced Nursing, 55*(4), 510–520. doi:10.1111/j.1365-2648.2006.03937.x PMID:16866846

Brooks, F., & Scott, P. (2006b). Knowledge work in nursing and midwifery: An evaluation through computer-mediated communication. *International Journal of Nursing Studies, 43*(1), 83–97. doi:10.1016/j.ijnurstu.2005.02.003 PMID:16326164

Casaló, L. V., Flavián, C., & Guinalíu, M. (2010). Determinants of the intention to participate in firm-hosted online travel communities and effects on consumer behavioral intentions. *Tourism Management, 31*(6), 898–911. doi:10.1016/j.tourman.2010.04.007

Chang, H. H., & Chuang, S.-S. (2011). Social capital and individual motivations on knowledge sharing: Participant involvement as a moderator. *Information & Management, 48*(1), 9–18. doi:10.1016/j.im.2010.11.001

Chen, C. J., & Hung, S. W. (2010). To give or to receive? Factors influencing members' knowledge sharing and community promotion in professional virtual communities. *Information & Management, 47*(4), 226–236. doi:10.1016/j.im.2010.03.001

Chen, I. Y. L. (2007). The factors influencing members' continuance intentions in professional virtual communities—A longitudinal study. *Journal of Information Science, 33*(4), 451. doi:10.1177/0165551506075323

Chen, I.Y.L., & Chen, N.S., & Kinshuk. (2009). Examining the Factors Influencing Participants' Knowledge Sharing Behavior in Virtual Learning Communities. *Journal of Educational Technology & Society, 12*(1), 134–148.

Cheung, C. M. K., & Lee, M. K. O. (2009). Understanding the sustainability of a virtual community: Model development and empirical test. *Journal of Information Science, 35*(3), 279–298. doi:10.1177/0165551508099088

Chiu, C. M., Hsu, M. H., & Wang, E. T. G. (2006). Understanding knowledge sharing in virtual communities: An integration of social capital and social cognitive theories. *Decision Support Systems, 42*(3), 1872–1888. doi:10.1016/j.dss.2006.04.001

Choi, S. Y., Kang, Y. S., & Lee, H. (2008). The effects of socio-technical enablers on knowledge sharing: an exploratory examination. *Journal of Information Science, 34*(5), 742–754. doi:10.1177/0165551507087710

Clarke, A., Lewis, D., Cole, I., & Ringrose, L. (2005). A strategic approach to developing e learning capability for healthcare. *Health Information and Libraries Journal, 22*(2), 33–41. doi:10.1111/j.1470-3327.2005.00611.x PMID:16279974

DeLone, W., & McLean, E. (1992). Information systems success: The quest for the dependent variable. *Information Systems Research, 3*(1), 60–95. doi:10.1287/isre.3.1.60

Docherty, C., Hoy, D., Topp, H., & Trinder, K. (2005). eLearning techniques supporting problem based learning in clinical simulation. *International Journal of Medical Informatics, 74*(7-8), 527–533. doi:10.1016/j.ijmedinf.2005.03.009 PMID:16043082

Doll, W. J., & Torkzadeh, G. (1991). The measurement of end-user computing satisfaction: Theoretical and methodological issues. *Management Information Systems Quarterly, 15*(1), 5–10. doi:10.2307/249429

Dubé, L., Bourhis, A., & Jacob, R. (2005). The impact of structuring characteristics on the launching of virtual communities of practice. *Journal of Organizational Change Management, 18*(2), 145–166. doi:10.1108/09534810510589570

Fang, Y. H., & Chiu, C. M. (2010). In justice we trust: Exploring knowledge-sharing continuance intentions in virtual communities of practice. *Computers in Human Behavior, 26*(2), 235–246. doi:10.1016/j.chb.2009.09.005

Fernandez, I., Gonzalez, A., & Sabherwal, R. (2004). *Knowledge Management, solutions, technology*. Prentice-Hall, Inc.

G-I-N. (2010). *G-I-N Emergency Care Community of Interest Annual Report*. Guidelines International Network.

Geoffery, G. (2008). *A community-based model for the production of ideas*. (Master Thesis). Simon Fraser University.

Ho, K., Jarvis Selinger, S., Norman, C. D., Li, L. C., Olatunbosun, T., Cressman, C., & Nguyen, A. (2010). Electronic communities of practice: Guidelines from a project. *The Journal of Continuing Education in the Health Professions, 30*(2), 139–143. doi:10.1002/chp.20071 PMID:20564704

Hsu, M. H., Ju, T. L., Yen, C. H., & Chang, C. M. (2007). Knowledge sharing behavior in virtual communities: The relationship between trust, self-efficacy, and outcome expectations. *International Journal of Human-Computer Studies, 65*(2), 153–169. doi:10.1016/j.ijhcs.2006.09.003

Jennex, M. E. (2008). Knowledge Management Success Models. In *Knowledge Management: Concepts, Methodologies, Tools, and Applications* (pp. 32–40). Hershey, PA: IGI Global.

Jennex, M. E., Smolnik, S., & Croasdell, D. (2008). Towards measuring knowledge management success. In *Proceedings of Hawaii International Conference on System Sciences*. IEEE.

Jin, X. L., Cheung, C. M. K., Lee, M. K. O., & Chen, H. P. (2009). How to keep members using the information in a computer-supported social network. *Computers in Human Behavior, 25*(5), 1172–1181. doi:10.1016/j.chb.2009.04.008

Kankanhalli, A., & Tan, B. C. Y. (2005). Knowledge Management Metrics: A Review and Directions for Future Research. *International Journal of Knowledge Management, 1*(2), 20–32. doi:10.4018/jkm.2005040103

Kankanhalli, A., Tan, B. C. Y., & Wei, K. K. (2005a). Contributing knowledge to electronic knowledge repositories: An empirical investigation. *Management Information Systems Quarterly, 29*(1), 113–143.

Kankanhalli, A., Tan, B. C. Y., & Wei, K. K. (2005b). Understanding seeking from electronic knowledge repositories: An empirical study. *Journal of the American Society for Information Science and Technology, 56*(11), 1156–1166. doi:10.1002/asi.20219

Kuo, B., Young, M. L., Hsu, M. H., Lin, C., & Chiang, P. C. (2003). *A study of the cognition-action gap in knowledge management*. Paper presented at the International Conference on Information Systems (ICIS) 2003. New York, NY.

Lin, H., Fan, W., Wallace, L., & Zhang, Z. (2007). An empirical study of web-based knowledge community success. In *Proceedings of the 40th Hawaii International Conference on System Sciences*. IEEE.

Lin, H. F. (2007). Effects of extrinsic and intrinsic motivation on employee knowledge sharing intentions. *Journal of Information Science, 33*(2), 135–149. doi:10.1177/0165551506068174

Lin, H. F. (2008a). Antecedents of virtual community satisfaction and loyalty: An empirical test of competing theories. *Cyberpsychology & Behavior, 11*(2), 138–144. doi:10.1089/cpb.2007.0003 PMID:18422404

Lin, H. F. (2008b). Determinants of successful virtual communities: Contributions from system characteristics and social factors. *Information & Management, 45*(8), 522–527. doi:10.1016/j.im.2008.08.002

Lin, H. F., & Lee, G. G. (2006). Determinants of success for online communities: An empirical study. *Behaviour & Information Technology, 25*(6), 479–488. doi:10.1080/01449290500330422

Lin, M. J. J., Hung, S. W., & Chen, C. J. (2009). Fostering the determinants of knowledge sharing in professional virtual communities. *Computers in Human Behavior, 25*(4), 929–939. doi:10.1016/j.chb.2009.03.008

Lin, T. C., & Huang, C. C. (2008). Understanding the determinants of EKR usage from social, technological and personal perspectives. *Journal of Information Science, 35*(2), 165–179. doi:10.1177/0165551508095780

Lubon, L. (2005). *Information by country*. UNICEF. Retrieved June 1, 2010, from http://www.unicef.org/infobycountry/malaysia_34164.html

Maier, R. (2007). *Knowledge Management Systems Information and Communication Technologies for Knowledge Management*. New York: Springer.

Merrill, J., & Hripcsak, G. (2008). Using social network analysis within a department of biomedical informatics to induce a discussion of academic communities of practice. *Journal of the American Medical Informatics Association, 15*(6), 780–782. doi:10.1197/jamia.M2717 PMID:18756000

Nahapiet, J., & Ghoshal, S. (1998). Social capital, intellectual capital, and the organizational advantage. *Academy of Management Review, 23*(2), 242–266.

Nistor, N., Schworm, S., & Werner, M. (2012). Online help-seeking in communities of practice: Modeling the acceptance of conceptual artifacts. *Computers & Education, 59*(2), 774–784. doi:10.1016/j.compedu.2012.03.017

Nonaka, I., & Takeuchi, H. (1995). *The knowledge-creating company: How Japanese companies create the dynamics of innovation*. Oxford University Press.

Parcell, G. (2005). *The Bulletin interview with Geoff Parcell*. World Health Organization. Retrieved June 13, 2012, from http://www.who.int/bulletin/volumes/83/10/interview1005/en/index.html

Preece, J. (2001). Sociability and usability in online communities: Determining and measuring success. *Behaviour & Information Technology, 20*(5), 347–356. doi:10.1080/01449290110084683

Rosenbaum, H., & Shachaf, P. (2010). A structuration approach to online communities of practice: The case of Q&A communities. *Journal of the American Society for Information Science and Technology, 61*(9), 1933–1944. doi:10.1002/asi.21340

Russell, J., Greenhalgh, T., Boynton, P., & Rigby, M. (2004). Soft networks for bridging the gap between research and practice: Illuminative evaluation of CHAIN. *BMJ (Clinical Research Ed.), 328*(7449), 1174. doi:10.1136/bmj.328.7449.1174 PMID:15142924

Shannon, C. E., & Weaver, W. (1949). *The mathematical theory of information*. Urbana, IL: University of Illinois Press.

Stergiou, N., Georgoulakis, G., Margari, N., Aninos, D., Stamataki, M., & Stergiou, E. et al. (2009). Using a web-based system for the continuous distance education in cytopathology. *International Journal of Medical Informatics, 78*(12), 827–838. doi:10.1016/j.ijmedinf.2009.08.007 PMID:19775933

Tremblay, D.-G. (2007). Communities of Practice (CoP), implementation challenges of e-working. *The Journal of E-Working, 1*, 69–82.

Tseng, F.-C., & Kuo, F.-Y. (2014). A study of social participation and knowledge sharing in the teachers' online professional community of practice. *Computers & Education, 72*, 37–47. doi:10.1016/j.compedu.2013.10.005

Urbach, N., Smolnik, S., & Riempp, G. (2010). An empirical investigation of employee portal success. *The Journal of Strategic Information Systems, 19*(3), 184–206. doi:10.1016/j.jsis.2010.06.002

Vavasseur, C. B., & MacGregor, S. K. (2008). Extending Content-Focused Professional Development through Online Communities of Practice. *Journal of Research on Technology in Education, 40*(4), 517–536. doi:10.1080/15391523.2008.10782519

Wang, H., Chung, J. E., Park, N., McLaughlin, M. L., & Fulk, J. (2012). Understanding Online Community Participation: A Technology Acceptance Perspective. *Communication Research, 39*(6), 781–801. doi:10.1177/0093650211408593

Wasko, M. M. L., & Faraj, S. (2005). Why should I share? Examining social capital and knowledge contribution in electronic networks of practice. *Management Information Systems Quarterly, 29*(1), 35–57.

Wasko, M. M. L., Teigland, R., & Faraj, S. (2009). The provision of online public goods: Examining social structure in an electronic network of practice. *Decision Support Systems, 47*(3), 254–265. doi:10.1016/j.dss.2009.02.012

Wenger, E. (1998). *Communities of practice: Learning, meaning, and identity*. Cambridge Univ Pr. doi:10.1017/CBO9780511803932

Wenger, E. (2004). Knowledge management as a doughnut: Shaping your knowledge strategy through communities of practice. *Ivey Business Journal, 68*(3), 1–8.

Wenger, E., McDermott, R., & Snyder, W. M. (2002). *Cultivating communities of practice: A guide to managing knowledge*. Cambridge, MA: Harvard University Press.

Yu, T. K., Lu, L. C., & Liu, T. F. (2010). Exploring factors that influence knowledge sharing behavior via weblogs. *Computers in Human Behavior*, *26*(1), 32–41. doi:10.1016/j.chb.2009.08.002

Zhang, W., & Watts, S. (2003). Knowledge adoption in online communities of practice. [ICIS.]. *Proceedings of ICIS*, *2003*, 96–109.

Zhang, Y., Fang, Y., Wei, K.-K., & Chen, H. (2010). Exploring the role of psychological safety in promoting the intention to continue sharing knowledge in virtual communities. *International Journal of Information Management*, *30*(5), 425–436. doi:10.1016/j.ijinfomgt.2010.02.003

Zviran, M., & Erlich, Z. (2003). Measuring IS User Satisfaction: Review and Implications. *Communications of the Association for Information Systems*, *12*(5), 81–104.

KEY TERMS AND DEFINITIONS

Human Dimension: The human dimension of online CoPs refers to the characteristics and senses of individuals who influence behaviour in online CoPs, consequently affecting knowledge sharing behaviour.

Knowledge Management: Knowledge management is considered as a systematic process of managing knowledge assets, processes, and environment to facilitate the creation, organiza-tion, sharing, utilization, and measurement of knowledge to achieve the strategic aims of an organization.

Online CoPs Evaluation: The Online CoPs evaluation refers to the process of assessing their value in managing knowledge by defining deter-minants of success and acceptance.

Online CoPs Outcomes: The outcomes of online CoPs refer to the actual benefits that par-ticipants receive from using online CoPs, including intangible benefits that can address subsequent effects of the utilization.

Online CoPs: The online CoPs consist of ex-perts in specific area, with a common interest who interact via ICTs to share skills and knowledge to solve problems in their area of expertise.

Semantic Dimension: The semantic dimen-sion refers to the success of the information in expressing its intended meaning and the user's expectations in terms of its usefulness and value.

Social Dimension: The social dimension refers to the strength of the relationships and communi-cation among members of online CoPs which is determined by individual's commitment, interper-sonal trust, reputation, and norm of reciprocity.

Technical Dimension: The technical dimen-sion of online CoPs refers to the influences that have an impact on how members of CoPs using the information and communication related tech-nologies within the online CoPs' environment in KM activities.

Chapter 3
Incorporating Usability Testing into the Development of Healthcare Technologies

Shilo H. Anders
Vanderbilt University, USA

Judith W. Dexheimer
Cincinnati Children's Medical Center, USA

ABSTRACT

The use of mobile devices in healthcare is increasing in prevalence and poses different constraints for use than traditional desktop computing. This chapter introduces several usability testing methods that are appropriate for use when designing and developing mobile technologies. Approaching the development of mobile technologies through a user-centered approach is critical to improve the interaction and use of the hardware and software that is implemented on a mobile platform in healthcare. User-centered design adds value by getting feedback about functionality, design, and constraints that need to be built into the system prior to its completion. Future work in this domain will require further tailoring and use of novel usability methods to evaluate and improve the design of mobile healthcare technologies.

INTRODUCTION

Standard mobile devices function frequently as more than just as cellular telephones, and include additional functionality such as email, Internet access, and application. Mobile technology is pervasive throughout the culture of the United States. As of 2012, approximately 326 million mobile devices are used (CTIA: The Wireless Association, 2012) with a wireless penetration of greater than 100%. (CTIA: The Wireless Associa-

tion, 2012) It leads from the saturation of mobile technology, that it will become very important not just in personal but also in professional settings.

The goal of this chapter is to provide an understanding of how the user-centered design process can be incorporated into the design and development of mobile applications. Especially as applications evolve to provide individuals with targeted and just-in-time interventions tailored to incorporate an individual's specific healthcare needs. In this chapter, we will discuss

DOI: 10.4018/978-1-4666-6150-9.ch003

the importance and strategies for implementing usability testing, and more broadly human factors engineering, into mobile healthcare technology design and development. We will discuss what user-centered design entails, why it is important to use when developing mobile Health IT, how it can be incorporated into system design and development, and finally we will discuss common barriers to the implementation of a user-centered design process and how these may be overcome. We will include an example of a mobile Health IT system that incorporated usability testing into its development process.

BACKGROUND

Mobile devices and associated technologies are transforming clinical healthcare systems, communication between patients and clinicians, and the utilization of personal health information. Advances in integrating mobile technology with the Internet, cloud computing, and clinical data systems provide unparalleled abilities to monitor, support, and motivate just-in-time clinical and patient-centered health decision-making. Examples of the potential of mobile technology transforming healthcare systems include providing low-cost, real-time means for assessing disease, behavior, environmental toxins, metabolites and other physiological variables, as well as integrating multiple sources of data from movement, images, social interactions, to inform health behaviors and healthcare decisions. With the increasing popularity of technologies, new issues arise that involve not just the accuracy of the medical advice but also the user's interaction with the system. It is important to involve the users in the design and implementation of any electronic system, but it is also important to ensure the system is well designed.

Mobile healthcare (mHealth) technology has the potential to bring data and contextually appropriate support to patients, clinicians and research-

ers in ways never before possible but only if they are efficient, effective and easy to use. Mobile technology encompasses cellular telephones and tablet computers. In two US surveys, approximately 90% of adults reported using mobile phones with 61% of them using smartphones (Sterling, 2013), and approximately one third of adults have a tablet computer. (Pew Internet & American Life Project & Zickuhr, June 2013) Mobile devices have the ability to store reams of information in a small, convenient and lightweight device that is highly portable for easy communication or reference. Devices are frequently wireless enabled that allow a user to access wireless or cellular networks. The devices have the potential to provide both data stored on the device along with external data that can be accessed through network, like cloud-based computing. This provides a mountain of information and support at each users almost instantaneous disposal.

What are some of the issues with using mobile devices and why are they difficult to use?

While the portability of mobile devices is valuable for the availability of information, the devices have some issues that hinder their usability. The security of mobile devices should be considered. Several key factors are important to consider including password protection, requiring 2-step authentication, and ensuring secure wireless transmissions. Devices are electronic and therefore users must be mindful of being charged, being available, as well as knowing where to find the appropriate data. If the data is available externally, network connectivity is an issue to overcome, especially in clinical care when immediate access may be necessary. Software included on mobile devices must be user-friendly and optimized to be viewed and digested on significantly smaller screens than may be currently used. Mobile devices are frequently small to optimize portability, which leads to a lessening of screen size. With this limited viewing area software needs to consider what is optimal to display, when it needs shown and how to display it.

Human factors engineering has been used to evaluate systems, design and evaluate new technology, analyze adverse events and catastrophic accidents. (Cook, Render, & Woods, 2000; Evans et al., 1998; Raschke et al., 1998; Reason, 1995; Salvendy, 2006) Health information technology (Health IT) intended for mobile technologies faces a unique set of challenges that are not a relevant to other platforms. In addition, Health IT design for a specific audience, be it clinicians or patients must accommodate multiple and diverse users; many, often complex tasks, and various contexts of use (e.g. at home, or in multiple locations throughout the hospital. Human factors engineering is a recognized approach to effectively address mobile Health IT design challenges because it is predicated on an empirical understanding of users, tasks, and contexts of use to design and test products rather than the developers perceptions of what users can, want and are capable of doing (Nielsen, 1993; Preece, 1995; Vicente, 2004). Specifically user-centered design, will allow for the development of technology that is useful, well designed and easy to use. This approach to mobile technology design has a demonstrable track record of useful and usable designs (Weinger, Gardner-Bonneau, & Wiklund, 2011), although it's emergence in mobile technologies has been limited (Mulvaney, Anders, Smith, Pittel, & Johnson, 2012). The human factors engineering approach is promoted in ISO standards for design and evaluation, FDA requirements for medical devices, and key publications (American National Standards Institute & Association For the Advancement of Medical Instrumentation, 2009; International Organization for Standardization, 2006, 2007, 2010). For example, a recent AHRQ report stated the Health IT projects should 'engage human factors experts in the design team' and use a user-centered design methodology; thus far this approach has seen minimal use in the development of Health IT products (Agency for Healthcare Research and Quality, 2011). Low adoption rates,

abandonment, workarounds, and use errors are testaments to this failure (Patterson et al., 2005; Wong et al., 2003).

In summary, mobile technologies hold great promise and potential to change how we engage, monitor and communicate about our health and health management. Mobile technologies have reached wide-spread use and will continue to be integrated in personal and professional settings. In order to sustain and improve the software design for mHealth, a recognized approach to design and evaluation is human factors engineering. is an approach that will be discussed further.

USER-CENTERED DESIGN FOR MOBILE TECHNOLOGIES

The design of user-centered sustainable mobile health IT requires a targeted and iterative approach. We will leverage the depth and breadth of current usability frameworks from the literature as they apply to mobile technologies in healthcare. Using current literature and authors' experience with usability in mobile technologies, we will systematically present usability aspects to consider during design including: 1) target user characteristics, 2) contexts, and 3) functional tasks in which technology will ultimately be used.

What is User-Centered Design (UCD)?

User-centered design (UCD) is an approach to the development of products, devices, or systems to be used to complete tasks efficiently, effectively, safely and satisfactorily by their intended users (International Organization for Standardization, 2010). This relies heavily on the application of knowledge about human physiology and behavior which is then applied to the design context.

The UCD approach is a rigorous set of methods in which to improve the design of systems including software/hardware, people, and process. For UCD, the system to be developed includes the mobile technology, people that will ultimately use that technology and the environment in which it will be used to achieve desired results (Woods & Hollnagel, 2006). For computer science often the software and hardware are typically the focus for system design, while UCD practitioners focus on the people and their interactions with the software and hardware. A core characteristic of UCD that differentiates it from other technology design processes is that the users are involved in the design of the technology throughout the development of the project. When considering mHealth technologies, future users should help shape the key information requirements and needs for the project since viewing space is limited. As the development cycle continues, users may provide additional requirements and feedback on usability aspects with early prototypes. This is especially true if they are able to use them in practice. Another characteristic of UCD is iterative and multiple approaches to the development

of a mobile technology may be taken. In fact, it is likely that UCD practitioners will use a number different methods to aid in design requirement development and evaluation. Prior to a UCD evaluation, clear goals and outcomes should be defined. For example, the focus of an evaluation may be to determine how best to represent a key pieces of information that practitioners require for their decision-making. The usability evaluation would what to test to criterion, which may be as defuse as the user could accomplish the task, or a specific time allocation may be specified.

Effective UCD (or redesign) depends on an in-depth understanding of the individuals that will ultimately use the mobile technology and its ability to integrate into the IT development cycle (Mayhew, 1999). Figure 1 shows a notional architecture for how this integration could occur. For UCD the initiating step in Health IT design requires a thorough understanding of frontline work and the perspective of health providers or patients and their caregivers depending on who will use the technology (it might be both!) and

Figure 1. Ideal user-centered design process integrated with software development process

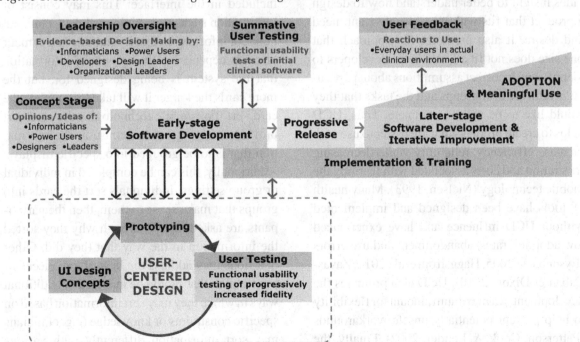

how that prospective might be obtained (Weinger, et al., 2011; Wiklund & Wilcox, 2005). This knowledge drives specific design requirements, which are then incorporated into the user interface (UI) design concepts. UCD includes the development of multiple alternative designs, followed by the development of higher fidelity prototypes in which these potential solutions are then evaluated through user testing. User testing may initially be informal and prior to deploy a summative usability evaluation of the designed system would ideally be conducted. Design evaluation then assesses whether users' needs were met as well as considers the contextual factors related to success or failure, and factors that will facilitate or prevent generalizability beyond the initial deployment site (Shilo Anders, Woods, Patterson, & Schweikhart, 2008; Wong, et al., 2003). After initial system implementation, facilitating and gathering user feedback is way to incorporate user driven changes into future system iterations.

Why is UCD Important?

Including UCD in the development process provides insight to better understand how to design a product that fits with what people want, need and desire. It also promotes the approach that one size does not fit all, and helps developers to identify any incorrect assumptions about particular healthcare user groups and the tasks that they would like to be able to complete. Thus, UCD helps to create products that are easier to use with increase efficiency, reliability while decreasing frustration and costs associated with learning the mobile technology (Nielsen, 1993). Many health IT tools have been designed and implemented without UCD influence and have experienced low adoption rates, abandonment and use errors (Eysenbach, 2005; Haggstrom et al., 2011; Zayas-Caban & Dixon, 2010). UCD also promotes the development of a maximum amount for flexibility to help prevent potentially unsafe workarounds (Patterson, Cook, & Render, 2002). Finally, the

UCD process allows individuals to evaluate and be involved in the actual design of the product or systems which may ease implementation burdens, increase user appeal and satisfaction (McCurdie et al., 2012), and provide individual champions in various hospital settings (Kortum & Safari Technical Books., 2008).

Approaches to UCD

UCD methodologies are varied in approach and can be modified according to the needs and challenges that a particular mobile technology is trying to achieve. The table lists the methodologies most utilized by UCD practitioners that are applicable to mHealth. Three of the ones that the authors have used most are subsequently described in more detail.

Card Sort

The card sort method is most utilized early in the UCD process, often prior to any interface design development. The researcher will create a number of paper cards that include the information to be included in the interface. This may consist of information such as physiological data, clinician notes, or information that is relevant. The number of cards depends on the amount of information that the system is being designed for, but the more cards the longer it will take to complete the card sort. For mobile technologies the card sort provides a way to parse and constrain the information that is to be grouped into specific displays. Additionally, this can be completed in individual or group settings. Individuals sort the cards into groups that make sense to them, then the participants are asked to talk through why they sorted the information in the way that they did. Other questions may address the lack of key pieces of information that should be included or additional ways in which they may sort information based on specific constraints or knowledge (e.g. clinicians may sort information differently with various patient diagnoses.) Across individuals patterns of information sets or groups can be found which can be used for the design of the system. The card helps to ensure that the information is organized in a manner that is consistent and logical for the individuals that will use the system.

For example, a project conducted by the authors involved using a card sort methodology to group physiological variables for ICU patients. The nurses that were asked to participate in the study grouped the variables according to how they monitored their patients and ordered the information by importance. The subsequent information display, while not specifically designed for a mobile platform grouped functional information together, which could be opened individually and ultimately displayed on a mobile platform. The subsequent design was further usability tested using numerous methods and culminated in a summative usability evaluation (S. Anders et al., 2012).

In mobile technology design, the use of the card sort affords the development of interfaces that group information in ways that make sense to the users. This can also help to constrain and put information on interfaces that assist in meeting the goals of the system thus minimizing extraneous information. For clinicians the card sort may contribute to the design of interfaces that provide the necessary information at a glance rather than having to navigate through multiple interfaces where data must then be synthesized. The limited screen size can be a detriment to ease of use of the system. When doing the card sort for mobile technologies it will be instrumental to limit the groupings to a manageable number that can easily be displayed on the interface. Additionally, in the mobile environment the researcher may also ask the user to consider a number of different situations for use (at home versus in the hospital) as this may influence the grouping of information.

Table 1. Summary of methodologies for UCD in mobile technology development

Methods	Definition
Card Sort	A technique that consists of individuals that will be users combining information found on cards in ways that make sense to them.
Expert evaluations	Review of the product or system by which a UCD or human factors expert preferably in conjunction with a product user (e.g. Heuristic evaluation).
Focus Groups	A skilled moderator leads 6-12 users in a discussion about a system or mobile technology. The moderator elicits answers to qualitative questions about use practices or envisioned system use.
Paper and pencil evaluations	Individual aspects of the user interface or system design are shown drawn on paper. The user is asked questions about how to operate and interact with the interface to accomplish task requirements.
Surveys	Questions about use and feedback about a system are generated and presented in a consumer friendly format. Traditional survey development involves validating the survey prior to widespread dissemination.
Cognitive Walk-through	A UCD professional leads a individual through actual user tasks. The user talks about their goals, feedback about the user interface and performance challenges.
Formative Usability Evaluation	Involves the development of problem statements or test objectives that are representative of the tasks that users engage. The user completes tasks where performance measures are collected. The outcome is improvement recommendations.
Summative Usability Evaluation	Test of the system just prior to implementation that usually involves the user performing tasks that test hypotheses. The user performs task unaided and any issues with the interface are noted, so improvements can be made.

Sources: (Dumas & Redish, 1999; Rubin, 1994; Wiklund & Wilcox, 2005)

Cognitive Walk-Through

A cognitive walk-through is a UCD method that involves the user and a moderator walking through the interface and subsequent user interaction of a mock-up or functioning prototype. The user talks out loud has he/she goes through the interface, explaining what they think a specific button, graphic or text means and how it links to other parts of the proposed system. This approach assists designers in helping to understand where there are uncertainties embedded in the interface that are likely to result in user confusion and errors. As the user walks through the interface they will provide feedback about their likes and potential improvements. Additionally, the user may suggest including information that was not previously considered as integral to the system and conversely information that is extraneous. The cognitive walk-through may be completed rapidly and iteratively with small incremental changes being made to the interface when participants suggest similar changes or encounter similar barriers. The walkthrough is conducted on an individual basis and may be conducted with prototype interfaces that are displayed as paper printouts. Conversely it may also be utilized with interfaces that are in production or close to production.

In a project involving the development of a mobile application to assist busy outpatient clinicians this method was employed to garner feedback from busy clinicians with minimal time available. The research team developed prototype interfaces that were printed and taken to users to provide feedback using this method (Figure 2). Participants were asked to walk through the elements in the interface and the expectation of how that element should behave was captured. After hearing feedback from a minimum of three users, the team improved upon the interface taking the user feedback into account (Figure 3). As can be seen in the figures below, over five iterations with a total of fifteen clinicians the interface changed dramatically to more accurately embody the clinicians work in

their environment (i.e. high volume clinics). It should be noted that initially this project was not specifically focused on designing for a mobile platform, however after initial feedback from clinicians the research team decided to include this in the requirements and platform flexibility became a key aspect of the design for subsequent iterations of the cognitive walkthrough.

For mobile technologies the cognitive walk-through is a quick and efficient way in which to gather feedback from users that can easily be incorporated into the design. If using paper printouts comments can be directly annotated onto the interface and there are numerous outlines for the various mobile technologies available. Online software exists in which prototypes may be tested in this manner and some even allow the user to enter comments into the interface. This is convenient if the population one wants to talk with are at a distance. Thus remote evaluations may be an alternative approach, and technologies exist in which these session may be video and audio recorded. The walk-through approach may be complicated if a prototype is use and the researcher and participant are both attempting to view the same interface. Finally, it may behoove the researcher and user to walk-through the interface in the context of use, such that potential issues with information viewing while on the go, sharing in the context of a visit or even connectively issues may be revealed.

Summative Usability Evaluation

A summative usability evaluation is an individual session involving a working prototype or beta version of the software, just prior to release. In the UCD process this is the final step before product implementation and if the UCD process is implemented, minimal use errors and user frustrations should exist. A total of 5-12 users will interact with the product completing the tasks that the functions of the product support. The researchers will create a realistic environment in which

Figure 2. Interface prior to numerous cognitive walk-through iterations

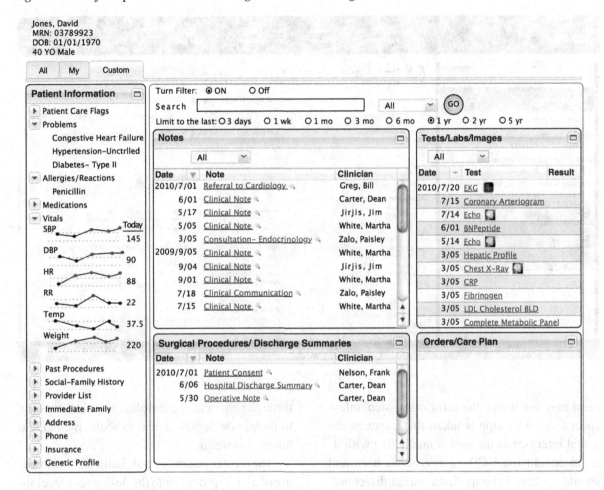

that practitioners will use the system although a usability lab setting may be utilized as well. The scenarios that each participant will work through should be representative of a set of tasks. Use errors, frustration, incomplete tasks and time on task are usually included in the evaluation that may be based on hypotheses about the system. In some cases, two diverse products are evaluated and compared for usability.

In a project that illustrates this type of evaluation, 19 nurses and 3 anesthesia providers utilized one of two patient identification devices for blood verification to complete a series of scenarios (S. Anders et al., 2011). The goal of the project was to assist hospital leadership in deciding which

technology to implement, thus the focus was on user satisfaction, use errors (e.g. did the provider give inappropriate blood products), and efficiency of use. The results revealed that both products had usability issues that included a lack of feedback to the user, limited information about required subtasks and lack of visibility about system state and limitation. These handheld devices both led to user frustration and workarounds during actual use.

Summative usability evaluations of mobile technologies especially when scenario driven can reveal usability issues and process errors that were previously unknown. The difficulty is in adequately capturing these events. If the scenario is in situ with a mobile device the UCD

Figure 3. Interface after numerous cognitive walkthroughs

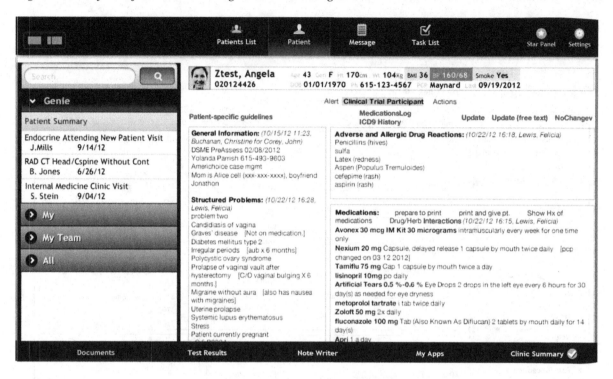

team may not notice the error or misstep unless special consideration is taken that captures the actual interface as the user is interacting with it.

In conclusion UCD methods have been and should continue to be applied to mHealth technology development. Special considerations regarding the viewing area and context of use should be considered when testing this technology. The next section presents a variety of barriers and challenges to incorporating UCD into the development process and recommendations to overcome these issues.

Challenges of Incorporating UCD into Development and Recommendations

Incorporating UCD into the Health IT design framework can be a daunting task. Some of the challenges that the authors have faced in doing this are described below as well as how these were overcome. Further, the challenges are illustrated

through generalized examples that relate not only to mobile devices, but also to social medial and hospital systems.

The most commonly cited challenges to including of a UCD process into the design and development of mobile technologies are presented below.

1. The UCD process will add more time than developers have allotted for project completion.

Overcoming this challenge involves the persistence and flexibility on the part of both the UCD team and the IT development process. The early that the UCD team can become involved in the development of the system, the easier it will be to incorporate these processes into the development cycle. UCD members should consider attending IT development meetings, especially if an agile software development cycle is used. Ideally the interface design should be ahead of the development team and be testing functionality prior to it being developed in the system. Countless redesigns of systems have occurred because UCD was not included in the system development process (Eysenbach, 2005; Haggstrom, et al., 2011; Zayas-Caban & Dixon, 2010).

2. There are not enough resources to include UCD.

Investment in UCD on the front end leads to greater user satisfaction, ease of use and sustained use. Depending on what you are designing, there may be room to creatively include UCD in the design process. Additionally, UCD processes can be as involved or minimally included as necessary and dependent upon what is being designed. Formal usability evaluations may not be necessary or desirable for some products, and some methods may be conducted with as few as three participants with minimal time involved. A mobile application may include UCD with minimal effort or incorporated into larger studies or as projects for students.

3. Limited access to users.

In mHealth, users can be highly varied and are usually all very busy; this seems to be especially true with clinicians. For UCD approaches to involve a number of participants the research must consider alternative ways to involve users. Having an advocate that regularly interacts with the users of interest to be your advocate may help to get time with users. Additionally, especially with physicians, alternative times, offering incentives, and limiting the amount of time that you are requesting can also help to get users. Finally, when the UCD team meets with the user they should be quick, direct and willing to visit at nontraditional times. For example, cognitive walk-throughs can use paper printouts and in 15 minutes get useful feedback about the interface, provided that questions are succinct and the interfaces included are not all possible options.

4. No expertise in UCD processes.

In this case, seek outside help and find the expertise that is needed. The IT department at a large academic medical center knew that implementing a UCD approach to its technology development was important. Thus, they sought and formed a relationship with UCD experts at the medical center that were conducting research in this area. The collaboration has been beneficial to both parties and to the users that are now using the products.

FUTURE RESEARCH DIRECTIONS

This chapter highlights the need for a UCD in mobile healthcare technology development and briefly describes some of the common methods. Currently UCD in healthcare organizations has been minimally incorporated in the development of technologies, although there are exceptions (Russ et al., 2012). Furthermore, applying UCD to mHealth has the potential to improve both the functionality and use of the mobile devices and their related applications.

To incorporate UCD into the design and implementation of new systems, an organizational change is required for adoption and integration. Including UCD requires extra time, planning, and money during the design phase of a project. While this investment will ultimately pay off, in user satisfaction and adoption of the technology, the importance of considering these design elements must be a priority to the organization. No application is created or used solely on it's own. Integration between devices and systems should be considering during the design, as should the integration between users of a system. If users are happy with the mHealth application, they are more likely to use it and suggest it to other interested users.

There is minimal research available in the literature regarding the impact of mobile health technologies on practice (Divall et al, 2013). Given the healthcare providers desire for hand-held devices, it is inevitable that more healthcare decisions and information will come from mobile devices. Future research should focus on the design, functionality, and availability of information through mHealth devices. Important topics such as connectivity, security, and accessibility should be addressed in both the literature and considered through the design process.

CONCLUSION

With the increase in mobile devices in everyday use and healthcare specifically, the importance of design is increasing. Overall the chapter used the framework of usability engineering to help capture how efforts to translate scientific evidence into clinical practice could be more successful. This chapter provides a human-centered design focus to the mobile health technical and intellectual literature. User-centered design can improve the functionality and use of applications on mobile devices. There is currently a dearth of information in the literature about using mobile devices for healthcare, future work should focus on employing usability methods in the design and evaluation of applications aimed to improve clinician performance and improve clinical care.

REFERENCES

Agency for Healthcare Research and Quality. (2011). Improving Consumer Health IT Application Development: Lessons from Other Industries-Background Report (AHRQ Publication No. 11-0065-EF). Rockville, MD: AHRQ.

American National Standards Institute & Association For the Advancement of Medical Instrumentation. (2009). ANSI/AAMI HE75, 2009 Ed. - Human factors engineering - Design of medical devices. Arlington, VA: American National Standards Institute.

Anders, S., Albert, R., Miller, A., Weinger, M. B., Doig, A. K., Behrens, M., & Agutter, J. (2012). Evaluation of an integrated graphical display to promote acute change detection in ICU patients. *International Journal of Medical Informatics*, *81*(12), 842–851. doi:10.1016/j. ijmedinf.2012.04.004 PMID:22534099

Anders, S., Miller, A., Joseph, P., Fortenberry, T., Woods, M., Booker, R., & France, D. (2011). Blood product positive patient identification: Comparative simulation-based usability test of two commercial products. *Transfusion*, *51*(11), 2311–2318. doi:10.1111/j.1537-2995.2011.03185.x PMID:21599676

Anders, S., Woods, D. D., Patterson, E. S., & Schweikhart, S. (2008). Shifts in Functions of a New Technology over Time: An Analysis of Logged Electronic Intensive Care Unit Interventions. *Proceedings of the Human Factors and Ergonomics Society Annual Meeting, 52*(12), 870-874.

Cook, R. I., Render, M., & Woods, D. D. (2000). Gaps in the continuity of care and progress on patient safety. *British Medical Journal*, *320*(7237), 791–794. doi:10.1136/bmj.320.7237.791 PMID:10720370

CTIA. The Wireless Association. (2012). *Wireless Quick Facts: Year-End Figures*. Retrieved September 30, 2013, from http://www.ctia.org/advocacy/research/index.cfm/aid/10323

Divall, P., Camosso-Stefinovic, J., & Baker, R. (2013). The use of personal digital assistants in clinical decision making by health care professionals: A systematic review. *Health Informatics Journal*, *19*(1), 16–28. doi:10.1177/1460458212446761 PMID:23486823

Dumas, J. S., & Redish, J. (1999). *A practical guide to usability testing* (Rev. ed.). Norwood, NJ: Intellect Books.

Evans, R. S., Pestotnik, S. L., Classen, D. C., Clemmer, T. P., Weaver, L. K., Orme, J. F. Jr, & Burke, J. P. (1998). A computer-assisted management program for antibiotics and other antiinfective agents. *The New England Journal of Medicine*, *338*(4), 232–238. doi:10.1056/NEJM199801223380406 PMID:9435330

Eysenbach, G. (2005). The law of attrition. *Journal of Medical Internet Research*, *7*(1), e11. doi:10.2196/jmir.7.1.e11 PMID:15829473

Haggstrom, D. A., Saleem, J. J., Russ, A. L., Jones, J., Russell, S. A., & Chumbler, N. R. (2011). Lessons learned from usability testing of the VA's personal health record. *Journal of the American Medical Informatics Association*, *18*(Suppl 1), i13–i17. doi:10.1136/amiajnl-2010-000082 PMID:21984604

International Organization for Standardization. (2006). *ISO 9241-110:2006 Ergonomics of human-system interaction -- Part 110: Dialogue principles*. Geneva, Switzerland: ISO.

International Organization for Standardization. (2007). [*Medical devices -- Application of usability engineering to medical devices*. Arlington, VA: AAMI.]. *IEC*, *62366*, 2007.

International Organization for Standardization. (2010). *ISO 9241-210:2010 Ergonomics of human-system interaction -- Part 210: Human-centred design for interactive systems*. Geneva, Switzerland: ISO.

Kortum, P., & Safari Technical Books. (2008). *HCI beyond the GUI design for haptic, speech, olfactory and other nontraditional interfaces*. San Francisco: Morgan Kaufmann.

Mayhew, D. J. (1999). *The usability engineering lifecycle: A practitioner's handbook for user interface design*. San Francisco: Morgan Kaufmann Publishers. doi:10.1145/632780.632805

McCurdie, T., Taneva, S., Casselman, M., Yeung, M., McDaniel, C., Ho, W., & Cafazzo, J. (2012). mHealth consumer apps: The case for user-centered design. *Biomedical Instrumentation & Technology*, 49–56. doi:10.2345/0899-8205-46.s2.49 PMID:23039777

Mulvaney, S. A., Anders, S., Smith, A. K., Pittel, E. J., & Johnson, K. B. (2012). A pilot test of a tailored mobile and web-based diabetes messaging system for adolescents. *Journal of Telemedicine and Telecare*, *18*(2), 115–118. doi:10.1258/jtt.2011.111006 PMID:22383802

Nielsen, J. (1993). *Usability engineering*. Boston: Academic Press.

Patterson, E. S., Cook, R. I., & Render, M. L. (2002). Improving patient safety by identifying side effects from introducing bar coding in medication administration. *Journal of the American Medical Informatics Association*, *9*(5), 540–553. doi:10.1197/jamia.M1061 PMID:12223506

Patterson, E. S., Doebbeling, B. N., Fung, C. H., Militello, L., Anders, S., & Asch, S. M. (2005). Identifying barriers to the effective use of clinical reminders: Bootstrapping multiple methods. *Journal of Biomedical Informatics*, *38*(3), 189–199. doi:10.1016/j.jbi.2004.11.015 PMID:15896692

Pew Internet & American Life Project, & Zickuhr, K. (2013, June). *Tablet Ownership 2013*. Retrieved September 30, 2013, from http://pewinternet.org/Reports/2013/Tablet-Ownership-2013.aspx

Preece, J. (1995). *Human-computer interaction.* Wokingham, UK: Addison-Wesley Pub. Co.

Raschke, R. A., Gollihare, B., Wunderlich, T. A., Guidry, J. R., Leibowitz, A. I., Peirce, J. C., & Susong, C. (1998). A computer alert system to prevent injury from adverse drug events: Development and evaluation in a community teaching hospital. *Journal of the American Medical Association, 280*(15), 1317–1320. doi:10.1001/jama.280.15.1317 PMID:9794309

Reason, J. (1995). Understanding adverse events: human factors. *Quality in Health Care, 4*(2), 80–89. doi:10.1136/qshc.4.2.80 PMID:10151618

Rubin, J. (1994). *Handbook of usability testing: How to plan, design, and conduct effective tests.* New York: Wiley.

Russ, A. L., Weiner, M., Russell, S. A., Baker, D. A., Fahner, W. J., & Saleem, J. J. (2012). Design and implementation of a hospital-based usability laboratory: Insights from a Department of Veterans Affairs laboratory for health information technology. *Joint Commission Journal on Quality and Patient Safety, 38*(12), 531–540. PMID:23240261

Salvendy, G. (2006). *Handbook of human factors and ergonomics* (3rd ed.). Hoboken, NJ: John Wiley. doi:10.1002/0470048204

Sterling, G. (2013). *Pew: 61 Percent in US Now Have Smartphones.* Retrieved September 30, 2013, from http://marketingland.com/pew-61-percent-in-us-now-have-smartphones-46966

Vicente, K. J. (2004). *The human factor: Revolutionizing the way people live with technology.* New York: Routledge.

Weinger, M. B., Gardner-Bonneau, D., & Wiklund, M. E. (2011). *Handbook of human factors in medical device design.* Boca Raton, FL: CRC Press.

Wiklund, M. E., & Wilcox, S. B. (2005). *Designing usability into medical products.* Boca Raton, FL: Taylor & Francis/CRC Press. doi:10.1201/9781420038088

Wong, D. H., Gallegos, Y., Weinger, M. B., Clack, S., Slagle, J., & Anderson, C. T. (2003). Changes in intensive care unit nurse task activity after installation of a third-generation intensive care unit information system. *Critical Care Medicine, 31*(10), 2488–2494. doi:10.1097/01.CCM.0000089637.53301.EF PMID:14530756

Woods, D. D., & Hollnagel, E. (2006). *Joint cognitive systems: Patterns in cognitive systems engineering.* Boca Raton, FL: CRC/Taylor & Francis. doi:10.1201/9781420005684

Zayas-Caban, T., & Dixon, B. E. (2010). Considerations for the design of safe and effective consumer health IT applications in the home. *Quality & Safety in Health Care, 19*(Suppl 3), i61–i67. doi:10.1136/qshc.2010.041897 PMID:20959321

ADDITIONAL READING

Anders, S., Albert, R., Miller, A., Weinger, M. B., Doig, A. K., Behrens, M., & Agutter, J. (2012). Evaluation of an integrated graphical display to promote acute change detection in ICU patients. *International Journal of Medical Informatics, 81*(12), 842–851. doi:10.1016/j.ijmedinf.2012.04.004 PMID:22534099

Anders, S., Miller, A., Joseph, P., Fortenberry, T., Woods, M., Booker, R., & France, D. (2011). Blood product positive patient identification: comparative simulation-based usability test of two commercial products. *Transfusion, 51*(11), 2311–2318. doi:10.1111/j.1537-2995.2011.03185.x PMID:21599676

Bevan, N. (2001). International standards for HCI and usability. *International Journal of Human-Computer Studies*, *55*(4), 533–552. doi:10.1006/ijhc.2001.0483

Carayon, P. (2010). Human factors in patient safety as an innovation. *Applied Ergonomics*, *41*(5), 657–665. doi:10.1016/j.apergo.2009.12.011 PMID:20106468

Chaudhry, B., Wang, J., Wu, S., Maglione, M., Mojica, W., Roth, E., & Shekelle, P. G. (2006). Systematic review: impact of health information technology on quality, efficiency, and costs of medical care. *Annals of Internal Medicine*, *144*(10), 742–752. doi:10.7326/0003-4819-144-10-200605160-00125 PMID:16702590

Eysenbach, G. (2011). CONSORT-EHEALTH: improving and standardizing evaluation reports of Web-based and mobile health interventions. *Journal of Medical Internet Research*, *13*(4), e126. doi:10.2196/jmir.1923 PMID:22209829

Grudin, J. (1994). Computer-supported cooperative work: history and focus. *IEEE Computer*, *27*(5), 19–26. doi:10.1109/2.291294

Hicks, J., Ramanathan, N., Kim, D., Monibi, M., Selsky, J., Hansen, M., & Estrin, D. (2010). *AndWellness: an open mobile system for activity and experience sampling*. Paper presented at the Wireless Health 2010, San Diego, California.

Hollnagel, E., & Woods, D. A. (2005). *Joint cognitive systems: foundations of cognitive systems engineering*. Boca Raton, FL: CRC Press. doi:10.1201/9781420038194

Johnson, C. W. (2006). Why did that happen? Exploring the proliferation of barely usable software in healthcare systems. *Quality & Safety in Health Care*, *15*(Suppl 1), i76–i81. doi:10.1136/qshc.2005.016105 PMID:17142614

Karsh, B. T. (2004). Beyond usability: designing effective technology implementation systems to promote patient safety. *Quality & Safety in Health Care*, *13*(5), 388–394. doi:10.1136/qshc.2004.010322 PMID:15465944

Karsh, B. T., Weinger, M. B., Abbott, P. A., & Wears, R. L. (2010). Health information technology: fallacies and sober realities. *Journal of the American Medical Informatics Association: JAMIA*, *17*(6), 617–623. doi:10.1136/jamia.2010.005637 PMID:20962121

Kientz, J. A., Choe, E. K., Birch, B., Maharaj, R., Fonville, A., Glasson, C., & Mundt, J. (2010). *Heuristic evaluation of persuasive health technologies*. Paper presented at the Proceedings of the 1st ACM International Health Informatics Symposium, Arlington, Virginia, USA.

Kjeldskov, J., Skov, M., Als, B., & Høegh, R. (2004). Is It Worth the Hassle? Exploring the Added Value of Evaluating the Usability of Context-Aware Mobile Systems in the Field. In S. Brewster, & M. Dunlop (Eds.), *Mobile Human-Computer Interaction - MobileHCI 2004* (Vol. 3160, pp. 61–73). Springer Berlin Heidelberg. doi:10.1007/978-3-540-28637-0_6

Koppel, R., Metlay, J. P., Cohen, A., Abaluck, B., Localio, A. R., Kimmel, S. E., & Strom, B. L. (2005). Role of computerized physician order entry systems in facilitating medication errors. *Journal of the American Medical Association*, *293*(10), 1197–1203. doi:10.1001/jama.293.10.1197 PMID:15755942

Kushniruk, A. (2002). Evaluation in the design of health information systems: application of approaches emerging from usability engineering. *Computers in Biology and Medicine*, *32*(3), 141–149. doi:10.1016/S0010-4825(02)00011-2 PMID:11922931

Middleton, B., Bloomrosen, M., Dente, M. A., Hashmat, B., Koppel, R., Overhage, J. M., & Zhang, J. (2013). Enhancing patient safety and quality of care by improving the usability of electronic health record systems: recommendations from AMIA. *Journal of the American Medical Informatics Association: JAMIA*, *20*(e1), e2–e8. doi:10.1136/amiajnl-2012-001458 PMID:23355463

Miller, R. A., & Gardner, R. M. (1997). Recommendations for responsible monitoring and regulation of clinical software systems. American Medical Informatics Association, Computer-based Patient Record Institute, Medical Library Association, Association of Academic Health Science Libraries, American Health Information Management Association, American Nurses Association. *Journal of the American Medical Informatics Association: JAMIA*, *4*(6), 442–457. doi:10.1136/jamia.1997.0040442 PMID:9391932

Mulvaney, S. A., Anders, S., Smith, A. K., Pittel, E. J., & Johnson, K. B. (2012). A pilot test of a tailored mobile and web-based diabetes messaging system for adolescents. *Journal of Telemedicine and Telecare*, *18*(2), 115–118. doi:10.1258/jtt.2011.111006 PMID:22383802

Nemeth, C. P. (2004). *Human factors methods for design: making systems human-centered.* Boca Raton, Fla.: CRC Press. doi:10.1201/9780203643662

Nielsen, J. (1993). *Usability engineering.* Boston: Academic Press.

Nilsen, W., Kumar, S., Shar, A., Varoquiers, C., Wiley, T., Riley, W. T., & Atienza, A. A. (2012). Advancing the science of mHealth. *Journal of Health Communication*, *17*(Suppl 1), 5–10. doi:10.1080/10810730.2012.677394 PMID:22548593

Patterson, E. S., Cook, R. I., & Render, M. L. (2002). Improving patient safety by identifying side effects from introducing bar coding in medication administration. *Journal of the American Medical Informatics Association: JAMIA*, *9*(5), 540–553. doi:10.1197/jamia.M1061 PMID:12223506

Rubin, J. (1994). *Handbook of usability testing: how to plan, design, and conduct effective tests.* New York: Wiley.

Saleem, J. J., Patterson, E. S., Militello, L., Anders, S., Falciglia, M., Wissman, J. A., & Asch, S. M. (2007). Impact of clinical reminder redesign on learnability, efficiency, usability, and workload for ambulatory clinic nurses. *Journal of the American Medical Informatics Association: JAMIA*, *14*(5), 632–640. doi:10.1197/jamia.M2163 PMID:17600106

Saleem, J. J., Russ, A. L., Sanderson, P., Johnson, T. R., Zhang, J., & Sittig, D. F. (2009). Current challenges and opportunities for better integration of human factors research with development of clinical information systems. *Yearbook of Medical Informatics*, 48–58. PMID:19855872

Shneiderman, B. (2011). Tragic errors: Usability and electronic health records. *Interaction*, *18*(6), 60–63. doi:10.1145/2029976.2029992

Svanaes, D., Alsos, O. A., & Dahl, Y. (2010). Usability testing of mobile ICT for clinical settings: methodological and practical challenges. *International Journal of Medical Informatics*, *79*(4), e24–e34. doi:10.1016/j.ijmedinf.2008.06.014 PMID:18789753

Svanaes, D., & Seland, G. (2004). *Putting the users center stage: role playing and low-fi prototyping enable end users to design mobile systems*. Paper presented at the Proceedings of the SIGCHI Conference on Human Factors in Computing Systems ACM, Vienna, Austria.

Weinger, M. B., Gardner-Bonneau, D., & Wiklund, M. E. (2011). *Handbook of human factors in medical device design*. Boca Raton, FL: CRC Press.

KEY TERMS AND DEFINITIONS

Card Sort: A data collection method that involves sorting and categorizing data so that it makes sense to the participant.

Cognitive Walk-Through: Method of data collection, where a participant is shown the candidate interface and asked to think aloud as they interact with the interfaces.

Health Information Technology: Area of information technology that involves the design, development, and use of information systems and tools for the healthcare industry.

Human Factors Engineering: The study of fitting the cognitive abilities and human body dimensions to the design of equipment and devices.

Mobile Healthcare Technology: Easily portable tools or applications that are pertain to well-being and management of illness.

Usability: How easy a system or technology is to use. Usability typically refers to how the efficiently, effectively, and error free a user interaction with a system is.

User-Centered Design: A process of system/tool development that emphasizes the involvement of who will be the user and is iterative.

Chapter 4
Mobile Technologies in the Emergency Department:
Towards a Model for Guiding Future Research

Judith W. Dexheimer
Cincinnati Children's Medical Center, USA

Elizabeth Borycki
University of Victoria, Canada

ABSTRACT

Hand-held and mobile technology is steadily expanding in popularity throughout the world. Mobile technologies (e.g. mobile phones, tablets, and smart phones) are increasingly being used in Emergency Departments (ED) around the world. As part of this international trend towards introducing mobile technologies into the ED, health professionals (e.g. physicians, nurses) are now being afforded opportunities to access patient information and decision supports anywhere and anytime in the ED. In this chapter, the authors present a model that describes the current state of the research involving mobile device use in the ED, and they identify key future directions where mobile technology use is concerned.

INTRODUCTION

Mobile technologies are increasingly being used in regional health authorities, health care systems, hospitals, and clinics throughout the world. Mobile technologies have afforded healthcare providers (e.g. physicians, nurses, therapists) the ability and opportunity to access patient information anytime and almost anywhere in and outside of health care organizations (i.e. in the hospital and in the com-

munity). This rapid access to patient information has made mobile technologies a valuable tool and provided health professionals with an aid in supporting patient care related decision making. When first implemented in health care organizations, mobile technologies provided limited access to health information on the World Wide Web. They were a significant contrast to desktop computers that provided access to electronic health records in hospitals. Electronic health records (EHRs) were

DOI: 10.4018/978-1-4666-6150-9.ch004

accessed via desktop computers that were located in specific areas of the health care organization (e.g. at the nursing station, at the end of a hallway). Desktop computers could not be easily moved from one location to another. With the development of varying types of mobile technologies, EHRs and their components including provider order entry, medication administration systems, laboratory information systems, and others can now be accessed anytime and anywhere.

There is a need to understand how these technologies are being used in EDs. Therefore, the researchers will present the findings of a scoping review addressing the current literature focusing on the use of mobile devices in the ED environment. In this chapter, we outline the current state of the research in using mobile devices and identify future research directions. We will also present a model. We will begin by providing background information about the ED, EHRs and Decision Support Systems (DSS) followed by information about mobile device technologies and software use in the ED.

BACKGROUND

The Emergency Department

The emergency department (ED) see patients needing critical or urgent care. Visits range from life-threatening to minor and non-acute complaints. From 1996-2006, ED visits increased by 3% annually (Pitts, Niska, Xu, & Burt, 2008) and utilization rate increased by 18% (Pitts, et al., 2008). The majority of visits occur in community EDs. A dedicated ED includes access to a wide-variety of specialists. The ED plays an important role in addressing, treating, and stabilizing life-threatening conditions. To address the unique needs of providing patient care there is a need to identify technologies that would best support

health professional work in these settings. These technologies include EHRs, DSS and mobile technologies.

Electronic Health Records and Decision Support Systems

Approximately 55% of hospitals have a comprehensive HER (Jamoom et al., 2012); 46% of EDs have EHRs (Geisler, Schuur, & Pallin, 2010) 34.3% have Computerized Provider Order Entry and 26.7% have clinical guideline support (Nakamura, Ferris, DesRoches, & Jha, 2010). Children's hospitals have a smaller rate of EHR implementation with approximately 2.8% of children's hospitals have a comprehensive EHR with 17.9% having some form of basic system (Nakamura, et al., 2010). However, EHRs are increasingly implemented in hospitals, with the adoption of EHRs doubling over the last two years (U.S. Department of Health & Human Services (HHS), 2011). EHRs are replacing paper-based processes and records. Computer-based decision support is provided to healthcare providers to support clinical decision making and standardize care. Decision support systems are integrated with EHRs to guide treatment decisions and to aid the decision-making process at the point of care. Decision support can be delivered in a variety of ways, such as suggesting medications, medication warnings, providing guideline recommendations, alerting about abnormal values, and many other suggestions.

Fifty-five percent of U.S. healthcare institutions have EHRs (Jamoom, et al., 2012); decision support is frequently part of implementation and is defined as "any program designed to help health-care professionals make clinical decisions (Musen, Shakar, & Shortliffe, 2006)." It can cover many aspects of care including patient-specific recommendations (Slagle et al., 2010), information management (Chute, Beck, Fisk, & Mohr, 2010), and guideline compliance (Bell et al., 2010). The framework for decision support (Miller, Waitman, Chen, & Rosenbloom, 2005) outlines the types of support and the options for ideal workflow integration. Decision support should be provided at the right place, to the right person, at the right time, and these ideas should be incorporated into the design (Sirajuddin et al., 2009). CDS should improve performance so that the computer is a tool not a hindrance (Friedman, 2009). Design elements of effective decision support have been reported in the literature (Garg et al., 2005; Kawamoto, Houlihan, Balas, & Lobach, 2005; Sittig et al., 2008). Three key axes to consider in the design and implementation of decision support are: the role, when to intervene, and the method of intervention (Miller, et al., 2005). CDS is frequently built on evidence-based guidelines that represent the expert consensus on the ideal ways to manage patients and decrease variation in practice (Bakken, Cimino, & Hripcsak, 2004). Such systems have demonstrated positive effects on patient outcomes (Dexter, Perkins, Maharry, Jones, & McDonald, 2004). However, barriers exist that limit the implementation and integration of these into clinical practice and one of these is accessibility.

Mobile devices can help overcome the accessibility issue. These devices are already integrated into health care facilities for general use by health professionals to input, access and review patient information, or even as a source of information. They have provided health professionals with ubiquitous access to DSS which can be used during care.

Mobile Devices and Software in the ED

Ideally, access to the EHR and DSS via mobile technologies such as a tablet and the Smartphone can influence how a healthcare provider delivers patient care. Through mobile technologies, providers have the ability to access EHR data

and decision supports in real time and virtually anywhere. This is vital in the ED, a location where having instantaneous access to information can be critical for patients with life threatening injuries or illnesses. Therefore, the ED context is ideal for mobile device use. In the ED, patients are treated by a variety of providers who move from one location to another. Over the past several years emergency departments (ED) have increasingly become more computerized with desktop computers, laptops, hand-held tablets, smartphones, and other portable devices.

The ED is conducive to the use of mobile devices as healthcare providers move constantly from room to room to treat patients. The episodic nature of the care visits lends itself to studying a clinician workflow or presentation of a disease instead of the chronic disease model, which is more patient-oriented. As part of this trend towards computerization of EDs, we have seen the introduction of mobile devices (e.g. tablets) as a way of providing health care professionals (e.g. physicians, nurses) with access to patient information and decision supports in the ED in real-time, anywhere and anyplace. In the next section of this book chapter the researchers will outline the findings of our scoping review.

METHODS AND PROCEDURES

Scoping Review of the Literature

The researchers conducted a scoping review to assess the state of mobile technology use in the ED. They systematically assessed the body of literature at the intersection of mobile devices and use of these technologies in the ED. Key studies were identified. Following this the studies were reviewed for key themes and findings. The researchers' inclusion criteria were broad as this area of research is only beginning to emerge (Arksey & O'Malley, 2005; Landa et al., 2011). The researchers reviewed studies that: (a) examined mobile devices such as wireless mobile computers, mobile work stations, personal digital assistants (PDAs), mobile handheld computers, tablets and smart phones, and (b) evaluated a software and mobile hardware intervention in the ED. Studies were excluded if they did not involve humans, focused on software design alone, lacked an evaluation component, studied a clinician or patient educational intervention only, took place outside of the ED or were a case report, abstract, survey, editorial, letter to the editor, or non-English language report. Articles were excluded when their focus was upon the use of a mobile device for only image-display purposes such as radiology report reading. Do you need to discuss the dates of the searches?

We searched the major electronic databases PUBMED® (MEDLINE®) ("PUBMED,"), OVID CINAHL® ("CINAHL®,"), ISI Web of Science™ ("ISI Web of Knowledge,"), and EMBASE ® ("EMBASE ®,"). Searches were performed from the databases' inception through July 18, 2012. In all databases, searched terms were classified as keywords. In PUBMED, search terms were defined as keywords and Medical Subject Headings (MeSH®) where appropriate. We based the search strategy on including emergency medicine facility, mobile devices, and medical informatics. Search terms included the following:

'emergency medicine' and any combination of the terms 'tablet computer,' 'phone,' 'medical informatics,' 'mobile,' 'tablet,' 'iPad,' or 'PDA' and relevant plurals.

A sample query is shown below:

(emergency medicine OR emergency services, hospital) AND (tablet computer OR phone OR medical informatics OR mobile OR tablet OR iPad OR PDA).

After completion of the first search, we performed an additional MeSH term search to be more inclusive. The results were included in the title and abstract review:

(medical informatics AND emergency medicine AND computers, handheld).

The two authors reviewed the titles and abstracts of all articles identified through the keyword searches. Disagreements between the authors were resolved through consensus. Articles meeting inclusion criteria were pulled for review. We removed any identified duplicate manuscripts describing the same study as another included manuscript. Duplicate results were removed. Included manuscripts were reviewed by both authors to ensure meeting inclusion criteria and references were examined for any missed manuscripts. Additional disagreements were resolved through consensus.

RESULTS

The literature search produced 6,672 articles, after exclusions, 38 articles were selected for inclusion. Of these, 28 articles were excluded for not meeting the inclusion criteria. Ten articles were included in the analysis. Several themes emerged from our reviews of the articles (see Figure 1).

Much of the research has focused on physician and nurse's use of mobile technologies in ED settings. Nurses were the focus of the research when a triage system was used. Alternatively, physician users were studied for all other types of systems. Physicians and nurses are not the only users of technology in a busy ED. Every person who has patient contact potentially uses technology from registration, to treatment, to discharge. In pediatric EDs, child-life specialists may use mobile technology to help entertain children during their visit. Additional research assistants are increasingly able to use mobile technology to screen patients, perform surveys, and collect basic research-related information on patients. We focused on physician and nurses as the users of the technology since they are most likely to use the tablet for situations that would benefit from decision support.

As physicians and nurses were the users of the mobile technology in conjunction with the software tools much of the research focused on how physician and nurse work was affected by

Figure 1. Overview of key themes emerging from the scoping review

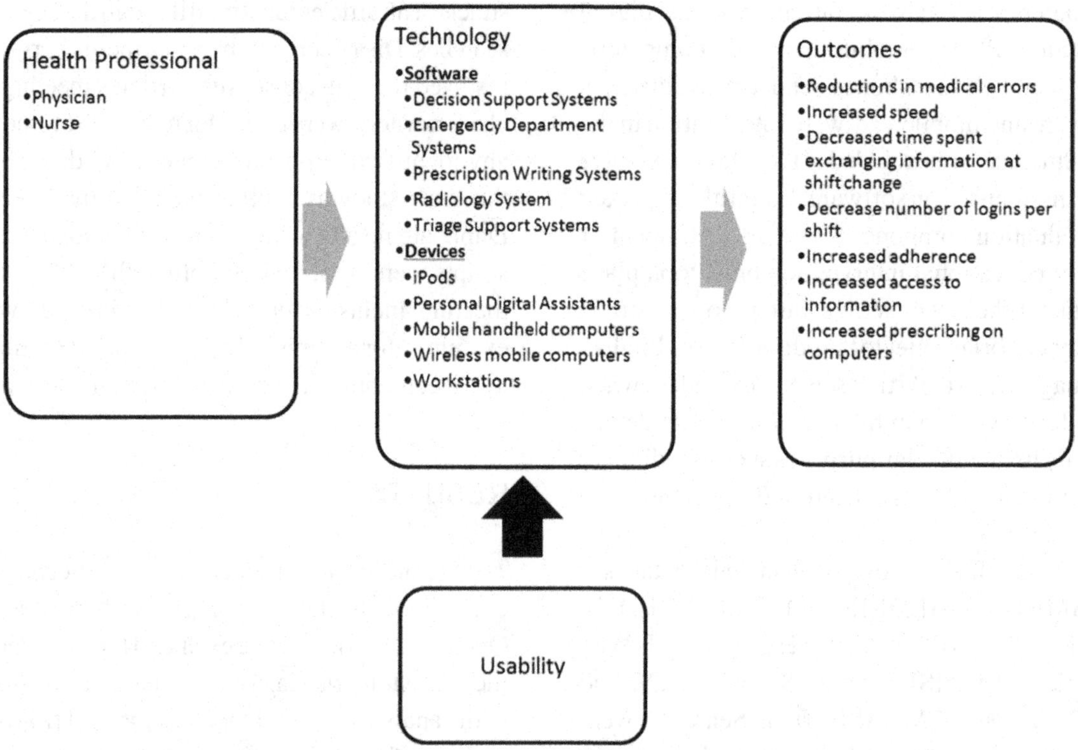
Health Professional
•Physician
•Nurse
Technology
•Software
•Decision Support Systems
•Emergency Department Systems
•Prescription Writing Systems
•Radiology System
•Triage Support Systems
•Devices
•iPods
•Personal Digital Assistants
•Mobile handheld computers
•Wireless mobile computers
•Workstations
Outcomes
•Reductions in medical errors
•Increased speed
•Decreased time spent exchanging information at shift change
•Decrease number of logins per shift
•Increased adherence
•Increased access to information
•Increased prescribing on computers
Usability

the introduction of an intervention (i.e. mobile device + a software tool) in the ED. We focused on mobile technology providing some form of decision support for providers. By limiting to decision support, the total number of studies was reduced, however given the large range of uses for mobile technologies from telephone calls to games, we wanted to focus on an area that had the potential to show direct clinical benefit (e.g. decision-making support).

As patients move through the ED during a visit, physicians or nurses lead their care predominantly in different areas and stages. In Figure 2, we present a simplified view of a patient's movement through the ED from arrival to discharge. In this figure, we have labeled where the nurse or physician is the predominant decision-maker. In a typical ED, the nurse would perform triage. This flow suggests the basic stages where mobile technology could be employed. Each of these steps is more complicated than it appears. A patient room may be changed during treatment, and there are other providers who participate in patient care who aren't mentioned. Mobile devices, however, can

Figure 2. Simplified view of patient movement through an Emergency Department

Patient Arrival
Triage - Nurse
Room Assignment
Treatment – Nurse, Physician
Disposition Decision - Physician
Patient Discharge - Nurse

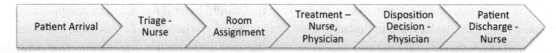

be employed at any of these steps to provide additional information, improve team communication, or provide decision support.

Mobile Devices

Mobile devices were treated as the primary intervention in all of the studies. Here, the researchers attempted to evaluate the impacts of introducing these mobile technologies upon nurse and physician work in the ED setting. Several differing types of mobile devices were studied by the researchers. Our findings identified that a range mobile devices were studied by researchers. The devices included iPods, Personal Digital Assistants (PDAs), Mobile Handheld computers, wireless mobile computers and mobile workstations. Only one study examined the implementation of a Smartphone, the current dominant technology in the global consumer market. The majority of the devices were studied were personal digital assistants (PDAs) (n=6) (See Figure 1). PDAs differ in terms of shape and size and have limited ability to run complex software applications.

Software Tools

The published articles we reviewed in this work documented that there were a range of software tools that were used in conjunction with mobile technologies in the ED setting. These tools included software that would allow health professionals to triage patients (i.e. a triage support system used by nurses), review patient data (i.e. radiology system software, emergency department system), write prescriptions (i.e. prescription writing software) and view information/guidelines (i.e. videos, guidelines) (See Figure). No one type of software tool predominated in the studies. Each study represented an evaluation of one type of software tool with no other study evaluating the same or a similar software tools; for example, there was only one study that focused on the use of prescription writing software use in the ED.

Instead a range of differing types of software were studied in conjunction with the above outlined mobile technologies. As a result, we found it difficult to make recommendations about the use of any particular software tool or type of software (e.g. prescription writing system or triage tool) for use in ED settings. According to the literature, differing types of software tools enable users to perform differing actions. As mentioned earlier in this scoping review, there were single study descriptions and evaluations of single software tools. Therefore, it was not possible to make comparisons across studies for an individual type of software or software tool (e.g. all prescription writing systems used on a PDA). More research is needed on specific types of software that are used in the ED and there is also a need for several studies using the same software tool as such research would also provide additional insights as to the utility of the tool in differing ED settings (e.g. adult and pediatric contexts).

As well, little information was provided about the software tools themselves. For example, the publications provided limited information to the reader about the features and functions of each of the software tools. Therefore, it was difficult for the readers to determine what features and functions should be present in ED software tools and if the tools themselves were fully effective in supporting ED work and workflows. We find it difficult to recommend that specific features and functions be present in specific software tools such as triage systems because of a lack of information about software features and functions.

Usability and Workflow of Software Tools and Mobile Devices

Research has found that the usability and workflows emerging from mobile devices and software tools can influence their use. In this scoping review, only one study examined the usability of the software tools that were deployed in the ED. In this study, the investigator attempted to evaluate users perceived usability of the software tool. The focus of this research was a triage support system used in conjunction with a PDA. The researchers surveyed the study participants about their perceived ease of use of the system. Research from the usability literature suggests surveys of users perceived usability of a technology often do not provide detailed information that could be used to rectify specific usability problems and that further usability testing involving real users in laboratory and naturalistic contexts would need to be conducted to fully understand how a technology's features and functions support or detract from work in ED contexts (Kushniruk & Patel, 2004). None of the studies looked specifically at the effects of providing software tools via a mobile device upon workflow. Recent publications suggest there is a need to fully understand the impacts of these technologies upon workflow as some software/device configurations may introduce new types of workflow that are more cumbersome and may not fully support work in specific health care contexts such as an emergency departments (Borycki, Kushniruk, Kuwata, & Watanabe, 2009; Kushniruk, Borycki, Kuwata, & Kannry, 2006).

Usability and workflow are increasingly being recognized in the health informatics literature as important aspects of evaluating mobile technology and software configurations prior to implementation in real-world settings (Kushniruk, Triola, Borycki, Stein, & Kannry, 2005). Poor usability and workflow have been implicated in reducing adoption rates among users (Kushniruk, Patel, & Cimino, 1997), introducing inefficiencies in the process of using the technology (Borycki, et al., 2009; Kushniruk, et al., 2006) and introducing new types of errors into clinical settings - technology-induced errors (Kushniruk, et al., 2005). Technology induced errors are "medical errors that arise from the: design and development of a technology; implementation and customization of a technology; and interactions between the operation of a new technology and the new work processes that arise from the technology's use.

(Borycki & Kushniruk, 2008)" As well, usability and workflow can have a significant impact on study outcomes. This is especially the case when the focus of these studies is to assess whether the mobile device and software tools when combined have an effect upon the ability of users to effectively and efficiently use the technologies to conduct their work (Borycki, et al., 2009; Kushniruk, et al., 2006). More research will be needed to identify the best mobile device and software tool combination for use by specific ED users and in differing ED contexts. As well, research is needed to determine the types of devices that will be needed in the ED and the features and functions that are needed for specific types of software used in the ED.

Outcomes

In our work, we found no one particular outcome of introducing a mobile device and software tool combination was studied, although several key themes emerged where outcomes were concerned. Much of the research focused upon how the software/mobile device combinations could reduce the amount of time spent undertaking specific ED activities as well as how these software/mobile device combinations could improve the quality of patient care that was provided. In terms of improving efficiency of work, the focus of this research was upon time spent performing activities (increasing the speed associated with performing tasks or decreasing the amount of time spend performing specific activities). Alternatively, other studies described how the mobile technology/software tool combination would improve access to patient information, improve adherence to guidelines and reduce medical error rates – all key indicators of improved healthcare quality. No one particular measure of efficiency or quality was used by the researchers. As a result it was difficult to compare across studies in terms of mobile device/software tool device combinations or their impacts on efficiency or quality of healthcare. Health informatics researchers need to identify key outcomes variables that should be used across studies so that there is an opportunity to make comparisons between mobile devices, software tools and mobile technology/device combinations. As well, there is a need to identify other potentially relevant outcome measures from the ED literature that can be used to compare mobile device/software tool measures to other types of interventions implemented in an ED setting such as the introduction of new paper based protocols to assess clinical and patient care impacts of the technologies across studies and interventions.

FUTURE TRENDS AND RESEARCH

Mobile devices are increasingly permeating work and home life. Mobile devices are in no way limited to providing decision support. Many studies used the mobile devices to view radiology images in the ED (http://www.ncbi.nlm.nih.gov/pubmed/23893749, http://www.ncbi.nlm.nih.gov/pubmed/23413062). This is an apt use for the devices but was not included in our research question. Before choosing a methodology, this would certainly bear examining and discovering. This did not provide any direct decision support help or advice but acted as an image-viewer only.

There were fewer studies of mobile devices in the ED than expected. With the great demand for mobile devices and the many options of downloadable applications, we expected more research on how well these systems performed during clinical care. We suggest more research to examine how much these systems do improve either care or clinician satisfaction. We understand that this is a rapidly moving field but mobile technology does have the potential to improve care if implemented and used properly.

CONCLUSION

In summary, ten studies were identified in our scoping review of the literature. Research examining the effects of introducing mobile devices and their associated software tools is in its infancy. To date few studies have focused upon any one type of mobile software tool in evaluating its interface design or workflow and its impact on health care outcomes in terms of efficiency and ability to improve the quality of care in the ED. Alternatively, although there are more studies specifically looking at the introduction of the PDA in the ED setting, the PDA itself has become obsolete as a technology that can be used in the ED. More recently, Smartphones have become popular among healthcare consumers and health professionals. Health professionals are increasingly demanding that the technology be used in ED settings. Yet, few studies have specifically explored the impact of the device upon health professionals working in the ED. There is a great deal of variability in the types of outcomes variables that were measured. There is a need to identify key indicators of mobile device/software tool quality that can be used to evaluate the impacts of introducing these technologies across differing types of hardware and software. Lastly, there is a need to conduct usability and workflow studies involving software and mobile devices used in the ED. Such work is necessary as there is little known about the qualitative impacts of the software features and functions as well as workflows emerging from the use of software and mobile devices on the quality of patient care, health professional work and medical error rates.

REFERENCES

Arksey, H., & O'Malley, L. (2005). Scoping Studies: Towards a Methodological Framework. *International Journal of Social Research Methodology, 8*(1), 19–32. doi:10.1080/1364557032000119616

Bakken, S., Cimino, J. J., & Hripcsak, G. (2004). Promoting patient safety and enabling evidence-based practice through informatics. *Medical Care, 42*(2Suppl), II49–II56. PMID:14734942

Bell, L. M., Grundmeier, R., Localio, R., Zorc, J., Fiks, A. G., Zhang, X., & Guevara, J. P. (2010). Electronic health record-based decision support to improve asthma care: A cluster-randomized trial. *Pediatrics, 125*(4), e770–e777. doi:10.1542/peds.2009-1385 PMID:20231191

Borycki, E., & Kushniruk, A. (2008). Where do technology-induced errors come from? Towards a model for conceptualizing and diagnosing errors caused by technology. In A. W. Kushniruk, & E. Borycki (Eds.), *Human, social, and organizational aspects of health information systems* (pp. 148–166). Hershey, PA: Information Science Reference. doi:10.4018/978-1-59904-792-8.ch009

Borycki, E., Kushniruk, A., Kuwata, S., & Watanabe, A. (2009). Simulations to assess medication administration systems. In B. Staudinger, V. Höss, & H. Ostermann (Eds.), *Nursing and clinical informatics: Socio-technical approaches* (pp. 144–159). Hershey, PA: Information Science Reference. doi:10.4018/978-1-60566-234-3.ch010

Chute, C. G., Beck, S. A., Fisk, T. B., & Mohr, D. N. (2010). The Enterprise Data Trust at Mayo Clinic: A semantically integrated warehouse of biomedical data. *Journal of the American Medical Informatics Association, 17*(2), 131–135. doi:10.1136/jamia.2009.002691 PMID:20190054

CINAHL®. (n.d.). Retrieved 1 August 2012, from http://web.ebscohost.com/ehost/search/selectdb?sid=a54fae89-7491-46d4-953c-958345858902%40sessionmgr4&vid=1&hid=28

Dexter, P. R., Perkins, S. M., Maharry, K. S., Jones, K., & McDonald, C. J. (2004). Inpatient computer-based standing orders vs physician reminders to increase influenza and pneumococcal vaccination rates: A randomized trial. *Journal of the American Medical Association, 292*(19), 2366–2371. doi:10.1001/jama.292.19.2366 PMID:15547164

EMBASE ®. (n.d.). Retrieved 6 November 2012, from http://www.embase.com/

Friedman, C. P. (2009). A fundamental theorem of biomedical informatics. *Journal of the American Medical Informatics Association, 16*(2), 169–170. doi:10.1197/jamia.M3092 PMID:19074294

Garg, A. X., Adhikari, N. K., McDonald, H., Rosas-Arellano, M. P., Devereaux, P. J., Beyene, J., & Haynes, R. B. (2005). Effects of computerized clinical decision support systems on practitioner performance and patient outcomes: A systematic review. *Journal of the American Medical Association, 293*(10), 1223–1238. doi:10.1001/jama.293.10.1223 PMID:15755945

Geisler, B. P., Schuur, J. D., & Pallin, D. J. (2010). Estimates of electronic medical records in U.S. Emergency departments. *PLoS ONE, 5*(2), e9274. doi:10.1371/journal.pone.0009274 PMID:20174660

ISI Web of Knowledge. (n.d.). Retrieved 1 August 2012, from http://apps.webofknowledge.com/UA_GeneralSearch_input.do?product=UA&search_mode=GeneralSearch&SID=2DPDdNGBCKHI7NPmmI5&preferencesSaved=

Jamoom, E., Beatty, P., Bercovitz, A., Woodwell, D., Palso, K., & Rechtsteiner, E. (2012). Physician adoption of electronic health record systems: United States, 2011. *NCHS Data Brief,* (98), 1-8.

Kawamoto, K., Houlihan, C. A., Balas, E. A., & Lobach, D. F. (2005). Improving clinical practice using clinical decision support systems: A systematic review of trials to identify features critical to success. *British Medical Journal, 330*(7494), 765. doi:10.1136/bmj.38398.500764.8F PMID:15767266

Kushniruk, A., Borycki, E., Kuwata, S., & Kannry, J. (2006). Predicting changes in workflow resulting from healthcare information systems: Ensuring the safety of healthcare. *Healthcare Quarterly, 9,* 114–118. doi:10.12927/hcq..18469 PMID:17087179

Kushniruk, A. W., & Patel, V. L. (2004). Cognitive and usability engineering methods for the evaluation of clinical information systems. *Journal of Biomedical Informatics, 37*(1), 56–76. doi:10.1016/j.jbi.2004.01.003 PMID:15016386

Kushniruk, A. W., Patel, V. L., & Cimino, J. J. (1997). *Usability testing in medical informatics: Cognitive approaches to evaluation of information systems and user interfaces.* Paper presented at the AMIA Annual Symposium: American Medical Informatics Association. Retrieved from http://www.ncbi.nlm.nih.gov/pubmed/9357620

Kushniruk, A. W., Triola, M. M., Borycki, E. M., Stein, B., & Kannry, J. L. (2005). Technology induced error and usability: The relationship between usability problems and prescription errors when using a handheld application. *International Journal of Medical Informatics, 74*(7-8), 519–526. doi:10.1016/j.ijmedinf.2005.01.003 PMID:16043081

Landa, A. H., Szabo, I., Le Brun, L., Owen, I., Fletcher, G., & Hill, M. (2011). An Evidence-Based Approach to Scoping Reviews. *Electronic Journal of Information Systems Evaluation, 14*(1), 46–52.

Miller, R. A., Waitman, L. R., Chen, S., & Rosenbloom, S. T. (2005). The anatomy of decision support during inpatient care provider order entry (CPOE), empirical observations from a decade of CPOE experience at Vanderbilt. *Journal of Biomedical Informatics, 38*(6), 469–485. doi:10.1016/j.jbi.2005.08.009 PMID:16290243

Musen, M. A., Shakar, Y., & Shortliffe, E. H. (2006). Clinical Decision-Support Systems. In E. H. Shortliffe, & J. J. Cimino (Eds.), *Biomedical informatics: Computer applications in health care and biomedicine* (3rd ed., pp. 698–736). New York: Springer. doi:10.1007/0-387-36278-9_20

Nakamura, M. M., Ferris, T. G., DesRoches, C. M., & Jha, A. K. (2010). Electronic health record adoption by children's hospitals in the United States. *Archives of Pediatrics & Adolescent Medicine, 164*(12), 1145–1151. doi:10.1001/archpediatrics.2010.234 PMID:21135344

Pitts, S. R., Niska, R. W., Xu, J., & Burt, C. W. (2008). National Hospital Ambulatory Medical Care Survey: 2006 emergency department summary. *National Health Statistics Reports,* (7), 1-38.

PUBMED. (n.d.). Retrieved 1 August 2012, from http://www.ncbi.nlm.nih.gov/pubmed/

Sirajuddin, A. M., Osheroff, J. A., Sittig, D. F., Chuo, J., Velasco, F., & Collins, D. A. (2009). Implementation pearls from a new guidebook on improving medication use and outcomes with clinical decision support: Effective CDS is essential for addressing healthcare performance improvement imperatives. *Journal of Healthcare Information Management, 23*(4), 38–45. PMID:19894486

Sittig, D. F., Wright, A., Osheroff, J. A., Middleton, B., Teich, J. M., Ash, J. S., & Bates, D. W. (2008). Grand challenges in clinical decision support. *Journal of Biomedical Informatics, 41*(2), 387–392. doi:10.1016/j.jbi.2007.09.003 PMID:18029232

Slagle, J. M., Gordon, J. S., Harris, C. E., Davison, C. L., Culpepper, D. K., Scott, P., & Johnson, K. B. (2010). MyMediHealth - Designing a next generation system for child-centered medication management. *Journal of Biomedical Informatics*, *43*(5Suppl), S27–S31. doi:10.1016/j.jbi.2010.06.006 PMID:20937481

U.S. Department of Health & Human Services (HHS). (2011). *We Can't Wait: Obama Administration takes new steps to encourage doctors and hospitals to use health information technology to lower costs, improve quality, create jobs*. Retrieved November 4, 2013, from http://www.hhs.gov/news/press/2011pres/11/20111130a.html

KEY TERMS AND DEFINITIONS

Decision Support or Clinical Decision Support: Using a system (computerized or paper-based) to help healthcare providers make care and treatment decisions.

Human Factors: A multidisciplinary field that studies the design of equipment and how it relates to a user's physical space and cognitive ability.

Medical Informatics: The field of study that broadly addresses information and computer science in healthcare.

Prospective Study: A type of analytic study that is designed to identify if there is a relationship between a condition and a selected characteristic that is shared by members of a particular group.

Scoping Review: A review that gathers information in the literature and presents a mapping of the results.

Usability: the study of the ease of use of a user interface typically in a computerized system. It evaluates the system's learnability, efficiency, memorability, errors, and user satisfaction.

User Interface Design: Aspects of a health information system which are seen by human users.

User-Centered Design: An approach to the development of products, devices, or systems to be used to complete tasks efficiently, effectively, safely and satisfactorily by their intended users.

Workflow: The the tasks and steps in a procedure that people and organizations undertake as part of a health care or business process.

Section 2
Overview of the Field

The focus of this section is on providing a high-level overview of the field of social media and mobile technologies in healthcare.

Chapter 5
Use Cases and Application Purposes of Social Media in Healthcare

Kerstin Denecke
Innovation Center for Computer Assisted Surgery, Germany

ABSTRACT

This chapter presents the current state and outlines future directions in the possibilities of applying and exploiting social media in supporting healthcare processes. Starting from the abstracts of the Medicine 2.0 conference in 2012, the authors identify categories of application purposes for social media-based healthcare applications. The applications of social media tools and data are categorized into five groups: 1) supporting the treatment process, 2) for information gathering and prevention, 3) for networking and information exchange, 4) for knowledge management, and 5) for research and monitoring. Use of social media for information gathering and disease prevention is most prevalent. Existing applications mainly concentrate on supporting treatment of chronic and mental diseases. Technology is ready for supporting such applications. To go further in that direction, organizational and legal issues need to be addressed, including developing concepts for integrating with clinical information settings, establishing financing models, and ensuring security and trust.

INTRODUCTION

Advances in Internet and mobile technologies changed the way how people access, use and share information. New ways of communicating came up, enabling for timeless and location-independent information exchange. These new media comprise instant messaging, blogs, social networking (e.g. Facebook) or video sharing (e.g. YouTube). While younger populations were fast in adopting these new technologies, the number of older adults using these tools is also growing fast. What does social media has to do with healthcare?

Social media can be both - tool and information source for healthcare applications in various perspectives. Tools are enabling communication, networking or information exchange. Social media is also an information source for patients and health carers. Hospitals and physicians are providing information on offered healthcare services;

DOI: 10.4018/978-1-4666-6150-9.ch005

physicians are further presenting information on latest biomedical research results and treatments and patients provide information on their experiences, but also seek help through social media. In particular people suffering from chronic conditions or from rare diseases use these new media. They can learn what others have to say about quality of care, or learn important issues regarding treatment and diagnosis. Social media leads to empowered patients equipped with sophisticated technological tools.

In fact, patients increasingly rely on the Internet when looking for medical information and advice which increases their ability to share personal experiences and opinions on health concerns (Lau, Siek & Fernandez-Luque, 2011). In a survey performed by the Pew Research Center and California Healthcare foundation it has been found out that 66% of internet users look online for information about a specific disease or medical problem and 56% search for information on a particular treatment (Fox, 2011). This shows that patients take over the responsibility on healthcare treatment decisions via actively seeking information and options on the web. Mayo Clinic researchers have opined that social media has begun a process of "revolutionizing healthcare" by improving healthcare and quality of life (Aase, Goldman, 2012). The Mayo Clinic Center for Social Media compiled a list of health-related organizations[1] that are actively using social networking sites. It shows that healthcare providers are also interested in using the social media for informing patients and to communicate with them. For example, medical centers inform in their YouTube channels on latest research achievements in clinical therapy (e.g. the YouTube channel of the Mayo clinic, http://www.youtube.com/user/mayoclinic). Advertising healthcare services via the internet is nowadays practiced by many healthcare providers[2].

Beyond, through social-media tools, new possibilities for collaboration and information exchange in healthcare come up. Further, applications are coming up that make use of this new

information source; they analyze and interpret the social-media data for example for disease surveillance purposes. Beyond, social-media tools can be applied to support healthcare processes. Bringing social-media tools into healthcare becomes more and more an issue.

The objective of this chapter is to categorize existing approaches and tools of making use of social media in healthcare, to present existing and future use case scenarios and to describe open issues including strengths and weaknesses. We will investigate how social-media data and tools can be used in the treatment process including therapy, diagnosis, and prevention. Existing application areas will be categorised. The following questions will be addressed:

- How can social-media data and tools be used in healthcare?
- Which application purposes can be distinguished?
- Which open research questions do exist?

The chapter will start with a scenario showing the potential use of social media in a treatment process. Then, social media will be defined and opportunities that social media provide for healthcare purposes will be collected. To study the research and current state in that field, we performed a review of abstracts accepted for the Medicine 2.0 conference in 2012. Review methodology and the identified categories of applications will be described. The last section presents future issues and discusses general questions related to the use of social media in healthcare.

SCENARIO: SOCIAL MEDIA USAGE IN HEALTHCARE TREATMENT

To motivate the application of social media in healthcare, consider the following scenario:

Tom, 48 years old, is suffering from Parkinson's disease (PD) since one year. He is working as an accountant in a small company and is quite busy with work. Remaining active in his job and in his social life, even with the difficulties because of the disease, is one of the major goals for Tom. Although he suffers from slight tremor in the right hand and a somewhat slowed gait, he refuses to abandon any activities of his previous life.

So far, he had to go to the outpatient department once every three months to get an update of his drug status and to allow his neurologist to judge his current health status. Especially in the beginning of the therapy, he had to schedule visits more frequently – sometimes every four weeks - because he was not supporting his medication very well. In addition to his motor symptoms (tremor and slowness of gait) he also developed constipation, which required the scheduling of an additional visit. This procedure was very time consuming for him. Because Tom lives in a small town at 50 km distance from his tertiary care center, he had to take one day off for every visit. In addition, Tom felt depressed, because he had to go to a hospital so often, which he never had to do before in his life. Besides having been diagnosed with Parkinson's he still considers himself an active and healthy person.

Happily, he signed up to STIMOCOP, a social-media-based system, that allows him to manage his disease without the need to visit the clinics every time he has a question about his medication or a symptom is not well controlled. Every Sunday night, Tom spends one hour in front of his computer, learning a new physical exercise, which was proposed by the physician and his physical therapist placed into his account and sometimes records them via his web cam. The video is stored in the STIMOCOP data repository, to which he can grant access for his carers. He continues performing the exercises several times during the week. Sometimes, he includes a small exercise in his lunch break at work.

There is one aspect about STIMOCOP, Tom likes much. It is the possibility to communicate through a message board with his neurologist and the therapists as often as possible and when he feels the need to do so. Tom also answers questions asked by his doctor or continues to work on specific exercises proposed by his physiotherapists. The exercises are available as a set of exergames that motivate Tom to exercise regularly from home. He can even play with other patients to collect group points required to access other missions. A public scoreboard displays his weekly goals and achievements. This motivates him to exercise even when he is tired or not feeling too well.

A few days ago, Tom found out at the STIMOCOP dashboard that another PD patient of similar age lives in a town close to where he lives. He now plans to meet this patient at the meeting of the local PD patient group. Conveniently, the meetings of the local patient groups are also announced at the STIMOCOP dashboard.

Recently, the treating physiotherapist observed an improvement in the usage of the right hand as video-recorded by the exercises Tom performed. The physiotherapist uses STIMOCOP to transmit this observation to the treating neurologist, who now is more confident that the adapted medication is beneficial for Tom.

This scenario shows that the application of social media technology can support among others in

- Connecting health carers to a patient,
- Connecting patients to each other,
- Engaging patients in actively participating in the treatment process, e.g. by doing exercises,
- Monitoring regularly patient's health status without time consuming face-to-face visits.

WHAT IS MEDICAL SOCIAL MEDIA?

This section will introduce social media in the context of medicine and health. We will characterize *medical social-media* and describe the various facets of its content, ranging from information on diseases, treatments and drugs to experiences of patients and physicians. This section will also collect and summarize the opportunities that social media could provide to healthcare processes. Why should we consider these tools and information in healthcare applications? What are the benefits? These questions will be addressed in this section.

Social media are digital media and technologies that enable users to exchange information and to create media content on their own or in community with others. Individuals are engaged by social media in one-to-many conversations using electronic communication tools. Social-media data includes various kinds of publicly available content that is produced by end-users, rather than by the operator of a Web site, and has been uploaded without a commercial, marketing or promotional purpose in mind. Medical social-media data is a subset of the social-media data space, in which the interests of the participants are specifically devoted to medicine and health issues. The content is characterized by a mixture between expert knowledge, lay knowledge and empirical findings (Wicks, Massagli & Frost, 2010).

The phenomenon social media and its increased importance in the private as well as in the public sector shows that there are many potentials. Even in the medical domain, an increased usage has already begun. In particular persons suffering from chronic diseases more and more use social-media tools to communicate with others, exchange information and experiences. At the same time,

individuals (patients) start to be better informed since information is available and accessible very easily in the Web (Eysenbach, 2008).

The types of medical social-media data can be broadly placed into two categories. Users can either generate their own content, or alternatively annotate the content created by others. To make the distinction clear, we refer to the former as (user-generated) *content*, and the latter as *metadata*. Consider the following examples: In a weblog, some individual person is providing content, e.g. a patient describes his experiences in living with a disease (e.g., Bitter-Sweet, http://www.bittersweetdiabetes.com/). In a wiki, content is produced collaboratively. In review and rating portals, opinions and experiences are assigned to products, i.e. metadata is generated.

Medical Video-Blogs (VLog) provide information on medical issues in an audio-visual manner. A huge source of videos is available within the YouTube portal. The variety of videos ranges from recorded surgeries, and educational videos for patients or medical students, to reports on medical issues in news channels. Authors of VLogs are usually health professionals, official health institutions and organizations, or universities.

Medical Podcasts are examples of audio data with medical content. Podcasts provided by physicians inform patients about concrete health questions. Patient information on treatments (e.g. endoscopy, coronary angiography) or explanations of symptoms or diseases (e.g. obstructive

Table 1. Types of medical social-media data

	Collaborative	Non-Collaborative
Content	**Medical Wiki** (e.g. http://askdrwiki.com)	**Weblog** (e.g. http://www.webmd.com), **Micro-blog** (e.g. http://twitter.com/tudiabetes), **Video-Blog** (e.g. http://www.youtube.com/CDCstreaminghealth), **Podcasts** (e.g. http://www2c.cdc.gov/podcasts/), **Personal Health Records** (e.g. https://www.healthvault.com/)
Metadata	**Social Bookmarking** (e.g. http://www.PeerClip.com) **Social Networks** (e.g. (http://www.patientslikeme.com/)	**Review and Rating Portals** (e.g. (http://www.PatientOpinion.org.uk), **Question and Answer Portal** (e.g. http://www.netdoctor.co.uk)

sleep apnoea) are provided through websites of official organizations such as the Mayo Clinic (http://www.mayoclinic.com). Podcasts directed to physicians help to inform them about general issues or latest news such as medical informatics or electronic prescription. In addition, podcasts and video lectures are available for medical education purposes (e.g., http://www.podmetrics.com).

Forums and Query-Answer Portals (e.g., Forum of Diabetes Daily http://www.diabetesdaily.com/forum/) with a medical focus offer the opportunity to post queries or engage in discussions. Expert forums enable users to get a qualified answer to a question regarding a disease or treatment. In such portals, people's objective of posting is mainly to receive information related to drugs and disorders, with some attention also given to treatment-related issues (Denecke & Nejdl, 2009). Depending on the portal, answers can be provided either by health professionals or by the general public.

Content communities and social networking sites related to health and medicine enable people with similar interests to connect. More specifically, patients can share health data in order to empathize with each other or to learn about new techniques or medications. Health professionals exploit social networking sites to connect with other professionals who also share common (medical) interests. Yet other social networking sites such as *HelloHealth* connect patients to physicians. PatientsLikeMe is a social network for patients that allows to share health-related experiences and compare treatments. The community currently comprises more than 115,000 patient members (March 28, 2013). Over 1,000 conditions are reported in the platform. Users of social network platforms such as PatientsLikeMe experience benefit from participating in the community (Wicks, Massagli & Frost, 2010) by an information gain and (informal) social or psychological support.

The technology behind all these social-media applications and tools comprises facilities to

- Exchange information between persons,
- Post information items such as images, messages, videos,
- Form groups,
- Work collaboratively on content.

This brief summary shows that social media has many facets. The potentials of social media will be addressed throughout the rest of the paper, when we are describing groups of existing or future healthcare applications that base upon social media.

METHODS

To identify and categorize applications that make use of social-media data and tools in healthcare, we studied the abstracts accepted for the research track of the Medicine 2.0 conference held in 2012. Medicine 2.0 is a conference series for internet, social media, and mobile apps in health that started in 2008 (http://www.medicine20congress.com/). In total, 167 abstracts accepted for the research tracks in 2012 were considered. We went through these abstracts and identified categories of reported applications. The following inclusion and exclusion criteria were applied:

Abstracts were *excluded* from the categorization when they

- Referred to panels or keynotes,
- Studied general aspects of internet usage (e.g. patient-doctor relationship),
- Referred to applications that are not making use of social media data or tools (e.g. GPS tracking for activity monitoring),

- Referred to advertisement applications, e.g. in pharmaceutical market,
- Referred to studies or applications in education of medical students.

Abstracts were *included into* the assessment when they

- Reported about tools or applications making use of social media in some way,
- Reported about studies that apply existing tools related to social media.

Abstracts describing case studies that applied social-media tools were categorized according to application purpose of the underlying tool. For example, an abstract reported on a study that analyzed the use of Facebook for smoking prevention. This abstract was categorized as application for prevention. In total, 104 abstracts were categorized after considering the mentioned inclusion and exclusion criteria. In the following section, we describe the categories and the results of the assessment in more depth.

The categorization forms the basis for additional considerations and assessments regarding potentials and requirements of applications using social media in healthcare. Our assessments center around the following questions: 1. Which are application potentials of social media in healthcare and medicine? 2. Which open research questions exist?

HEALTHCARE APPLICATIONS MAKING USE OF SOCIAL MEDIA

By going through the research work reported in Medicine 2.0 conference abstracts, we could identify five categories of healthcare applications where social media is exploited. The percentage in brackets indicates the percentage of assessed abstracts that describe an application falling into the category. The categories are:

1. Applications supporting the treatment process (21%),
2. Applications for information gathering, prevention, health activity promotion, self assessment (50%),
3. Networking, information exchange, forums in healthcare (19%),
4. Knowledge management applications (2%),
5. Applications for research and monitoring (8%).

Most of the abstracts (50%) describe applications of social media to support information gathering and prevention. Further, many abstracts refer to applications supporting treatment processes as well as to applications for networking and exchanging information. Many applications and studies introduced in the texts concentrated on two main groups of diseases: chronic diseases (mainly diabetes) and psychological/mental diseases (e.g., depression, stress symptoms). In the following, we describe the various application categories in more detail. Table 2 summarizes the categories.

Social Media to Support the Treatment Process

As treatment process in healthcare, we consider all interactions between a patient and a physician or another healthcare provider starting with an initial meeting and an examination, followed by diagnosis and interactions or treatments. In a simple case of patient treatment, a patient gets some drugs and he is cured after some days without any additional interactions; he can even stay at home. For complex or chronic diseases, the treatment process can take several weeks, months or even years during

Table 2. Categories of social media applications in healthcare

Application Purpose	Description	Examples
Support of treatment process	**What?** Support of information exchange and communication	Diabetes self-management tools, pain management apps (Stinson, Jibb & Nathan, 2012), symptom diaries, or apps for glucose level reporting (Khairat, & Garcia, 2012)
	Who? Care team, patient	
	Why? Closer monitoring, reduce face-to-face consultations (increased independency of patient)	
	How? Online diaries, self-management tools, exchange and collaboration platforms	
Information gathering, prevention, health activity promotion	**What?** Information provision and search, health activity programs	Information retrieval, Smoking prevention (Struik, Bottorff, Jung & Budgen, 2012)
	Who? Healthcare provider, patient	
	Why? Exercising time and location independent, self-motivation, patient empowerment, making exercises in known environment (➜ acting more freely)	
	How? Information provision through web sites and blogs, activity programs realized as games, questionnaires, self-assessment tools	
Networking, information exchange	**What?** Exchanging experiences and knowledge with other patients or carers	Online support group for depression, http://www.dailystrength.org/c/Depression/support-group
	Who? Care team, patient	
	Why? Psychological support, get expertise from others	
	How? Social networking sites, discussion boards, chat rooms	
Knowledge management	**What?** Sharing information	Wikis, Google Docs (Archambault, Van De Belt & Grajales, 2012)
	Who? Researcher	
	Why? Easy access, generate content collaboratively	
	How? Wikis, Blogs	
Research and Monitoring	**What**? Monitoring health behavior or population health, experiences, opinions, learn about experienced outcomes of treatments and medications	Public Health Threat Detection (Denecke, Krieck & Otrusina, 2013)
	Who? Researcher, health organizations	
	Why? Additional, rich source of subjective information, timeliness	
	How? Mining of data provided via social media	

which monitoring of symptoms, of the progress of treatment or of the health status in general is necessary. Several healthcare providers including specialized physicians and therapists are involved in the treatment process. In traditional healthcare scenarios, monitoring requires the patient going to the physicians regularly. Anyway, such face-to-face visits are time-consuming for all involved persons, the healthcare team and the patient.

Social media-based tools are exploited to support the treatment process, in particular to enable

a continuous monitoring and self-management of diseases. Consider the following example, where social media supports a patient in self-managing his disease.

- George, suffering from chronic pain, keeps regularly an online diary where he records the strength of his pain, its location and other relevant information related to his disease. The diary has options for free-textual entries, provides scales, where George simply has to select a value as well as checkboxes to answer questions. George's physician and healthcare team can access his diary via a secure login. This allows them to monitor the symptoms and health status. The questions in the diary were put together by George's physician and his carers. To facilitate the analysis and continuous screening of the diary content, automatic tools pre-filter the content or even analyze it and provide notifications to the physician or other carers automatically when the health status changes according to the diary entries of George.

The example shows: Exploiting social-media tools during the treatment process can allow for a continuous, close health monitoring by reducing time-consuming face-to-face visits at the physician.

Beyond, social media is exploited for documenting or reporting observations on health status changes. For example, diabetes self-management tools, pain management apps (Stinson, Jibb & Nathan, 2012), symptom diaries, or apps for glucose level reporting (Khairat & Garcia, 2012) were introduced already. Further, social-media based collaboration platforms enable patients and health carers to communicate with each other, to regularly report and to exchange information during the treatment process (Ho, Weinstein & De Sousa, 2012). Online psychological support during treatment or internet-based nurse support can be provided through such platforms.

A main characteristic or benefit of exploiting social media to support the treatment process is that time- and location-independent communication. Another benefit of such technical support is that patient and carer, both, can monitor health data and have access to its interpretation. For the patient, self-management and active participation in the treatment process becomes possible.

Social Media for Information Gathering, Prevention, and Health Activity Promotion

The internet in general and social media in particular is a rich source of information. Thus, another application purpose of social media is to gather and provide information on diseases, symptoms and treatments. This kind of usage is already very common for patients (Fox, 2011). Studies showed that between 59 and 66% of person use the Internet to search for information on diseases and treatments. Physicians and healthcare providers started to go in-line with this development and provide information on treatment programs, or on disease prevention. Hospitals are providing information on their healthcare offers; physicians keep blogs where they inform patients about vaccination campaigns or new treatment options. Healthcare providers offer YouTube videos for patient education. Further, learning packages for specific diseases are suggested. Information search and access through the internet supports patient empowerment. On the other hand, physicians and other carers can use the social media to get latest research results by going through the information provided by their colleagues.

Beyond information provision and search, applications are developed that exploit social media for disease prevention, i.e. it supports in guiding health behavior, such as increasing physical activity by internet-based interventions. For example, the use of social networking sites for smoking prevention directed specifically towards young women was investigated to reply to smoking promotion activities of tobacco companies performed via social networking sites selected person groups, e.g., young women (Struik, Bottorff, Jung & Budgen, 2012).

The following scenario shows an example of a social-media based physical activity program.

- Fred, a 49 year-old man suffering from Parkinson's disease accesses through a web portal videos and descriptions of physical activity exercises his therapists prepared and selected particularly for him and his current health status. The exercises are provided through an individualized online portal to Fred. He performs the activities on an individual basis, but with support of online tutorials or videos provided by the therapists. Fred records once a week the exercises and stores them back to the portal where the carer can access them and provide feedback, see the progress and possibly, in case the health status decreased, ask the patient to come to an appointment via a messaging function built into the portal. Fred can also leave questions or comments for his therapists in the portal reflecting comments, experiences or difficulties that help the therapists and physician to monitor the health status.

The benefit of online-based health activity programs is that the patient can decide when to do the exercise. The barriers of making the exercises are reduced since no direct observation by a physician or therapist takes place. At the same time monitoring and feedback by a health carer is possible through recordings.

Applications falling into this category enable patients (and also health carers) to independently inform about a disease and related treatment options, but also to provide information and experiences. Patients are becoming in this way more empowered for making decisions concerning their health. Their motivation and compliance to medical treatments increases. Prevention and health promotion through social media can help in reaching the relevant persons.

Networking, Information Exchange, Forums in Healthcare

Self-help groups exist already for a long time. With social media, self-help received a new dimension: Patients can interact and communicate with each other over long distances, even if they cannot move from home. They exchange their experiences via social media tools such as networking platforms or forums, ask for help and get support by others who have similar problems. There are online patient communities that organize themselves, i.e. without any support from healthcare providers content is exchanged. Other patient networks are upcoming that are explicitly designed for patient education or allow for interactions with physicians (e.g. an online support group for depression, http://www. dailystrength.org/c/Depression/support-group). Networking sites, discussion boards or chats are social media tools exploited for networking and information exchange. We can also distinguish disease-specific networks, patient social communities and patient's blogs. The scenario describes such application:

- Fred, who is using the online activity program (see scenario in the previous section), connects to other patients with Parkinson's disease via a platform and online message board. He gets information on scheduled meetings of the self-help group and other interesting information posted by the others. From time to time, he posts his experiences with the activity games or asks others for their experiences with the disease. Once a week, an online chat is organized where he gets in contact with the others. They also invite sometimes healthcare providers to join the chat and to answer the questions of the group on specific topics.

In this way, Fred learns more about his disease, gets in contact with other persons suffering from the same medical condition. In particular, when his health status worsens, he gets support by other network participants. He benefits from their experiences.

In addition to patient networks and forums, platforms exist where healthcare provider can exchange their experiences on treatment and healthcare processes.

Again, the benefit of this application group is that experiences can be exchanged independently from time and location of the user. In particular for rare diseases, connecting with other patients or other physicians via social media becomes easier. For patients, networking has also a dimension of psychological and emotional support (i.e. by reducing feelings of loneliness) (Tarasenko, 2012). The content of social networks increases the patient's sense of control and the ability to manage their own illness.

Social Media for Knowledge Management

Social media is also exploited for knowledge management in medical research and science. Departments, research consortia etc. are using collaborative writing tools such as Wikis or Google Documents for making knowledge available or for managing knowledge (Archambault, Van De Belt, & Grajales, 2012). Social media can further provide a tool for collecting experiences on treatments made by physicians. As described in the section before, physicians and hospitals are also using blogs for providing knowledge on diseases and treatments to patients. Consider the following scenario:

- Dr. Harris is neurologist and specialized on treatment of patients with multiple sclerosis. There is a lot of research on this disease ongoing. He regularly posts his experiences with treatment options and on latest research results he became aware of, on a wiki dealing specifically with treatment of patients suffering from multiple sclerosis. Only physicians are allowed to contribute to this wiki. Dr. Harris also checks the entries from others and learns more about their experiences and new treatment options. In this way, he and his colleagues exchange experiences and knowledge and stay up to date.

The benefit of using social media tools for collecting and managing knowledge is the time- und location independent access; even simultaneous access is possible. Knowledge is continuously available and in particular experiences from various perspectives can be contrasted. The benefit of collaborative writing is that knowledge can be continuously extended and shared by several experts. However, such applications require active participation in information provision. Outdated information need to be marked or even be removed. An additional problem is to ensure quality of the provided content. In general, collaborative writing is also possible for patient communities (e.g. a wiki with patient experiences on drugs or treatments). In the UK, the service Patient Opinion (https://www.patientopinion.org.uk) collects experiences from patients to improve healthcare. However, applications of social media for managing knowledge for treatment and healthcare processes are still rare.

Social Media for Research and Health Monitoring

There are many research questions that can be addressed when analyzing social media data. The information provided through this channel is unique in a sense that there is no other written source of experiences from patients and health carers. For this reason, social-media content becomes more and more subject of research and monitoring in the field of healthcare and medicine.

The motivation behind grounds among others upon the fact that social-media data provides a new information source for researchers to learn about experiences of patients (and of physicians). Feelings, perceptions, experiences are often unconsidered in the treatment process given the short amount of contact time between physician and patient. Patient experiences with treatments and drugs reported in social media can be analyzed for studying efficiency of treatments or treatment preferences; risks can be identified from patient case data provided online for pharmaceutical research. There is for example Treato.com, a social health site that analyses online patient discussions to provide insights from patients' opinions and attitudes, helping to answer questions about a medication. Through the study of social-media data, for example of illness narratives, healthcare providers and the research community can learn how and what patients wish to share with their online health community, how patients view their illness and treatment, and what patients consider as gaps or success (Walters, 2012).

Another application area in this context is the recruitment of patients for clinical trials based on their social-media profiles or performing epidemiological studies grounding on the social media data available (Brownstein, Brownstein, & Williams, 2009). Further, potential health risks can be identified based on social-media data and a population's health status can be monitored (Denecke, Krieck & Otrusina, 2013).

Additionally, researchers examine how the value of patient online ratings reflects physician quality. It has been found out that there exist statistically significant correlations between the value of ratings and physician experience, board certification, education, and malpractice claims, suggesting positive correlation between online ratings and physician quality (Gao, McCullough & Agarwal, 2012).

DISCUSSION AND CONCLUSION

The previous section showed that there is a large variety of applications centered on social media tools and data. Some of them are already tested or even in regular use (e.g. information gathering). However, in all categories there is still room for improvement and further research. In this section, we will summarize the requirements for such applications as they were described before. Further, we discuss strengths and weaknesses of social media-based applications in healthcare and outline future directions.

Strengths and Weaknesses

By studying the content of abstracts accepted for the Medicine 2.0 conference in 2012, we identified several application fields of medical social-media data. Current research mainly concentrates on social media as information source. Beyond, applications to support in treatment processes are arising. Even though recognized as useful, knowledge management applications using social media are not yet well established in the healthcare domain. A reason might be the difficulty in getting active participating contributors. Exploitation and analysis of social-media data for monitoring and studying purposes is an upcoming field where research just begins.

Chronic and mental diseases are the main focus of current applications of social media, probably for several reasons: 1) Many people are concerned by chronic or mental diseases, 2) close progress monitoring is required for a long period, 3) to a certain extent self-help is possible; 4) compliance of the patient is crucial, which requires involvement in his treatment.

In the following, we summarize the general potentials of social-media usage in healthcare. They include:

1. Location-independent support,
2. Participation in decision making processes,
3. Integrated healthcare processes,
4. New research possibilities.

Social media allows to *shift information, communication and health monitoring from the social and healthcare sector into the private environment.* It thus allows for a *location-independent support.* By regularly entering data into web platforms, consistent health monitoring is enabled. Problem situations can be detected better or earlier, which is of high relevance, in particular for patients with chronic diseases. Patients can get information on diseases, engage in discussions with others including the healthcare team. This indirect, location-independent communication can increase the personal convenience and helps in preserving personal independence by simultaneously enabling continuous monitoring. A better risk awareness can be achieved. Social media provides also new possibilities for healthcare prevention, for example through social games for health activities or online health status monitoring during the treatment process.

A second potential of social media in healthcare processes is the possibility for patients in actively *participating in decision making processes.* Patient-centered care or participatory care is an upcoming trend in healthcare (Weitzel, Smith, Lee, de Deugd, & Helal, 2009). Nowadays, a patient has to take over more individual responsibility and is considered as partner in the medical decision making process. Social media supports this process by providing facilities for communicating and information exchange. People can for example ask in patient-doctor forums for information and explanations. Taking over individual responsibility can increase the compliance and supports ongoing treatment success.

An additional value of social media is connected to usage scenarios for realizing *integrated healthcare* processes. For a long time, healthcare processes lack of sufficient communication and information exchange among health carers. So far, the patient is the medium of communication, bringing information, reports and images from one carer to another. A social network among carers could overcome this lack. All involved carers can stay informed and communicate easily, not only via a patient but through the social network (which should be of course restricted in access). Even an information exchange with additional actors (e.g. nursing services, therapists) could be enabled through social-media technology. This could support in optimizing healthcare processes. For example, there is AmbulanzPartner (http://www.ambulanzpartner.de), a network established by a research group of the Charité in Berlin that coordinates the healthcare process and all involved persons (patients, physicians, therapists, healthcare provider etc.) through a social network-like platform.

Further, social media provides *new research possibilities* and insights for example by getting information on the course of therapy from different perspectives, from the patient and the physician. A large amount of information on patient behavior, patient experiences with treatments and drugs are available in the web, ready to be used for research and studies.

Several challenges exist when using social-media tools or data in healthcare: The participatory aspect of social media is its strength, but also a big challenge. Inaccurate information can be distributed through social-media channels and have related implications regarding patient health and safety. Reaching populations with lower socioeconomic status might be a challenge as well.

Requirements

For future developments of applications as described before and to integrate them into healthcare processes, several requirements need to be considered. They can be categorized into four groups: technical, functional, formal and organizational requirements.

Technical requirements comprise among others:

- Privacy and security aspects,
- Trust (technical, systemic, interpersonal),
- Access rights,
- Data storage,
- Integration with data from clinical information systems (e.g. electronic health records),
- Availability of data and textmining methods for information processing.

When social-media tools are exploited to support the treatment process, it needs to be ensured that - in case patient data is exchanged through such tools - privacy and security issues are considered. This includes among others access rights for the various persons that are involved in the process. Within the context of applications supporting the treatment process, integration with clinical information systems would be crucial for the health carers. Considering the example described at the beginning of the chapter, the patient-recorded activity sequences could become part of the electronic health record to document the progress of treatment. Additional technical requirements concern the recording and data processing capabilities of the tools to enable the described applications. These go hand in hand with *functional requirements* that include among others:

- Filtering or information selection facilities,
- Interactions and visualizations of data,
- Video recording facilities,
- Structured information exchange and communication,
- Availability of data and services,
- Information quality.

Patients should be enabled and encouraged through the use of social media to describe their experiences with treatments and drugs. Simultaneously, methods need to be available that support the physician in identifying the most relevant pieces of the chatter of their patients, or to get even alarms when the patient's health status seems to worsen. Thus, filtering facilities are crucial in order to avoid information overload with the health carers. This could also be realized by a structured information exchange (e.g., patient has to answer concrete questions). To facilitate interpretation and interaction with the data, appropriate visualizations and interaction facilities need to be available. Use cases need to be described and realized to identify realistic scenarios of using social media in healthcare and to communicate them to the stakeholders. Mainly in the context of information gathering from the internet and social media, ensuring information quality is crucial. To support users in identifying relevant information in the medical web, standards for medical web content were already defined to allow certification of quality health information (e.g. the HONcode certification (http://www.hon.ch)).

There are also *formal requirements* to be considered when exploiting social-media tools and data in healthcare. They comprise among others:

- Ethical and legal issues,
- Clarification of responsibilities,
- Quality of content, reliability of content,
- Payment models.

Payment models need to be established in order to include the usage of social media into the treatment process. The working time a physician spends in monitoring and interacting with his patients through social-media tools need to be reimbursed accordingly. This is crucial to successfully include such tools into the treatment process. Ethical and legal issues are related to the usage of data posted through social-media tools. Such questions mainly arise in the context of applications for monitoring and analyzing the data posted in social media. In this context, it is also important to clarify responsibilities. Imagine a health status monitoring tool exploited by a health organization identifies a group of sick persons based on their social-media chatter. In which manner should the health organization react? This and similar questions need to be answered.

Finally, *organisational requirements* of social-media applications concern:

- Integration into existing workflows or adaptation of workflows,
- Avoiding additional work and information overload,
- Social-media applications as mean to support or simplify existing treatment processes,
- Acceptance and active participation of involved parties.

It is crucial to make clear that the consideration of social media in the healthcare treatment process should not replace any face-to-face visits, but could enable a close monitoring by giving the patient the chance for self-managing his disease, taking over responsibility and on the other hand, enable physicians to monitor the health status more closely. Thus, the tools need to be integrated in existing workflows and will also require adaptation of workflows. However, this workflow integration is important to foster the acceptance of the tools and active participation of involved stakeholders.

FUTURE DIRECTIONS

This chapter showed that there are many ways where internet and social media can support healthcare and treatment. Applications are still under development and there are many open research questions to be addressed.

Important research questions concern the information gathering from social media: How can content be collected, stored, structured, fil-

tered, analysed (linguistically and content-wise) automatically? In Web Science, relevant methods are already introduced – for medicine, these methods still need to be extended. Mapping of social-media content to clinical ontologies is still limited (Denecke & Soltani, 2013). As soon as the social-media data is available in a structured manner, questions could be addressed such as:

- Which content is communicated? Which topics are discussed?
- How can subjective information be received from social-media data?
- Can social media be used for detecting disease outbreaks, (health) risk factors?

Given the results from the review of Medicine 2.0 abstracts, it becomes clear that social-media-based applications for supporting treatment are starting to become available.

The requirements listed before are not yet completely addressed and remain open for the future research. For example the integration of social-media data with the clinical data or electronic health records is still a big issue.

Social media makes it considerably more likely that patients, but also physicians and other health carers, learn about innovative and unproven therapies. It allows participants of a healthcare to improve communication and information exchange and also provides potentials for improving existing workflows in treatment.

REFERENCES

Aase, L., Goldman. D., Gould, M., Noseworthy, J., & Timimi, F. (2012). *Bringing the Social-media Revolution to Health Care*. Mayo Clinic Center for Social-Media.

Archambault, P. M., Van De Belt, T. H., Grajales, F. J., III, Eysenbach, G., & Aubin, K. (2012). *Wikis and Collaborative Writing Applications in Health Care: Preliminary Results of a Scoping Review.* iPROCEEDINGS Medicine 2.0 Boston. Retrieved from http://www.medicine20congress.com/ocs/index.php/med/med2012/paper/view/994

Brownstein, C. A., Brownstein, J. S., Williams, D. S., Wicks, P., & Heywood, J. A. (2009). The power of social networking in medicine. *Nature Biotechnology*, *27*, 888–890. doi:10.1038/nbt1009-888 PMID:19816437

Denecke, K., Krieck, M., Otrusina, L., Smrz, P., Dolog, P., Nejdl, W., & Velasco, E. (2013). How to Exploit Twitter & Co. for Public Health Monitoring? *Methods of Information in Medicine*. doi:10.3414/ME12-02-0010

Denecke, K., & Nejdl, W. (2009). How valuable is medical social media data? Content Analysis of the Medical Web. *Journal of Information Science*, *179*, 1870–1880. doi:10.1016/j.ins.2009.01.025

Denecke, K., & Soltani, N. (2013). The Burgeoning of Medical Social-Media Postings and the Need for Improved Natural Language Mapping Tools. In *Where Humans Meet Machines - Innovative Solutions for Knotty Natural-Language Problems*. Springer. doi:10.1007/978-1-4614-6934-6_2

Eysenbach, G. (2008). Medicine 2.0: Social networking, collaboration, participation, apomediation, and openness. *Journal of Medical Internet Research*, *10*(3), e22. doi:10.2196/jmir.1030 PMID:18725354

Eysenbach, G. (2011). Infodemiology and Infoveillance: Tracking Onlline Health Information and Cyberbehaviour for Public Health. *American Journal of Preventive Medicine*, *40*(5), 154–158. doi:10.1016/j.amepre.2011.02.006

Fox, S. (2011). *Health Topics*. Pew Research Center's Internet & American Life Project. Retrieved from http://www.pewinternet.org/~/media//Files/Reports/2011/PIP_Health_Topics.pdf

Fox, S., & Duggan, M. (2013). *Tracking for Health*. Pew Research Center's Internet & American Life Project. Retrieved from http://pewinternet.org/Reports/2013/Tracking-for-Health.aspx

Gao, G., McCullough, J. S., Agarwal, R., & Jha, J. K. (2012). *A Changing Landscape of Physician Quality Reporting: Analysis of Patients' Online Ratings of Their Physicians.* iPROCEEDINGS Medicine 2.0 Boston. Retrieved from http://www.medicine20congress.com/ocs/index.php/med/med2012/paper/view/954

Ho, W. H., Weinstein, P., De Sousa, D., Husain, J. T., Wu, R. A., Cafazzo, J. A., & Armour, K. (2012). *A Mobile Clinical Collaboration System for Inter-Professional Team Based Care in an Outpatient Setting.* iPROCEEDINGS Medicine 2.0 Boston. Retrieved from http://www.medicine-20congress.com/ocs/index.php/med/med2012/paper/view/1243

Khairat, S., & Garcia, C. (2012). *Introducing a Wireless Mobile Technology to Improve Diabetes Care Outcomes among Specific Minority Groups.* iPROCEEDINGS Medicine 2.0 Boston. Retrieved from http://www.medicine20congress.com/ocs/index.php/med/med2012/paper/view/900

Lau, A. Y., Siek, K. A., Fernandez-Luque, L., Tange, H., Chhanabhai, P., & Li, S. Y. et al. (2011). The Role of Social Media for Patients and Consumer Health: Contribution of the IMIA Consumer Health Informatics Working Group. *Yearbook of Medical Informatics*, *6*(1), 131–138. PMID:21938338

Lupiáñez-Villanueva, F., Mayer, M. A., & Torrent, J. (2009). Opportunities and challenges of Web 2.0 within the health care systems: An empirical exploration. *Informatics for Health & Social Care, 34*(3), 117–126. doi:10.1080/17538150903102265 PMID:19670002

Stinson, J., Jibb, L., Nathan, P. C., Maloney, A. M., Dupuis, L. L., Gerstle, J. T., et al. (2012). *Development and Testing of a Multidimensional IPhone Pain Assessment Application for Adolescents with Cancer.* iPROCEEDINGS Medicine 2.0 Boston. Retrieved from http://www.medicine-20congress.com/ocs/index.php/med/med2012/paper/view/910

Struik, L. L., Bottorff, J. L., Jung, M., & Budgen, C. (2012). *Facebook Me: The Use of Social Networking Sites for Gender-Sensitive Tobacco Control Messaging.* iPROCEEDINGS Medicine 2.0 Boston. Retrieved from http://www.medicine-20congress.com/ocs/index.php/med/med2012/paper/view/785

Tarasenko, E. (2012). *Facebook Me: Russian Social Media for Patients and Physicians: Problems and Perspectives.* iPROCEEDINGS Medicine 2.0 Boston. Retrieved from http://www.medicine-20congress.com/ocs/index.php/med/med2012/paper/view/1025

Walters, B. H. (2012). *Telling Tales: Treatment Stories on an Eating Disorder Support Website.* iPROCEEDINGS Medicine 2.0 Boston. Retrieved from http://www.medicine20congress.com/ocs/index.php/med/med2012/paper/view/924

Weitzel, M., Smith, A., Lee, D., de Deugd, S., & Helal, S. (2009). Participatory Medicine: Leveraging Social Networks in Telehealth Solutions. In *Ambient Assistive Health and Wellness Management in the Heart of the City (LNCS)* (Vol. 5597, pp. 40–47). Berlin: Springer. doi:10.1007/978-3-642-02868-7_6

Wicks, P., Massagli, M., Frost, J., Brownstein, C., Okun, S., & Vaughan, T. et al. (2010). Sharing Health Data for Better Outcomes on PatientsLikeMe. *Journal of Medical Internet Research, 12*(2), e19. doi:10.2196/jmir.1549 PMID:20542858

ENDNOTES

[1] Healthcare social media list: http://network. socialmedia.mayoclinic.org/hcsml-grid/

[2] This kind of application is not considered in this paper. We rather focus on applications where social media tools and data are exploited to support healthcare processes and treatment.

Chapter 6
The Past, the Present, and the Future:
Examining the Role of the "Social" in Transforming Personal Healthcare Management of Chronic Disease

Elizabeth Cummings
University of Tasmania, Australia

Leonie Ellis
University of Tasmania, Australia

Paul Turner
University of Tasmania, Australia

ABSTRACT

This chapter examines how the rapid diffusion of social media and Mobile Web is impacting personal healthcare management amongst those living with chronic disease. Despite a recent increase in research in this area (Moorhead, et al., 2013), evaluating the "social" still poses challenges to conventional notions of the "Internet empowered" patient and the best ways to support the management of chronic disease (Østbye, et al., 2005). The chapter argues that there is a need for advancing conceptual thinking on how health and IT are now interacting at the level of individual patients/citizens and how this is continuing to transform health professional-patient interactions (Glasgow, et al., 2008). By drawing on examples of e-health research, the chapter illustrates how notions of the "social" and "technology" have evolved over time from medically centred e-health through to patient-centred e-health. The chapter considers how this evolution may lead to a future focus on community-centred personal healthcare of chronic disease supported by "social" e-health tools, applications, and services that continue to blur the more conventional boundaries between health professionals, patients, and their social networks.

DOI: 10.4018/978-1-4666-6150-9.ch006

INTRODUCTION

The term social media covers a wide array of technologies, applications and services including social networking sites like Facebook, media-sharing platforms like YouTube, BitTorrent and Flickr, and an array of user content including Wikis, Blogs and micro-blogging services like Twitter. Despite some continuing definitional ambiguity in the literature, there is general agreement that social media involves interaction on-line around the generation, communication and exchange of user-generated content (Kaplan & Haenlein, 2010; Kietzmann et al, 2011). Simultaneously growth in the use of mobile devices (mobiles, tablets, laptops etc.) and mobile networks to access content on the internet has also expanded rapidly particularly during the last five years (Kelly, 2013). While

this trend is uneven globally, it is noticeable that some of the most rapid adopters of 'mobile web' are countries with rapidly developing economies including Brazil, Russia, India and China (BRICs). These countries are also increasingly aware of the need to address the changing healthcare challenges arising within their increasingly affluent populations (Bhaumik, 2013). The diversity of analysis on growth social media uptake is evident with graphs and tables presenting data according to social media types, user timelines, size, duration and by companies or industries. As an example Figure 1 presents social media penetration by country as at March 2013.

Combined, the near exponential growth in the adoption and use of social media and mobile web (Qualman, 2013) has, perhaps not surprisingly, led to the their deployment by a range of healthcare

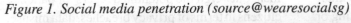

Figure 1. Social media penetration (source @wearesocialsg)

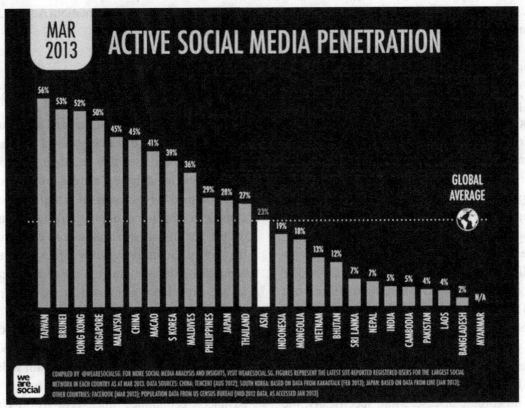

stakeholders including governments and public & private sector healthcare provider organisations; healthcare professionals and researchers; and patients/citizens (Thackeray et al, 2008; Moen et al, 2009; Colineau & Paris, 2010). Noticeably, the primary aims and objectives for using these 'social' technologies have varied considerably across the different stakeholders and have also changed over time. Governments and healthcare provider organisations have tended to have a strong focus on health information dissemination that has more recently given rise to trends that use social technologies for broader community engagement and awareness raising. Clinicians initially tended to focus on their own professional networks and on keeping their expertise up-to-date, but more recently some have been reaching out to their patients through these technologies to extend their services e.g. <www.ozdocsonline.com.au>.

For patients these social technologies primarily emerged as a way of either complementing or *by-passing* conventional sources of health related information. These technologies continue to be used to seek/share health information/advice, personal experiences and knowledge of medications/medical services, and to offer support and/or track personal healthcare (Househ, 2013). More recently there have been a number of other trends related to patient use of these social technologies. One major trend has been the emergence of private sector providers entering the social media market to support patients on-line health activities, for example, <www.patientslikeme.com> (Ellis, Showell, Turner, 2013). Another has been evidence of negative impacts on health arising from misinformation (Syed-Abdul et al, 2013) and/or reinforcement of negative behaviours (Hanson et al, 2013) as a result of 'social' networking.

The focus of this chapter is to examine how these different trends are impacting on personal health care management amongst an increasingly significant group of healthcare users – those living with chronic disease. More specifically, the chapter aims to examine how these different trends

challenge conventional thinking about those living with chronic disease and the best ways to support their personal healthcare management (Kuijpers et al, 2013; Østbye et al, 2005). In this context, by drawing on examples of e-health research into management/self-management of chronic disease, the chapter illustrates how notions of the 'social' and 'technology' are being transformed by social media and mobile web.

The chapter argues that there is a need for advancing conceptual thinking on how health and ICTs (e-health) are now interacting at the level of individual patients/citizens and how these changes require improved sophistication in approaches to the management of chronic disease by health professionals and health informatics specialists. Critically, the chapter argues that the challenge for the future is how best to ensure that social media benefits for personal healthcare management outweigh the potential dangers for patients/citizens in terms of privacy breaches, data misuse, exploitation and/or misinformation (Adams, 2010; Corea et al, 2010).

BACKGROUND

This section provides background on how approaches to both the management of chronic disease and the use of e-health in supporting this management have changed over time. To contextualise these changes it is useful to briefly consider current and future predicted pressures on the health care environment as the result of the increase in chronic and complex conditions, ageing populations and the sustained increase in life expectancy exhibited in most countries around the world.

In one sense, current and predicted pressures on health care budgets, systems and resources are the direct result of the successful delivery of healthcare services that has occurred in most advanced economies since post-World-War 2. Developments in medicines, clinical practices, health technologies and increasing social affluence have all contributed significantly to a reduction in infectious diseases and injury as the major causes of premature death or disability. Simultaneously with these changes however, has been the emergence of increases in the prevalence of risk factors leading to chronic disease (Wagner et al., 2001). As increasing numbers of citizens' live longer, increasing numbers also live with complex chronic conditions or disability. In many developed countries this trend has been compounded by a reduction in the overall birth rate such that for at least another twenty years the ratio of aged citizens living with one or more chronic disease relative to the population as a whole will continue to rise. These factors have combined to make finding cost effective and efficient solutions to the management of chronic disease a priority. They have also put considerable pressure on the health budgets of most developed countries with the percentage of GDP spend on health continuing to rise in ways predicted to be unsustainable in the near future.

As an example, Australia is trying to address its rapidly ageing population by approaches that promote healthy ageing as part of strategies to support the maintenance of high quality health-care services into the future. Current estimates are that between 2010 and 2050 the number of people between the ages of 65 and 84 will more than double, and the number of very old (85 years and over) will more than quadruple. In Australia, chronic conditions already contribute to more than 80% of the total health burden and contribute significantly to decreased quality of life for many patients/citizens and their carers. Based on the national health survey for 2007-08, an estimated 75% of Australians already had a long-term condition. It is also known that the number of long-term conditions that people report increases with age such that 50% of those aged 65 years or older are likely to have five or more long-term conditions (AIHW, 2010).

Chronic conditions are ongoing in nature and are rarely, if ever, completely cured (AIHW, 2012).

Given the variety of chronic diseases/conditions it can be difficult to provide a single definition however it is clear that most chronic conditions exhibit the following characteristics:

- They have complex and multiple causes;
- They usually have a gradual onset, although they can have sudden onset and acute stages;
- They occur across the life cycle, although they become more prevalent with older age;
- They can compromise quality of life by causing physical and/or mental impairment or disability;
- They are long term and persistent, leading to a gradual deterioration of health; and
- They tend initially not to be immediately life threatening, but they are the most common and leading cause of premature mortality.

The increasing costs and the increasing incidence of chronic conditions have placed emphasis on ensuring the patient journey is proactive, planned, coordinated, and efficient (Coleman et al., 2009). It has also led to awareness that existing models of chronic disease management were not sustainable and that alternatives needed to be examined.

CHRONIC DISEASE MANAGEMENT AND CHRONIC DISEASE SELF-MANAGEMENT

Traditional approaches to chronic disease management rely on a health care model that positions the clinician-patient relationship as one in which the clinician is the sole source of expertise and decision making authority (Charles, Gafni, & Whelan, 1997). With the growth in the incidence of chronic disease, it has now been recognized that this approach is both unsustainable and inappropriate (Wagner et al, 1996; <www.improving-chroniccare.org>).

As a result, a number of more integrated and collaborative approaches have emerged that aim to variously support improved continuity of care, use of evidence based practices and direct involvement of patients and their carers. These include collaborative management (Von Korff, Gruman, Schaefer, Curry, & Wagner, 1997), patient empowerment (Funnell et al., 1991), shared decision making (Charles, Gafni, & Whelan, 1997), the partnership model (Holman & Lorig, 2000), and the chronic care model (Wagner, 1998; Wagner et al., 2001). Following Wagner et al, the chronic care model provides a general framework for these approaches and highlights that for successful self-management interventions there are a number of essential elements including: Collaborative problem definition; Targeting, goal setting and planning; Self-management training and support services; and Active and sustained follow-up.

These elements aim to ensure the development of self-management initiatives that enable patient's to define their problems in conjunction with their health professionals. This includes identifying the issues that are of greatest importance to the patient and clinician as the basis for the setting of realistic goals and the development of personalised care plans. To enhance the probability of success it is important that any processes are guided by the patient's readiness to change and the development of their self-efficacy skills. Ensuring that patients are provided with instruction about disease management, behavioural support, and physical activity and that they also have the emotional demands of living with a chronic condition addressed appear to be also be very important success factors (Coleman, 2009; IoM, 2012)

While these approaches vary in emphasis, all share a common perspective that clinicians, patients and their carers should share information and where possible make choices together (Barrett, 2005). Of course, underlying this focus on collaboration is the assumption that patients have the right to take part in all health decisions (Charles, Gafni, & Whelan, 1997), and that they are capable, with appropriate support, of making valuable contributions to these decisions (Wagner et al., 2001). This assumption has been criticized because of the fact that many patients living with chronic conditions may be unwilling or unable to take on these new responsibilities and that furthermore, even if they do, that the result will necessarily be improved quality of care (Cummings & Turner, 2010).

There is however a growing body of evidence reporting positive outcomes from attempts to 'empower' some patients and engage in more integrated care practices in relation to chronic disease (Coleman et al, 2009). But it is also clear that these outcomes are not evenly spread amongst those living with chronic conditions and that other socio-economic and educational factors are important in contributing to the capacity of patients to achieve positive health outcomes (Showell & Turner, 2013). This stated, for many patients the opportunity to engage in self-management is a positive development. Self-management being defined here as simply the active participation of patients/citizens in the own personal health care management. Clearly self-management does not mean patients managing their conditions in isolation. It requires an effective partnership between patient, carer and health service provider. Working together to ensure that essential care requirements are available when needed and that the various people involved in the care are informed and work together to ensure the best possible outcomes for patients (Harvey, Battersby, & Misan, 2003).

Evidence highlights that many patients engaged in self-management make better use of health care professionals' time and particularly where they have developed effective self-management skills (Barlow, Turner, & Wright, 2000; Lorig et al., 1999). Systematic reviews indicate clear clinical benefits for patients with conditions such as diabetes and hypertension through self-management programmes. However, such reviews are limited by the heterogeneity of interventions and outcomes (Chodosh et al., 2005; Warsi, LaValley, Wang, Avorn, & Solomon, 2003; Warsi, Wang, LaValley, & Avorn, 2004). The increased ability to self-manage conditions and prevent or mitigate deterioration are linked to improving patient control of their condition (Cummings, 2008). However, this requires a more patient centred system based upon a deep understanding of both the patient and their perceptions of health care (Simborg, 2010).

As will be discussed below in relation to the use of technology this implies that what works for one patient may not work for another and this does create difficulties for health care systems that tend towards 'one-size fits all' approaches as they attempt to move towards patient centred care (Novak et al., 2013)

E-HEALTH AND CHRONIC DISEASE SELF-MANAGEMENT

As highlighted in the previous section of this chapter there is already a considerable body of health research in the areas of chronic disease management, self-management, active ageing, and independent living (Lorig et al., 2006, Jessup et al., 2006, Camarinha-Matos and Afsarmanesh, 2011).

Much of this work has utilised information and communication technologies (ICTs) to support interventions (Lorig et al, 2006, Cummings et al, 2010; Kuijpers et al, 2013). Many of these technology supported health interventions have been critiqued for their overly simplistic assumptions about the relationships between information provision and improved health outcomes (Cummings & Turner, 2010). In parallel with these types of disease specific technology supported health interventions, there has also been research focused on broader lifestyle change and wellness management amongst those with chronic diseases. However, as indicated previously, a major challenge how to ensure the sustainability of these lifestyle changes, which is an area of research that continues to receive limited attention (Freyne et al, 2011).

From a technological perspective, it is evident that there are significant differences amongst older people in the adoption and use of ICT. In Australia, where internet access and the penetration of computing technology is relatively high, a number of studies have confirmed that lack of internet access or computing technology continues to be correlated with a range of factors including low incomes, living in rural areas, low educational levels and old age (Fox, 2011, Gilhooly et al. 2009). To avoid accentuating this e-health divide, increased digital inclusion and use of assistive technologies can deliver benefits for the elder and those with chronic conditions such as increased independence and social participation (Gilhooly et al., 2009). However, there is also significant potential for the further isolation of already marginalised groups as more and more social, political and commercial services are transferred onto the Internet and those without ICT skills or access are further marginalized through a digital divide (Gilhooly et al., 2009; Niehaves and Plattfaut, 2010).

Following Niehaves and Plattfaut (2010), the single most important predictor of whether older people used ICT was their expectation of the benefits that ICT could bring them. Other factors identified as barriers to the adoption of ICT by older people include lack of interest, feeling too old, fear of new technology (fear of breaking it), lack of resources and access, lack of IT skills and experience, cost and concerns about security and privacy (Olphert et al., 2005; Charness & Boot, 2009). These factors are compounded by age-related decline as loss of vision, dexterity and motor skills make it more difficult for older or disabled people to use technologies (Olphert et al., 2005). Most of these impairments are directly correlated with chronic conditions.

Another dimension of these barriers relates to differences in people's health literacy. Following, Pearce-Brown et al. (2009) and Jordan et al. (2008) it has become evident that health literacy and the capacity to self-management are correlated. Personal capacity to seek, access, understand and use health information and services directly influences participation in treatment decisions. People with lower health literacy are those most likely to have chronic conditions and in turn they are the least able to manage those conditions (Hawkins et al. 2010; Pearce-Brown et al. 2009). Improved self-management may help compensate for lower levels of health literacy and improve health-related behaviours (Hibbard et al. 2007). However, currently there is little evidence on the costs of poor health literacy and the cost-effectiveness of interventions to improve health literacy (Eichler et al. 2009).

Clearly it is highly complex and challenging to genuinely understand individual patient's capacities and experiences in interacting with these technologies per se, as well as how they may contribute to improved self-management (Cummings and Turner, 2010). In recognition of this complexity, more recent approaches to the use of e-health to support chronic disease self-management have become more patient-centred and attempted to involve patients directly in the design of the solutions (Roehrer et al, 2013).

Two of the author's on this chapter have been directly involved in the design, implementation and evaluation of e-Health systems to support chronic disease self-management programs with a range of patient cohorts living with one or more chronic conditions including COPD and CF (Cummings, Chau, & Turner, 2009; Cummings et al., 2010; Cummings & Turner, 2007, 2008; Cummings & Turner, 2010; Roehrer, Cummings, Beggs et al., 2013; Roehrer, Cummings, Ellis, & Turner, 2011; Roehrer, Cummings, Turner et al., 2013). Below is a brief summary of some of this research work relating to one major project.

The Pathways Home project sought to support daily self-monitoring and recording of symptoms by patients suffering from two chronic respiratory conditions: chronic obstructive pulmonary disease (COPD), and cystic fibrosis (CF). The main purpose was to test the hypothesis that by assisting patients in the processes of identification, and comprehension about their condition they can initiate early action in relation to changes in their condition and so decrease the severity of exacerbations and slow their decline. The project was premised on the view that where possible patients should play a central role in decisions about their own health and that providing evidence-based knowledge to patients would enhance their ability to participate in self-management of their condition.

The COPD arm aimed to assist older people with COPD to achieve self-management skills, mediated through the development of self-efficacy for patient-identified health behaviours. The project supported self-management through self-monitoring and recording of symptoms (preferably in an electronic format) with a graphical longitudinal feedback report provided to participants and their mentors. Evaluation of this project appeared to indicate that the use of the online patient diary impedes or limits the development of self-efficacy for self-management in people suffering from moderate to severe COPD but that other social benefits can be achieved as the participants become more housebound by their condition (Cummings, 2008; Cummings et al, 2010).

The CF arm of the Pathways project was an investigation to see if an ICT tool, in this case a mobile phone application, could be developed for the use of daily symptom monitoring. The study hoped to discover if individuals with CF would use the tool and if the use of the ICT tool made a difference to the self-management behaviours and quality of life for individuals with CF. This was undertaken by was the support of mentoring activity through ICT, feedback from participants also indicated that further research was needed

(Cummings et al., 2011). Pathways Home demonstrated that mentoring assisted with developing self-efficacy for self-management behaviours, but the pilot study was too small to make definitive conclusions on the ICT arm (Cummings et al., 2011).

The Pathways Home CF project was then extended to explore the effect of its implementation for a group of adolescents and older children with CF based in Queensland. The aim of this project was to examine task-specific self-efficacy and self-monitoring and the project was designed to improve self-management behaviours and quality of life amongst CF patients (Roehrer et al., 2013). The project ran for six months, with a further six months of follow up. Data collection involved both quantitative and qualitative assessments collected at commencement, 3, 6 and 6 months post completion. Again this consisted of an electronic diary and participants were able to view a summary of their feedback to monitor changes in their symptoms. The project mentors were also able to review their patients remotely. The outcomes of this project provided sufficient positive response from the qualitative data and usage statistics to indicate that further investigation with a broader scope encompassing a more sophisticated suite of products to support the CF community may be beneficial. Useful information was also obtained

on aspects of self-monitoring that were not viewed favourably by these younger CF patients such as the need to enter diary data on a daily basis, which not surprisingly was not an attractive option for young adolescents (Roehrer et al., 2013).

This resulted in the development of a final project, the myCF project, which utilised web based resources that could also be accessed via mobile devices. This project had three proposed outcomes: development of a web based information portal which contained expert reviewed health information sheets and links to other relevant sites; Increasing the availability of community support from peers and other families through a secure online chat room; and introduction of a health mentor system of trained health professionals to encourage the development of self-monitoring and increase self-awareness about their condition.

What the above examples highlight is the complexity of using e-health to sustainably support chronic disease self-management in a manner that produces benefits recognized by both the patients and the health professionals (Kuijpers et al, 2013). A major conceptual challenge is addressing the implicit info-centrism that emerges within these types of intervention i.e. the prioritization of the importance of information provision per se. The implicit assumption that axiomatically through the provision of additional information patients

Figure 2. Timeline and relationship between projects

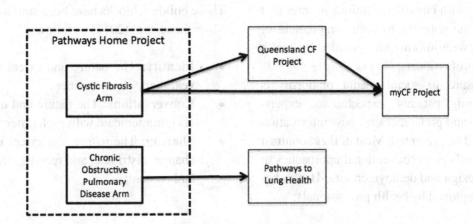

will achieve better outcomes ignores the psychosocial, attitudinal and contextual factors that are important for good healthcare and the capacity to self-manage.

It is in this context that the emergence of social media and mobile web are transforming personal health care management of chronic disease and challenging some key assumptions that are embedded in health systems and health informatics approaches to support self-management.

CHRONIC DISEASE AND THE 'SOCIAL'

The above discussion has highlighted the complexity of supporting personal health care management of chronic disease. This situation has become even more complex as increasing numbers of patients and their carers adopt social media and mobile web in relation to their health.

This chapter argues that the impact of this 'social' use of information and communication technologies in personal healthcare management amongst many of those living with chronic conditions is further transforming conventional health professional – patient interactions, attitudes and expectations. In particular, it is evident that:

- Patient to Patient interactions through social media and mobile web are changing the nature and flow of information available on living with chronic conditions in ways that have the potential to both complement or *clash* with information provided by health care professionals;
- Exposure to social media platforms is changing patients' expectations, experiences and preferences for how information should be presented. Most of these contrast markedly with conventional approaches to the design and deployment of e-Health being deployed by health professionals;

- The dramatic adoption and diffusion of social media and mobile web across the population of those living with chronic conditions has already started to challenge many of the assumptions held by health professionals and health informatics specialists about who their service users are, what they need and want and how services should be provided, as more patients access alternative and more readily available information, peer-support and advice through social media and mobile web.

It is argued that these changes require advancement in conceptual thinking on how health care systems and health informatics solutions can be used to optimize the benefits of for individual patients/citizens engage in personal health care management of chronic disease. More critically, looking to the future, health professionals and health informatics specialists need to ensure that social media benefits for personal healthcare management outweigh the potential dangers for patients/citizens in terms of privacy breaches, data misuse, exploitation and/or misinformation (Adams, 2010; Corea et al, 2010).

In trying to understand how social media and mobile web are transforming the nature of health communications it is useful to consider the Keitzmann et al (2011) framework that describes seven major building blocks in terms of form and function exhibited by different social media. These building blocks have been summarized by Moorehead et al (2013) as follows:

- **Identity:** The nature and extent users reveal themselves on-line;
- **Conversations:** The nature and extent users communicate with each other;
- **Sharing:** The nature and extent users exchange, distribute, and receive information and content;

- **Presence:** The nature and extent users are aware of each other's availability on-line;
- **Relationships:** The nature and extent users socially relate to one another;
- **Reputation:** The nature and extent users are aware of and understand the social standing and trustworthiness of information, content and other users;
- **Groups:** The nature and extent users are aligned, structured and/or form identifiable communities.

What this framework highlights is how social media and the mobile web are changing the nature of spatial and temporal interactions between health content and patients. As Fox (2011) reports while health professionals remain the most important source of information increasing numbers of 'highly-engaged patients and caregivers' are playing an active role in sharing with others what they are learning through social media. Fox (2011) latest results indicate that of the 74% of USA adults who use the internet surveyed:

- 80% looked on-line for information concerning any of 15 health topics such as a specific disease or treatment.
- 34% read someone else's commentary or experience about health or medical issues on an online news group, website, or blog.
- 18% have gone online to find others who might have health concerns similar to theirs.
- 62% use social media platforms: and of these,
    - 23% of social network site users followed their friends' personal health experiences or updates on the site;
    - 17% of social network site users have used social networking sites to remember or memorialize other people who suffered from a certain health condition.

Significantly, while younger users still dominate social media platforms, increasing numbers of older and lower income users are using these platforms to find health related information (Chou et al, 2009; Kontos et al, 2010). This simultaneously challenges conventional thinking on the e-health divide and also raises concerns about the types of information these users are obtaining, its reliability and trustworthiness as well as the types of behavior interactions through these 'social' channels create? To date, these questions have remained under-explored. Indeed, as the most recent review of research into social media in health highlights, despite considerable optimism about the benefits of social media in healthcare the quality of evidence validating its impact remains low. This is especially the case in relation to the impact of social media amongst specific patient groups for example, those living with chronic disease (Moorhead et al, 2013).

DISCUSSION

This chapter has highlighted the reality that social media and the mobile web are now being adopted and used by increasing numbers of patients including those living with chronic conditions. This continuing trend and its impacts pose several questions for how health professionals and health informaticians should best respond given that major concerns are beginning to emerge about the quality and reliability of health information available through these 'social' channels, the potential for breaches of patient privacy and confidentiality and the dangers of inaccurate, misleading or harmful information being consumed by vulnerable user groups such as those living with chronic conditions (Adams, 2010a; Adams, 2010b).

For health professionals the first step in responding to the 'social' is to acknowledge that it is happening! Thereafter, exploring ways that social media can be leveraged to enhance health communications with patients and improve the quality and reliability of information and advice accessed will be important. Critically, health professionals must recognise that evidence that their patients are accessing social media for health information does not imply that these patients have necessarily high levels of health literacy (Jordan et al, 2010). Indeed, there is some evidence to suggest that using social channels to find health information is precisely because many patients find health information provided through conventional health service channels to be unhelpful or unusable. It is important for health professionals to recognise that without attempts to reach out to patients using these social channels there is a real danger that 'untethered social media use' may accentuate rather than mitigate existing health care challenges and inequalities amongst patients/citizens in terms of healthcare services (Simborg, 2010).

For health informaticians it is evident that the rapid adoption and use of social media and mobile web by patients is both simultaneously an opportunity and a challenge. For those living with chronic conditions the diversity of impairments and co-morbidities make it extremely challenging to ensure systems, applications and services are appropriate, user-friendly and useful for all users. However, that increasing numbers of patients are now on-line, presents greater opportunities to build applications and services to engage directly with them as part of the design, implementation and evaluation of 'social' health services. Indeed, it can be argued that the growth in use of social media for health amongst patients reveals an unmet appetite to engage on-line that is not being met by conventional healthcare channels. Certainly the emergence of private sector providers in this space supports this perspective (Ellis et al, 2013).

While it is important to avoid simply replacing patient dependency on health professionals for patient dependency on e-health systems, applications or services, there may be an opportunity to support and facilitate greater community-centred applications and services that leverage patients

'social' appetites. These types of applications and services open up the possibility of developing ways to mitigate the dangers of information overload and/or of patients receiving conflicting advice that may inhibit their ability to engage in self-management. In these more community-centred models social media and mobile web become platforms to complement other channels and as mechanisms to provide emotional, psycho-social and peer support amongst patients moderated by a range of health professionals working collaboratively (Frost et al, 2008). These emerging models do however suggest the need for a fundamental shift in thinking by health professionals in relation to their use of e-health and support of chronic disease self-management (Cummings & Turner, 2010; Kuijpers et al, 2013).

More broadly this community-centred approach leveraging social media platforms connects with a large body of published research that approaches self-management by investigating mechanisms to support positive lifestyle changes amongst a diverse range of users (Webb et al, 2010). While much of this research is focused on interventions with specific diseases, mechanisms to support prevention through wellness management have started to emerge as an important area of investigation. These types of intervention are focused on modifying problematic behaviours and/or promoting healthy lifestyles tailored to individual's context (Portnoy et al, 2007). While some of these investigations have critiqued the value of 'stages of change' models (Trans-theoretical models) for guiding interventions (Adams & White, 2005), most view the deployment of personalised interactive information services as useful tools to support these types of lifestyle change interventions (Yardley et al, 2010). Although it is acknowledged that user studies still point to significant challenges in how best to design these services and evaluate their impact across different types of users and contexts of use.

In attempting to enhance personal health care management amongst those living with chronic disease another challenge continues to be how to ensure sustainability of self-management and life-style changes and to reduce subsequent behaviour regression or reversal (Demiris et al, 2008). In this context, patients' adoption and use of social media opens up the possibility of finding new ways to personalise health systems, applications and services. More specifically, community-centred models leveraging peer communication and support may generate new ways of:

- Making health interventions 'sticky' in terms of maintaining interest in use amongst different types of users and in terms of being able to adapt to changing user needs in personal health care management (Baghaei et al, 2011);
- Making interventions persuasive in terms of enhancing sustainability of initiated health and lifestyle changes over time (Torning & Oinas-kukkonen, 2009).

Looking to the future this chapter suggests that responding to the growth of social media for health may lead to more community-centred personal e-health. In this vision, the community is dynamically formed in multiple different ways – patients communicating with and advising each other, patients and health professionals working in partnerships, and patients, carers, families and healthcare professionals communicating in a more fluid and integrated manner to form genuinely supportive communities (local or virtual) to aid patients to self-manage their conditions and live longer independently in their respective communities.

FUTURE RESEARCH DIRECTIONS

There are multiple opportunities for future research in the area of social media use in relation to transforming personal health care management of chronic disease. Whilst to date most of the research

the authors have undertaken has been exploratory, and the results mixed, it is understood that there is a need to develop more explanatory research and undertake robust evaluation. Certainly longitudinal studies will be of use to determine whether the use and engagement with social media and mobile web changes patient behaviours in a sustained manner. These will require larger sample sizes than have previously been used and so a mixed methodological approach may be appropriate.

There is also further evidence required into how differentials in health literacy, cultural and linguistic diversity, gender, age, level of educational attainment and socio-economic affluence interact with the use of social media and patient's abilities to gain or sustain positive changes in their self-management behaviours.

Finally, different countries have different health care systems and also data protection standards. An investigation of the risks and issues that may arise through the on-line sharing of health information across jurisdictions would be beneficial. This could then be used to develop methods of providing education to users regarding methods of assessing risks and maintaining their privacy and confidentiality when using on-line social media for health care.

CONCLUSION

This chapter has examined the emerging impact of the increasing adoption of social media and mobile web on personal health care management amongst those living with chronic diseases and conditions. It has highlighted that to engage in this examination is challenging and complex as is the result of the diversity of factors and types of users, applications and health systems involved. The chapter has argued that one impact of the increasing adoption and use of social media and mobile web is to challenge many current notions about who and how patients are engaging with management of their own health. This has included insights how some patients are complementing and/or by-passing health professionals to obtain peer support, advice and insight from other patients. While from one perspective these changes appear to support the idea of 'internet empowered patients', it was also highlighted that many users of social media for health may have limited health literacy and may be obtaining health information that is inaccurate, misleading or even harmful from their peers. It was also highlighted that in the internet space many users may be inexperienced in terms of understanding how their on-line behaviours may jeopardise their privacy and confidentiality.

This chapter has also considered how this complexity also poses challenges for healthcare systems and health informatics solutions. It has tried to examine these impacts and to explore what types of tailored/personalised information technology solutions might complement/leverage these social media and mobile web trends. One suggested approach is a move towards more community-centred solutions that leverage peer communications and the 'social' to more meaningfully tailor solutions to the attributes and lifestyles of those living with chronic disease. The future is certainly developing rapidly and we need to recognise the changing landscape that is transforming patients – health professional interactions, attitudes and expectations around the personal management of chronic disease.

It is anticipated that this chapter has contributed to advancing conceptual thinking on how health and IT are now interacting at the level of individual patients/citizens as a result of the emergence of social media and mobile web. It is hoped that the case has been made for the need for improved sophistication in the approaches to the management of chronic disease being developed by health professionals and health informatics specialists. Critically, the chapter has pointed out that the challenge for the future is how best to ensure that the benefits of social media benefits for personal healthcare management outweigh the potential dangers for patients/citizens in terms of privacy breaches, data misuse, exploitation and/or misinformation (Adams, 2010; Corea et al, 2010).

REFERENCES

Adams, S. A. (2010a). Blog-based applications and health information: Two case studies that illustrate important questions for Consumer Health Informatics (CHI) research. *International Journal of Medical Informatics*, *79*(6), e89–e96. doi:10.1016/j.ijmedinf.2008.06.009 PMID:18701344

Adams, S. A. (2010b). Revisiting the on-line health information reliability debate in the wake of web 2.0: an inter-disciplinary literature and website review. *International Journal of Medical Informatics*, *79*(6), 391–400. doi:10.1016/j.ijmedinf.2010.01.006 PMID:20188623

Andersen, N. B., & Söderqvist, T. (2012). *Social Media and Public Health Research* (Working Paper/Technical Report). Faculty of Science, University of Copenhagen.

Australian Institute of Health and Welfare (AIHW). (2010). *Australia's health 2010. Australia's health series no. 12. Cat. no. AUS 122*. Canberra, Australia: AIHW.

Australian Institute of Health and Welfare (AIHW). (2012). *Risk factors contributing to chronic disease chronic disease, Cat. no. PHE 157*. Canberra, Australia: AIHW.

Baghaei, N., Kimani, S., Freyne, J., Brindal, E., Berkovsky, S., & Smith, G. (2011). Engaging Families in Lifestyle Changes through Social Networking. *International Journal of Human-Computer Interaction*, *27*(10), 971–990. doi:10.1080/10447318.2011.555315

Bhaumik, S. (2013). BRICS nations agree to collaborate on research and public health challenges. *BMJ (Clinical Research Ed.)*, *346*, f369. PMID:23335476

Camarinha-Matos, L. M., & Afsarmanesh, H. (2011). *Collaborative Ecosystems in Ageing Support*. Paper presented at PRO-VE'11. São Paulo, Brazil.

Charness, N., & Boot, W. R. (2009). Aging and information technology use: Potential and barriers. *Current Directions in Psychological Science*, *18*(5), 253–258. doi:10.1111/j.1467-8721.2009.01647.x

Chou, W., Hunt, Y., Beckjord, E., Moser, R., & Hesse, B. (2009). Social media use in the United States: implications for health communication. *Journal of Medical Internet Research*, *11*(4), 48. doi:10.2196/jmir.1249 PMID:19945947

Coleman, K., Austin, B. T., Brach, C., & Wagner, E. H. (2009). Evidence on the Chronic Care Model in the new millennium. *Health Affairs*, *28*(1), 75–85. doi:10.1377/hlthaff.28.1.75 PMID:19124857

Colineau, N., & Paris, C. (2010). Talking about your health to strangers: Understanding the use of online social networks by patients. *New Review of Hypermedia and Multimedia*, *16*(1-2), 141–160. doi:10.1080/13614568.2010.496131

Correa, T., Willard Hinsley, A., & de Zúñiga, H. G. (2010). Who interacts on the Web? The intersection of users' personality and social media use. *Computers in Human Behavior*, *26*(2), 247–253. doi:10.1016/j.chb.2009.09.003

Cummings, E. (2008). *An investigation of the influence of an online patient diary on the health outcomes and experiences of people with chronic obstructive pulmonary disease (COPD) participating in a mentored self-management clinical controlled trial*. (PhD Thesis). University of Tasmania, Hobart, Australia.

Cummings, E., Chau, S., & Turner, P. (2009). Assessing a Patient-Centered E-Health Approach to Chronic Disease Self-Management. In E. V. Wilson (Ed.), *Patient-Centered E-Health*. Hershey, PA: Medical Information Science Reference.

Cummings, E., Robinson, A., Courtney-Pratt, H., Cameron-Tucker, H., Wood-Baker, R., & Walters, E. et al. (2010). Pathways Home: Comparing Voluntary IT and Non-IT Users Participating in a Mentored Self-Management Project. *Studies in Health Technology and Informatics*, *160*, 23–27. PMID:20841643

Cummings, E., & Turner, P. (2007). Considerations for deploying web and mobile technologies to support the building of patient self-efficacy and self-management of chronic illness. In L. Al-Hakim (Ed.), *Web Mobile-Based Applications for Healthcare Management*. Hershey, PA: Idea Group, Inc. doi:10.4018/978-1-59140-658-7.ch011

Cummings, E., & Turner, P. (2008). Considerations for Deploying Web and Mobile Technologies to Support the Building of Patient Self-Efficacy and Self-Management of Chronic Illness. In S. Clarke (Ed.), *End-User Computing: Concepts, Methodologies, Tools, and Applications* (Vol. 2, pp. 1053–1064). Hershey, PA: Information Science Reference. doi:10.4018/978-1-59904-945-8.ch076

Cummings, E., & Turner, P. (2010). Patients at the Centre: Methodological Considerations for Evaluating Evidence from Health Interventions Involving Patients use of Web-Based Information Systems. *The Open Medical Informatics Journal*, *4*, 188–194. PMID:21594007

Demiris, G., Afrinb, L., Speedie, S., Courtney, K. L., Sondhie, M., & Vimarlund, V. et al. (2008). Patient-Centered Applications: Use of Information Technology to promote Disease management and Wellness. *Journal of the American Medical Informatics Association*, *15*(1), 8–13. PMID:17947617

Dickerson, S. S., Reinhart, A., Boemhke, M., & Akhu-Zaheya, L. (2011). Cancer as a Problem to Be Solved: Internet Use and Provider Communication by Men With Cancer. *Computers, Informatics, Nursing, 29*(7), 388–395. doi:10.1097/NCN.0b013e3181f9ddb1 PMID:20975535

Eichler, K., Wieser, S., & Brügger, U. (2009). The costs of limited health literacy: A systematic review. *International Journal of Public Health, 54*(5), 313–324. doi:10.1007/s00038-009-0058-2 PMID:19644651

Ellis, L., Showell, C., & Turner, P. (2013). Social Media and patient self management: Not all sites are created equal. In *Proceedings of Information Technology and Communications in Health (ITCH) Conference*. IOS Press.

Fox, S. (2011). *The Social Life of Health Information*. Retrieved from http://www.pewinternet.org/Reports/2011/Social-Life-of-Health-Info.aspx

Freyne, J., Berkovsky, S., Baghaei, N., Kimani, S., & Smith, G. (2011). Personalised Techniques For Lifestyle Change. In *Proceedings of the 13th International Conference on Artificial Intelligence in Medicine in Europe*. Bled, Slovenia: AIME.

Gilhooly, M. L., Gilhooly, K. J., & Jones, R. B. (2009). Quality of life: conceptual challenges in exploring the role of ICT in active ageing. In Information and Communication Technologies for Active Ageing – Opportunities and Challenges for the European Union. IOS Press.

Glasgow, N. J., Jeon, Y.-H., Kraus, S. G., & Pearce-Brown, C. L. (2008). Chronic disease self-management support: The way forward for Australia. *Med J, 189*(10), 14.

Hanson, C. L., Cannon, B., Burton, S., & Giraud-Carrier, C. (2013). An Exploration of Social Circles and Prescription Drug Abuse Through Twitter. *Journal of Medical Internet Research, 15*(9), e189. doi:10.2196/jmir.2741 PMID:24014109

Hawkins, A. O., Kantayya, V. S., & Sharkey-Asner, C. (2010). Health literacy: A potential barrier in caring for underserved populations. *Disease-a-Month, 56*(12), 734–740. doi:10.1016/j.disamonth.2010.10.006 PMID:21168579

Hibbard, J., Mahoney, E., Stock, R., & Tusler, M. (2007). Self-management and health care utilization: Do increases in patient activation result in improved self-management behaviors? *Health Services Research, 42*(4), 1443–1463. doi:10.1111/j.1475-6773.2006.00669.x PMID:17610432

Hopgood, A. A. (2005). The State of Aritificial Intelligence. *Advanced in Computers, 65*, 1–75. doi:10.1016/S0065-2458(05)65001-2

Househ, M. (2013). The Use of Social Media in HealthCare: Organisational, Clinical and Patient Perspectives. In *Proceedings of Information Technology and Communications in Health (ITCH) Conference*. IOS Press.

Huber, J., Ihrig, A., & Peters, T. et al. (2011). Decision-making in localized prostate cancer: Lessons learned from an online support group. *BJU International, 107*(10), 1570–1575. doi:10.1111/j.1464-410X.2010.09859.x PMID:21105988

Institute of Medicine (IoM). (2012). *Living well with chronic illness: A call for public health action*. Washington, DC: The National Academies Press.

International Telecommunications Union (ITU). (n.d.). *ICT data and statistics*. Retrieved from http://www.itu.int/ITU-D/ict/statistics/

Jessup, M., Courtney-Pratt, H., Robinson, A., Cameron-Tucker, H., Walters, H., & Wood-Baker, R. et al. (2006). Cementing Pathways Home: Enhancing quality of life for people with chronic obstructive pulmonary disease (COPD). *Ageing International, 31*, 232–240. doi:10.1007/BF02915231

Jones, J., Hook, S., Park, S., & Scott, L. (2011). Privacy, security and interoperability of mobile health applications. In *Proceedings of the 6th international conference on universal access in human-computer interaction*. Orlando, FL: Springer-Verlag.

Jordan, J. E., Briggs, A., Brand, C., & Osborne, R. H. (2008). Enhancing patient engagement in chronic disease self management support initiatives in Australia: The need for an integrated approach. *The Medical Journal of Australia, 189*(10). PMID:19143585

Jordan, J. E., Buchbinderb, R., & Osbourne, R. H. (2010). Conceptualising health literacy from the patient perspective. *Patient Education and Counseling, 79*(1), 36–42. doi:10.1016/j.pec.2009.10.001 PMID:19896320

Kaplan, A. M., & Haenlein, M. (2010). Users of the world, unite! The challenges and opportunities of social media. *Business Horizons, 53*(1), 59–68. doi:10.1016/j.bushor.2009.09.003

Kelly, N. (2013, June 6). 7 Trends in Global Internet Growth You Can't Afford to Ignore. *Huffington Post*. Retrieved from http://www.huffingtonpost.com/nataly-kelly/seven-trends-in-global-in_b_3382907.html

Kietzmann, J. H., Hermkens, K., McCarthy, I. P., & Silvestre, B. S. (2011). Social media? Get serious! Understanding the functional building blocks of social media. *Business Horizons, 54*(3), 241–251. doi:10.1016/j.bushor.2011.01.005

Kontos, E. Z., Emmons, K. M., Puleo, E., & Viswanath, K. (2010). Communication inequalities and public health implications of adult social networking site use in the United States. *Journal of Health Communication, 15*(Suppl 3), 216–235. doi:10.1080/10810730.2010.522689 PMID:21154095

Korda, H., & Itani, Z. (2013). Harnessing Social Media for Health Promotion and Behavior Change. *Health Promotion Practice, 14*(1), 15–23. doi:10.1177/1524839911405850 PMID:21558472

Kuijpers, W., Groen, W. G., Aaronson, N. K., & Van Harten, W. (2013). A Systematic Review of Web-Based Interventions for Patient Empowerment and Physical Activity in Chronic Diseases: Relevance for Cancer Survivors. *Journal of Medical Internet Research, 15*(2), e37. doi:10.2196/jmir.2281 PMID:23425685

Lorig, K., Ritter, P., Laurent, D., & Plant, K. (2006). Internet-Based Chronic Disease Self-Management: A Randomized Trial. *Medical Care, 44*, 964–971. doi:10.1097/01.mlr.0000233678.80203.c1 PMID:17063127

Moen, A., Smørdal, O., & Sem, I. (2009). Web-based resources for peer support-opportunities and challenges. *Studies in Health Technology and Informatics, 150*, 302–306. PMID:19745318

Moorhead, S. A., Hzlett, D. E., Harrison, L., Carroll, J. K., Irwin, A., & Hoving, C. (2013). New Dimension of Health Care: Systematic Review of the Uses, Benefits, and Limitations of Social Media for Health Communication. *Journal of Medical Internet Research, 15*(4), e85. doi:10.2196/jmir.1933 PMID:23615206

Neiger, B. L., Thackeray, R., Van Wagenen, S. A., Hanson, C. L., West, J. H., Barnes, M. D., & Fagen, M. C. (2012). Use of Social Media in Health Promotion Purposes, Key Performance Indicators, and Evaluation Metrics. *Health Promotion Practice, 13*(2), 159–164. doi:10.1177/1524839911433467 PMID:22382491

Niehaves, B., & Plattfaut, R. (2010). *T-Government for the Citizens: Digital Divide and Internet Technology Acceptance among the Elderly*. Paper presented at the T-Gov Workshop. London, UK.

Olphert, C. W., Damodaran, L., & May, A. J. (2005). *Towards digital inclusion – Engaging older people in the 'digital world'*. Paper presented at the Accessible Design in the Digital World Conference. Dundee, UK.

Østbye, T., Yarnall, K. S. H., Krause, K. M., Pollak, K., Gradison, M., & Lloyd Michener, J. (2005). Is There Time for Management of Patients With Chronic Diseases in Primary Care? *Annals of Family Medicine*, *3*(3), 209–214. doi:10.1370/afm.310 PMID:15928223

Pearce-Brown, C., Glasgow, N., Jeon, H., Jenkins, S., & Douglas, K. (2009). *Health literacy and self management in COPD: The same, different or misunderstood?* Paper presented at the PHC Research Conference. New York, NY.

Portnoy, D. B., Scott-Sheldon, L. A., Johnson, B. T., & Carey, M. P. (2008). Computer-delivered interventions for health promotion and behavioural risk reduction: A meta-analysis of 75 randomized controlled trials, 1988 – 2007. *Preventive Medicine*, *47*, 3–16. doi:10.1016/j.ypmed.2008.02.014 PMID:18403003

Qualman, E. (2013). *Socialnomics: How Social Media Transforms the way we live and do business* (2nd ed.). John Wiley & Sons.

Roehrer, E., Cummings, E., Beggs, S., Turner, P., Hauser, J., & Micallef, N. et al. (2013). Pilot evaluation of web enabled symptom monitoring in cystic fibrosis. *Informatics for Health & Social Care*. doi:10.3109/17538157.2013.812646 PMID:23957685

Roehrer, E., Cummings, E., Ellis, L., & Turner, P. (2011). The role of user-centred design within online community development. *Studies in Health Technology and Informatics*, *164*, 256–260. PMID:21335720

Roehrer, E., Cummings, E., Turner, P., Hauser, J., Cameron-Tucker, H., & Beggs, S. et al. (2013). Supporting cystic fibrosis with ICT. *Studies in Health Technology and Informatics*, *183*, 137–141. PMID:23388270

Schwarzer, R. (1999). Self-regulatory Processes in the Adoption and Maintenance of Health Behaviours. *J Health Psychol March*, *4*(2), 115-127.

Showell, C., & Turner, P. (2013). The PLU problem: are we designing personal ehealth for People Like Us? In *Proceedings of Information Technology and Communications in Health (ITCH) Conference*. IOS Press.

Simborg, D. (2010). Consumer empowerment versus consumer populism in healthcare IT. *Journal of the American Medical Informatics Association*, *17*, 370–372. doi:10.1136/jamia.2010.003392 PMID:20595301

Syed-Abdul, S., Fernandez-Luque, L., Jian, W.-S., Li, Y.-C., Crain, S., & Hsu, M. et al. (2013). Misleading Health-Related Information Promoted Through Video-Based Social Media: Anorexia on YouTube. *Journal of Medical Internet Research*, *15*(2), e30. doi:10.2196/jmir.2237 PMID:23406655

Thackeray, R., Neiger, B. L., Hanson, C. L., & McKenzie, J. F. (2008). Enhancing promotional strategies within social marketing programs: Use of web 2.0 social media. *Health Promotion Practice*, *9*(4), 338–343. doi:10.1177/1524839908325335 PMID:18936268

Torning, K., & Oinas-Kukkonen, H. (2009). Persuasive system design: State of the art and future directions. In *Proceedings of the 4th International Conference on Persuasive Technology*. New York: ACM.

Wagner, E. H., Austin, B. T., Davis, C., Hindmarsh, M., Schaefer, J., & Bonomi, A. (2001). Improving chronic illness care: translating evidence into action. *Health Affairs*, 20(6), 64–78. doi:10.1377/hlthaff.20.6.64 PMID:11816692

Wagner, E. H., Austin, B. T., & Von Korff, M. (1996). Improving outcomes in chronic illness. *Managed Care Quarterly*, 4(2), 12–25. PMID:10157259

Webb, T. L., Joseph, J., Yardley, L., & Michie, S. (2010). Using the Internet to promote Health Behaviour Change: A systematic review and meta analysis of the impact of theoretical basis, use of behaviour change techniques, and mode of delivery on efficacy. *Journal of Medical Internet Research*, 12(1). doi:10.2196/jmir.1376 PMID:20164043

Yardley, L., Morrison, L. G., Andreou, P., Joseph, J., & Little, P. (2010). Understanding reactions to an Internet delivered healthcare intervention: Accommodating user preferences for information provision. *BMC Medical Informatics and Decision Making*, (1): 52. doi:10.1186/1472-6947-10-52 PMID:20849599

KEY TERMS AND DEFINITIONS

Info-Centrism: This refers to prevalence of thinking that prioritises the role of information over other factors. This type of thinking presumes that the provision of information axiomatically is the answer to any problem addressed.

Chapter 7
Synopsis for Health Apps:
Transparency for Trust and Decision Making

Urs-Vito Albrecht
Hannover Medical School, Germany

Oliver Pramann
Hannover Medical School, Germany

Ute von Jan
Hannover Medical School, Germany

ABSTRACT

Unfortunately, many users are unaware of the risks and limits that arise from the use of health-related and medical apps in a medical context. Often, problems arise from insufficient, misleading, or false information, but they also arise from errors within the app or inappropriate hardware that is used for running the app. Provided information is often inadequate to enable users to assess whether a medical or health app is reliable and safe. Laws and regulations that are meant to provide consumer safety (for patients and medical professionals alike) only apply to a limited number of apps with a specific medical purpose. For non-regulated apps used in a health context, there are various projects and initiatives, for example relating to app certification, but not all of these provide the information they collect about an app in a comprehensible and verifiable manner. The app synopsis presented in this chapter aims at alleviating the situation. The authors propose that manufacturers and developers use its clear structure for providing users with information about an app, ideally in a place where they commonly look (e.g. the app stores).

INTRODUCTION

"I will do no harm" is a promise to be found as an integral part of the Hippocratic Oath (National Library of Medicine, 2014. Ever since this timeless phrase was coined, for sake of the patient's safety, physicians have been called upon to follow it. The line drawn by this simple ethical principle forces the physician to estimate the costs and benefits of every action taken on the patient. In this context, every new method to be used on patients, including new procedures used for prevention, diagnostics,

DOI: 10.4018/978-1-4666-6150-9.ch007

or therapy must be carefully evaluated – in the last instance by the performing physician who is guided by regulations and guidelines as well as experience and his conscience. The use of smart devices and apps for medical purposes does not allow for exceptions from this rule: although these technologies are rapidly being adopted in the medical field, their effects on health care processes and thus also on the outcome of the patients' treatment are still not fully understood: mobile devices as well as the software they run on are relatively new players in the field and in their enthusiasm for such exciting technologies, developers as well as users – medical professionals and laypersons alike – often do not acknowledge that while such devices certainly offer new opportunities, there are also many pitfalls that may not always be obvious at first glance.

In the past, the process of distributing software to a large audience often required considerable efforts on the part of the developers and distributors. In contrast, the advent of the app stores offered for many mobile platforms considerably simplified the process of rapidly developing and easily distributing a software product – even for individual developers or small companies – to a large audience that includes billions of potential users. The barriers for publishing a product are very low and the quality standards that an app must conform to in order to gain admission into an app store are often reduced to checking whether the app is not in violation of the distributor's policies, e.g. due to undesirable content or by using the functionality of the target device in some way that is not sanctioned by the distributor. If at all, aspects such as safety and privacy are often only causally evaluated before an app is admitted into an app store. Another problem that must be considered in this context is that mobile devices are often brought from the private sector – where users may accept lower standards (or simply do not think of the consequences) – into professional application settings, where more strict standards need to be applied, especially when it is health

that could be affected. Already, there are about 97,000 "health apps" and "medical apps" on the market and this number grows by about a thousand apps every month (Research2Guidance, 2013).

Definition

What makes an app a "health app" or a "medical app"? There is often no clear distinction between these two terms and they are also used with variation in different countries. To better define the term "health app", we would like to suggest using the definition provided by the World Health Organization (WHO) in 1946 that defined health as "a state of complete physical, mental, and social well-being and not merely the absence of disease or infirmity" (WHO, 1948). Therefore, applications (apps) that are in accordance with this definition of health – including apps that deal with wellness and fitness – can be summarized as "health apps". Apps dealing with the prevention of or aid with diagnostics and treatment of diseases as well as injuries could also be added to this category, but since they touch on areas typically covered by medical professionals (Merriam-Webster, 2014), assigning the label "medical app" seems more appropriate to underline the diagnostic and therapeutic aspects of such apps (Figure 1).

The Potential of Health Apps

Medical apps have the potential of supporting both the patient and his physician: They may be valuable for diagnostic as well as therapeutic purposes and for performing general health care related tasks, since they support users in obtaining (individualized) information, aid them in recording, storing and evaluating any health related data. Often, they also simplify access to an individual's datasets for other partners participating in the health care process. These features also open up new possibilities for better integrating patients in their own care, e.g. by using feedback mechanisms to actively inform them about changes in their health

Figure 1. Definition of "health app" and "medical app"

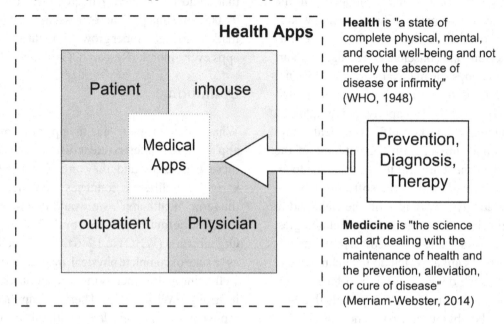

status and/or by providing them with general or individualized information. If used appropriately, an increase in efficiency may become possible and may potentially result in lowering the cost of health care.

In contrast to medical apps that usually target healthcare professionals as well as patients that have already been diagnosed with a specific – often chronic – problem, health apps generally address healthy individuals who are simply interested in obtaining general information about their body and health status and want to keep fit and stay healthy. Often, persons with an acute health issue also try to use apps (or related information sources such as health related web pages) that fall into this category for "diagnostics" or to search for information. This problem will be described in more detail in the following section.

Risks and Limits

Especially when used in a medical context, smart devices and the apps that run on them have the potential to significantly harm patients. For casual users, this may not be immediately obvious

(Table 1). For example, lay persons often do not have sufficient background to judge whether the presented information is correct or misleading. In the worst case, using such an app may lead to patients not seeking help when necessary or to seeking help with considerable delay. This was shown in a study (Wolf et al., 2013) on apps that tried to classify suspicious skin lesions by evaluating images acquired via the devices' camera: almost none of the apps had an acceptable recognition rate. If such an app falsely gives an "all clear", treatment for a malignant lesion, e.g. a melanoma, might be delayed and a still treatable problem might turn into one with considerably lower chances of being cured. The app giving the most reliable results (although there were still some limitations) did not perform the evaluation on the device itself but rather transferred the images to be evaluated by a (remote) expert. This is a prime example of why – in spite of all recent developments for health apps as well as medical apps – certain tasks should always remain in the hands of qualified professionals.

Nevertheless, false classifications that may cause real harm to users (and possibly those

Table 1. App limitations

1. Apps *do not do* what they should:	2. Apps *do more* than they should:
The promised functionality is not available or only limited functionality is provided.	The app contains functions that are *not necessary* for fulfilling its purpose.
• Technical deficiencies. • Too little or erroneous content. • Problems with the implementation. • Usage restrictions.	• Data collection. • Data storage. • Data transfer. • Data processing.
General adverse effects on the user and/or his environment: Disappointment or even endangerment	General adverse effects on the user and/or his environment: Advertising and personal tracking

they interact with) are only one of the pitfalls one may encounter when using mobile technologies and apps in medicine and for general health related applications. Other problems may range from users becoming disappointed with an app because it does not live up to its promises, i.e. does not provide all expected functionality, to disinformation (intentional or due to information sources being unreliable), or problems with the integrated algorithms or the way they are implemented within the app. For example, an app that aims at calculating the dose of a drug based on some parameters that the user enters may use an algorithm that is inappropriate for this specific calculation, e.g. by not considering all necessary parameters or a faulty implementation of the correct algorithm, which could result in the dose being either too low or too high. Additional problems might arise if an app makes use of some feature, e.g. a sensor or another component directly integrated into the mobile device or an external sensor connected to the device: aside from being broken and simply giving erroneous results, different models of mobile devices may make use of sensors that only appear similar at first glance but may give dissimilar results. All this may lead to misinterpretations.

Moreover, many apps communicate more than they should; often, apps "only" make use of the acquired data to provide specially tailored advertisements to their users. However, if apps start to track users and combine this information

with the medical and health related data entered into the application, which is of a highly sensitive nature, this is very disturbing.

Current Status

In 2008, Apple started its iTunes app store with a "starting capital" of 500 apps and the slogan "There's an app for that". Meanwhile, more than 850,000 apps can be found within the store and every second, customers are downloading around 800 apps, amounting to a volume of about 2 billion apps per month. Recently, the historical mark of 50 billion downloads was exceeded (James, 2013). Currently, there are 23 app categories to allow customers to more easily find what they are looking for. Games are the largest category and have a share of approximately 16% of all available apps; their sales volume amounts to 50% of all app sales. The categories "medicine" and "fitness" are comparatively small with a volume of approx. 2%. In 2013, Research2Guidance (Research2Guidance, 2013) counted over 97,000 apps for these two categories and estimates are that roughly 1000 new medicine and health related apps are being published per month. Numbers for other app stores, e.g. Google's Play Store, are not much different. Altogether, these numbers make it clear that – independent of the platform – it is hard not to lose the overview over the market for apps in general and medical as well as health apps in particular. The consumer can easily become overwhelmed by the quickly expanding market and it is particularly difficult for him to differentiate whether an app satisfies his needs as well as professional demands for a safe and secure usage in a medical context.

OBJECTIVE

Due to the rapid development and distribution processes described above, it is not easy for average users to assess the safety of an app in a medical context. Official regulatory processes, e.g. via notified bodies and regulatory authorities such as the Food and Drug Administration (FDA, 2013) are only relevant for a small number of apps. Private certification processes offered by various initiatives and institutions, for example as provided by Happtique (2014) or Healthon (2014) are usually targeting larger companies or professional developers that already have reached a certain sales volume instead of smaller companies. Also, since both official regulation processes as well as those offered by private institutions are often time consuming and expensive, even for those who are willing to conform to certain standards, they are not attractive.

Certificates issued by private initiatives are usually based on tests the institutions carry out themselves. They are quick in publishing their results but often they do not disclose their testing standards. Thus, quality control of the processes such initiatives employ for certifying an app may be an additional issue, which recently became apparent when Happtique had to temporarily halt their certification program after serious flaws were found in some apps that had just received certification (Dolan, 2014). Users also need to be careful about blogs posts and user comments that can often be found on various web pages or directly in the app stores if they want to base their decision about trusting an app on information published on such media, since in most cases, there is little to no background information about these sources.

Nevertheless, to leverage the high potential of apps and accompanying smart devices for all sectors, including medical and health related applications, it is important to provide users with apps that are trustworthy and well adapted for the settings they are to be applied to in order not to gamble away the trust of users, as this would have a negative influence on the overall market and thereby also hinder (future) innovations. The big question is in which way users can be aided in their assessment while still keeping costs and effort for developers and distributors low.

One potential solution might be to establish a "standard reporting" mechanism for apps, which could be a comparatively cheap and easy way that also allows for comparability of and discussions about apps that are to be used in the eHealth sector (Albrecht, von Jan, and Pramann, 2012; Albrecht, Matthies, and Pramann, 2012). This "standard reporting" should present all necessary information about the app in a standardized and transparent way. Based on this, users may more easily check whether an app meets their requirements and whether they can trust this app. As an example and to promote the discussion about standard reporting, we developed an app synopsis that will be presented in the following sections.

METHODS

The app synopsis mentioned above makes use of the results that were obtained from an evaluation of pre-existing efforts with a similar aim, i.e. providing users with detailed and transparent information about apps that might interest them. In some cases, such projects and proposals are instigated by review institutions or official organizations such as the FDA that already have expertise in similar areas of application, e.g. medical devices. In addition to the information acquired from our evaluation, we also included various aspects already mentioned in data protection policies that some, but unfortunately not all, manufacturers provide for their apps. Additional resources, e.g. established standard reporting tools like the PRISMA-statement (Moher et al., 2009) and CONSORT-statement (CONSORT, 2010) as well as Health-On-Net (Health On the Net Foundation, 2010), were also considered by the authors of this chapter, whose professional backgrounds include medicine and public health (UVA), medical law (OP) as well as medical informatics (UvJ). During the information gathering phase, the authors tried to identify pre-existing publications, projects and initiatives that were either directly targeted at medical and health apps in general or at least at similar areas of application such as medical web pages or other sources of medical information (Ozdalga, Ozdalga, Ahuja, 2012, Health On the Net Foundation, 2010, Eysenbach et al., 2000). We also made use of some items that were collected for appreciem, an initiative started by some members (Albrecht, von Jan, Gonnermann, 2013, Albrecht, Gonnermann, 2013) of our working group. The appreciem statement specifically aims at apps that make use of or provide evidence based medicine content, although there was an exchange of information and collected items between both appreciem and the app synopsis since they were at least partially developed in parallel.

Based on the information collected during the gathering phase and their professional experience, each of the authors tried to identify the points he or she thought important. In a second step, the collected items were evaluated in a collaborative process with respect to whether they have potential to aid users in assessing an app, i.e. whether they provide information about product functionality, an app's limitations as well as details about the quality of the included content or any methods employed by an app. Since, by nature, medical and health apps often deal with highly sensitive data, points pertaining to safety and security, i.e. measures taken for protecting access, transmission and storage of any data, as well as available information about data protection and privacy policies were also closely scrutinized. As a last

point, policies dealing with potential conflicts of interest were also added to the list of points that should be considered when dealing with apps in a highly sensitive area of application, which is certainly the case for medical apps as well as health apps.

RESULTS

We identified several items for inclusion into the app synopsis and grouped them in 5 main categories: 1. basic information that should be available in form of an imprint, 2. the rationale behind the app, 3. details about its functionality, 4. information about its validity and reliability and, finally, 5. a description of methods used for data acquisition, storage and transmission:

1. **Imprint:** Items falling within this category should provide users with information about who they are dealing with, i.e. who developed the app or who distributes it and thus who should be contacted or held responsible in case of problems. Where applicable, information should also be provided about third parties that might potentially have an influence on the app, e.g. sponsors in order to let users more easily determine whether there are any potential conflicts of interest that may have an undue influence on information and functionality included in an app.

2. **Rationale:** Descriptions interested users are confronted with, e.g. on the app stores, are often kept very general. Based on these descriptions, users can often not be quite sure whether an app fits their needs. It should be clearly stated whether an app is a medical product with a diagnostic or therapeutic purpose and thus had to undergo official regulatory processes before being distributed (if so, additional information should be given about when and where these were carried out). Other items of this category include

specific information about the apps purpose and targeted user group(s) (e.g. lay persons interested in health issues vs. patients with a specific condition vs. medical professionals) and usage scenarios (e.g., "at home", "clinical use") for each of these groups should also be provided.

3. **Functionality:** Items belonging within this category serve to clarify the functions included within an app. It is important to not simply list all functions integrated in an app but also to provide basic background information, for example, what were the sources and methods used for developing a specific function, are they up-to-date etc. In addition to describing what the app can do, it should also be clearly stated what its limitations are, i.e. what an app cannot do. And finally, to enable users to assess usability before installing the app, methods used for ensuring a quality user experience should be listed along with results of usability tests if these were performed.

4. **Validity and Reliability:** In this category, items have the purpose of providing users with aggregated information about the app's validity and reliability. While some sources relating to specific functionality may already have been listed under the previous category, this is primarily the place to provide additional information, not only about these sources, but also about the experts who selected the information, i.e. about their professional background and qualifications. It should also be specified which information sources were used (and their level of quality), whether any studies were conducted to ascertain the effectiveness of the app (and how these studies were done), and these should be listed. For apps making use of evidence based medicine content, this might also be a place to include information gathered according to the previously mentioned appreciem statement (Albrecht, Gonnermann, 2013).

5. **Data Requisitioning and Management:** Information included here should cover mechanisms employed for data protection as well as data integrity and privacy, not only for data stored on the device but also – where applicable – for transmission and remote storage. This also includes a statement about specific data items are requested to let the user assess whether the collected amount is adequate for the stated purpose of the app.

A more detailed description of the main categories we used as a basis for building a clear structure for the items that were identified as being important during our analysis of pre-existing assessment projects is shown in Table 2. In summary, the app synopsis gives a description of what the app has to offer as well as its limitations.

The detailed synopsis in the form of a checklist, including explanations of the items, is presented in Table 3.

While collecting the aforementioned items, another important aspect we became aware of during the research phase is the way information collected using standard reporting mechanisms such as the proposed app synopsis should be distributed in order to have an impact on potential users to allow them to make a well-informed decision about whether they want to use an app or not. Many initiatives only provide the collected information in central places such as on specific web pages or even specialized app stores that may or may not be easy to access for casual users. A very recent example of such an approach is work published by Lewis (2013), who also collected a set of standard criteria similar to those published by the Health on the Net foundation (2010), and proposed the use of a central platform, e.g. the United Kingdom National Health Service App Store, to allow registered developers to publish information about their app's conformance to these criteria.

Although these ways for disseminating information seem promising at first glance, in casual

Table 2. Criteria for assessing health apps and medical apps (Albrecht, 2013)

Criteria	Content	Rationale
Imprint	Information about the manufacturer/distributor and associates	To get in touch, to identify conflicts of interest (influence) of the sponsor and all associated parties.
	Meta data of the app	To get basic information about the actuality of the app.
Rationale	Description of the app's intended purpose(s), targeted user(s), group the dedicated setting of the app, its categorization as a medical/ non-medical app	To understand the idea behind the app, its categorization on a professional level and its ideal deployment setting and field of application.
Functionality	Description of the functionalities and features of the app and its restrictions and limits	To understand the underlying functions to achieve the app´s purpose(s) and its limits and risks to estimate whether the app is safe for usage.
	Details about what measures have been taken to assure good usability of the app	To be informed about methods that were employed during the development cycle regarding the app's usability for specific target groups.
Validity and Reliability	Description and reliability of information sources the app is based on	To assess whether the content and its authors are reliable and whether the functionality is based in reliable and valid information sources.
	Description of quality assurance methods	To estimate the level of quality in the production process of the app.
Data requisitioning & management	Description of the amount and types of data that are being collected and processed	To be able to determine whether the app's data collection & processing are adequate to fulfill the stated purpose.
Data protection & privacy	Information about the manufacturer's adherence to data protection and privacy laws and regulations and the involved jurisdictions	To find out whether the manufacturer provides a privacy statement and data protection policy that is well adapted to the app's purpose.
Data transmission & storage	Description of all measures taken to protect data entrusted to the app	To assess whether data transmission & storage is protected adequately.

discussions with some colleagues at Hannover Medical School (both medical professionals as well as medical IT experts), we noted that aside from those who had explicitly researched information about medical apps, often only relating to their own area of expertise, many of them were unaware of specialized information portals for medical as well as health apps. Partially due to time constraints, most of them simply referred to information already available on the app store(s) for their chosen mobile platform – including ratings assigned by other users. If even professional users are not always aware of specialized information platforms for medical or health apps, the same will probably hold true for laypersons. Another factor to consider is that even in professional settings such as a hospital, users often tend to bring their own mobile devices to the workplace, and often, use these devices for their work. As long as the apps they use do not access the hospital's IT systems, which is often the case for "standalone" apps such as medical calculators or reference apps, this is often done without knowledge or oversight by the organization's IT staff or superiors, unless there is a firm policy in place regarding BYOD (Meneghetti, 2013). Without knowing about what these private devices are used for, it is not easy for IT departments to provide specific information and users are pretty much left on their own, although there may be serious repercussions for both the users themselves as well as for their employer if they make an error in judgment. Altogether, this emphasizes that information should be provided in places where users tend to look first in order

Table 3. Proposed structure and detailed description of items of the app synopsis for health apps and medical apps (Albrecht, 2013)

Item Category	Checklist Item	Sub Items
1. Imprint	1.1 Meta Data	1. Operating system. 2. Version number. 3. Web link (project pages and link to the app store). 4. **Category:** Commercial project, non-commercial project, other. 5. **Category:** public access via an app store, only available to a restricted number of users/experts (in-house), other (please specify).
	1.2 Developer/Distributor	1. Information about the manufacturer/developer. 1.1. Name, address, web page, contact person(s), email address, phone and fax number. 2. Information about the distributor. 2.1. Name, address, web page, contact person(s), email address, phone and fax number.
	1.3 Sponsoring/Advertising	1. Information about the funding used for developing the app. 1.1. **Category:** Sponsoring, advertisements, other.
2. Rationale	2.1 Category	1. **Category:** Medical product or not, if yes: which class; has the app been certified voluntarily (by whom?), uncertified app.
	2.2 User group	For each user group: 1. Specific disease / condition (or as an alternative/addition: which health care professions are targeted, etc.). 2. Gender, age (range), other descriptive items.
	2.3 Setting	1. Clinical, outpatient setting, at home, other. 2. Short description of a typical "use case".
	2.4 Purpose	1. Short description of the purpose of the app. 2. **Category:** Information, reference work, educational resources, documentation, diagnostics, therapy, prevention, research, other. 3. Basic description of what the app is to be used for including specific information for the user group(s)
3. Functionality	3.1 Functions and features	For each available function / feature: 1. Function (designation). 1.1 Example. 1.2 Source(s). 1.3 **Category:** Scientifically accepted, up-to-date content and reflects the current state of science and technology, evidence level if applicable.
	3.2 Restrictions and Limits	1. Restrictions and limits of the app. 1.1. Specific description of the app's restrictions and limits. 1.2. Description of potential or existing risks for the user group(s). 1.3. Measures that have been implemented to avoid risks for the user group(s). 2. Already known undesirable effects. 2.1. Detailed description of undesirable effects, if any.
	3.3 Usability	1. Methods that were employed during the development cycle 1.1. Results of usability testing

continued on following page

Table 3. Continued

Item Category	Checklist Item	Sub Items
4. Validity and reliability	4.1 Content	1. Information about the expert(s) responsible for the app's content. 1.1. Name of the author(s). 1.2. Description of the qualification of the expert(s). 1.3. Description of potential or actual conflict of interest. 2. Information about source(s)/reference(s) for all content and algorithms integrated into the app. 2.1. Specific information about the source(s). 2.2. Evidence level of the source(s). 3. Studies that have been performed concerning the app. 3.1. Type of the study, references/literature, other evidence. 4. Additional material about the app (test reports, etc.). 4.1. Type of additional material, reference links, ...
	4.2 Quality assurance	1. Information about quality assurance measures that were used during development.
5. Data requisitioning & management	5.1 Data handling	1 Data processing. 1.1 Information about data collection mechanisms integrated into the app. 2 Data protection & privacy. 2.1 Voluntariness of participating in any data collection. 3 Data transmission & storage. 3.1 Purpose of the data collection. 3.2 Who profits from the collected data. 3.3 What kind of and how much data are being collected, at what times (including time intervals where applicable)? In which country is the data being stored? This is especially important considering the differences between data privacy laws and regulations in different countries. 3.4 Which methods are being used for storing and evaluating the data? 3.5 Specifics about user's rights to obtain information about any data that are stored about him; in addition, there must be means to revoke an already given permission to store data. For this purpose, a contact address must be specified. 3.6 It must also be possible to delete data that have already been stored and the user must be informed about the time span that is needed until the data are really deleted. 3.7 Encryption methods and level used for protecting the user's data during transmission, storage and evaluation. It should also be specified whether it is possible to connect a specific user to the stored data or whether the data are being stored anonymously or pseudonymized. 3.8 An indication about whether it is possible to prevent data collection and/or transmission and if yes, how this is possible.

to better enable them to make an informed decision, which is why we propose publishing the information accumulated using our app synopsis directly in the descriptions in the respective app stores: ideally in full, or – if that is not possible due to constraints of the respective app store (e.g., Google's Play Market has a limit of 4000 characters (Google, 2014), in an abbreviated version with an online link to the full version.

DISCUSSION

In its current form, the app synopsis is not meant as a replacement for existing (private) certification or regulatory processes. Instead, its aim is to provide users as well as developers and distributors with an easy to use method in cases where certification and regulation do either not apply or still leave some questions unanswered. The proposed synopsis includes many aspects that were previously already used by other projects and initiatives, but it has a broader aim. Some of the pre-existing projects that were evaluated target an entirely different area of application. The HONCode (Health On the Net Foundation, 2010), which is a code of conduct for web pages specifically targeted at medical and health websites, is a prime example of this. Although its eight principles certainly also apply to medical and health apps, there are some differences between how users do or should interact with web pages or apps on their smartphone. Users often do not perceive an app as an extension that would warrant caution but rather as an integral part of their device. Thus, they may entrust information to an app that they would commonly not enter on a web page. There are also some technological differences that have to be kept in mind. On principle, (native) apps running on a personal mobile device have a considerably higher potential to access information that should better be kept private, including information gathered using the device's sensors or information stored by other apps that are also installed on the device.

The targeted audience is also a point where many projects and initiatives differ from our proposal in the way they provide the information about an app. Many such projects are only meant for a single, more or less exclusive group of users such as healthcare professionals while leaving interested laypersons (who may very well be experts when it comes to a specific disease they may suffer from) out of the picture. This may be done either intentionally or due to the fact that without a more or less extensive search, many users – especially those that are causally installing an app they may just have found – are simply not aware of the fact that this additional information is available and where. Also, users interested in medical as well as technical background information may sometimes have to resort to using more than one source of information.

The proposed app synopsis aims at alleviating some of the aforementioned issues. Its primary purpose is to provide comprehensive information that addresses the concerns of a very broad audience in a location where interested users usually look anyway, i.e. on the app stores, corresponding web pages or (for later reference) directly within the respective app. All these are locations that users are already familiar with and where they tend to look for the information they want. And although one might raise concerns that – since the manufacturers / developers themselves collect and provide the information made available in this way, it might be somewhat biased or important facts might be left out without official review processes, we do not think many will risk to intentionally publicize misleading or outright false information in this way since – due to its open availability – the information can easily be scrutinized by its users and also competitors in the field. Intentionally providing false information might also very well lead to legal consequences and competitive disadvantages, which professional companies will probably try to avoid at all costs.

Another potential use of the clearly structured app synopsis can be its integration into certification processes. For example, currently, a certification process for "Trusted Medical Apps" is being developed by a joint venture between the Hannover Medical School and an institute for data protection and data security. Its focus is on ensuring patient safety based on content validity and data security. The app synopsis is an integral part of this certification process and is used as a basis for the analysis of the health related content. As part of the certification of an app, developers and distributors are required to hand in the completed checklist, which in turn will serve as a basis for a further evaluation that is being performed by experts of the relevant medical specialties. Thus, based on the app synopsis, a standardized review process is triggered. The standardized documentation obtained by applying the app synopsis also helps to identify the intended use, possible application settings and the target audience as well as accompanying risks and limitations that might otherwise have been ignored by the developers/ distributors. The certification process is kept transparent since the results are made available for all interested parties, thus providing an insight into the certification process for both manufacturers and users.

Regarding evaluation of the concept, there are several possibilities that come to mind. One possibility would be to set up a central database and to ask developers and distributors who make use of the app synopsis to kindly provide a link to the location where they publish their information, i.e. app stores as well as additional information or to (ideally) also directly enter the information they compiled for the synopsis into this database. In addition to entering their information, developers or distributors will also be asked to fill out a short questionnaire about the usability of the synopsis, i.e. whether any items were missing in their opinion or whether there were any items that they think need refinement or perceived as superfluous. To give others an example, the synopsis has already been filled out and published for recent mobile apps developed by our group (e.g. for deBac-app, an app meant for providing users in the medical field with a standardized guide for disinfection their devices, see Albrecht, von Jan, Sedlacek Groos, Suerbaum, Vonberg, 2013 for a corresponding study). Once the aforementioned database has been set up, we plan on entering the information for our apps. As soon as a sufficient number of participating developers and companies have provided their information, experts from the fields of medicine as well as computer science and medical law – not necessarily members of our group – will then be asked to assist in evaluating the provided information. Part of this evaluation will be to compare the provided information directly to each respective app to determine whether the synopsis fits its purpose or to identify problems. In addition to the information gathered from companies and developers, plans also include asking users – depending on the focus of the evaluated apps, stratified for specific user groups – about their opinions. This survey should be performed in an anonymous manner and could for example be started via a link that is published along with the synopses provided by participating developers and distributors.

Using these approaches, we hope to get sufficient feedback for an evaluation that can compare in quality to evaluations of other initiatives such as CONSORT (Altman, Moher & Schulz, 2012 and Plint et al., 2006) or PRISMA.

CONCLUSION

The app synopsis we propose is so far unique and may offer benefits for all parties concerned; while only requiring little additional effort on the developer's and distributor's side, it would nevertheless provide users with detailed information to aid them in their assessment of whether they deem an app trustable or not (Albrecht, von Jan, and Pramann, 2013).

Providing adequate information to users of an app, especially if these users are patients, goes hand in hand with the way patients are (or at least should be) treated in today's medical settings. Only a well informed patient can judge whether a proposed therapy meets his needs and give his consent. The same holds true when dealing with apps that are to be used in a medical context. Just as for conventional therapies, the benefits, limits and risks should be known beforehand.

The proposed standardized app synopsis provides a solution for users as well as manufacturers and distributors: users benefit from receiving a complete and easily understandable set of information that they can use to make their informed decision, while manufacturers can follow the simple structure of the synopsis to easily compile the necessary information.

To ensure a high impact, once the app synopsis has been completed, the results should be published prominently, e.g. in the description of the app provided in the respective app store (or other distribution channels if applicable). It should also be included on web pages that provide information about the app or in marketing materials that are being distributed. Thus, by providing extensive and transparent information, consumer confidence in medical and health apps could be significantly increased and many current problems could be alleviated. Since the app synopsis is not an officially sanctioned method, there is no guarantee for the viability of the published results. However, once it has been published, it can nevertheless serve as a reference in case of any disputes between users and the developers or distributors. Practicability, acceptance and value of the proposed concept are currently being evaluated for developers and distributors as well as potential users alike.

REFERENCES

Albrecht, U. V. (2013). Transparency of health-apps for trust and decision making. *Journal of Medical Internet Research*, *15*(12), e277. doi:10.2196/jmir.2981 PMID:24449711

Albrecht, U. V., & Gonnermann, A. (2013). *Appreciem – Appropriate reporting of EbM content in electronic media*. Retrieved January 21, 2014 from http://www.appreciem-statement.org

Albrecht, U. V., Matthies, H., & Pramann, O. (2012). Vertrauenswürdige Medical Apps. In H. Reiterer, & O. Deussen (Eds.), *Mensch & Computer 2012 – Workshopband: Interaktiv informiert – allgegenwärtig und allumfassend!?* (pp. 261–266). München: Oldenbourg Verlag.

Albrecht, U. V., von Jan, U., & Gonnermann, A. (2013). *Appropriate reporting of EbM content in electronic media – APPRECIEM*. Paper presented at Medicine 2.0 ´13. London, UK.

Albrecht, U. V., von Jan, U., & Pramann, O. (2013). Standard reporting for medical apps. *Studies in Health Technology and Informatics*, *190*, 201–203. PMID:23823422

Albrecht, U. V., von Jan, U., Pramann, O., & Matthies, H. (2012). *I, app: Trustworthy medical apps*. Paper presented at T11 – Village of the Future – Pillar 5: Social and Policy Incentive Framework. Pisa, Italy.

Albrecht, U.-V., von Jan, U., Sedlacek, L., Groos, S., Suerbaum, S., & Vonberg, R.-P. (2013). Standardized, app-based disinfection of ipads in a clinical and nonclinical setting: Comparative analysis. *Journal of Medical Internet Research*, *15*(8), e176. doi:10.2196/jmir.2643 PMID:23945468

Altman, D., Moher, D., & Schulz, K. F. (2012). Improving the reporting of randomised trials: The CONSORT Statement and beyond. *Statistics in Medicine*, *31*(25), 2985–2997. doi:10.1002/sim.5402 PMID:22903776

CONSORT. (2010). *CONSORT Statement*. Retrieved January 21, 2014 from http://www.consort-statement.org/consort-statement/overview0/

Dolan, P. L. (2014). *Health app. certificiation program halted*. Retrieved January 21, 2014 from http://exclusive.multibriefs.com/content/health-app-certification-program-halted

Eysenbach, G., Yihune, G., Lampe, K., Cross, P., & Brickley, D. (2000). Quality management, certification and rating of health information on the net with medcertain: Using a medpics/rdf/xml metadata structure for implementing ehealth ethics and creating trust globally. *J Med Internet Res*, *2*(2 Suppl), 2E1.

FDA. (2013). *Mobile Medical Applications - Food & Drug Administration (FDA): Draft Guidance for Industry and Food and Drug Administration Staff – Mobile Medical Applications*. Retrieved January 21, 2014 from http://www.fda.gov/medicaldevices/productsandmedicalprocedures/connectedhealth/mobilemedicalapplications/default.htm

Google. (2014). *Android developer – Help: Upload applications*. Retrieved January 21, 2014 from https://support.google.com/googleplay/android-developer/answer/113469?hl=en

Happtique. (2014). *App. certification: Draft standards*. Retrieved January 21, 2014 from http://www.happtique.com/app-certification/

Health on the Net Foundation. (2010). *Operational definition of the HONcode principles*. Retrieved January 21, 2014 from http://www.hon.ch/HONcode/Webmasters/Guidelines/guidelines.html

HealthOn. (2014). *App-Testberichte – HealthOn-Apps*. Retrieved January 21, 2014 from http://tests.healthon.de/app-testberichte.html

James, J. (2013). *Apple's app. store marks historic 50 billionth download*. Retrieved January 21, 2014 from http://www.apple.com/au/pr/library/2013/05/16Apples-App-Store-Marks-Historic-50-Bill

Lewis, T. L. (2013). A systematic self-certification model for mobile medical apps. *Journal of Medical Internet Research*, *15*(4), e89. doi:10.2196/jmir.2446 PMID:23615332

Meneghetti, A. (2013). Challenges and benefits in a mobile medical world: Institutions should create a set of byod guidelines that foster mobile device usage. *Health Management Technology*, *34*(2), 6–7. PMID:23469466

Merriam-Webster. (2014). *Definition of medicine*. Retrieved January 21, 2014 from http://www.merriam-webster.com/dictionary/medicine

Moher, D., Liberati, A., Tetzlaff, J., & Altman, D. G.The PRISMA Group. (2009). Preferred reporting items for systematic reviews and meta-analyses: The PRISMA statement. *PLoS Medicine*, *6*(7), e1000097. doi:10.1371/journal.pmed.1000097 PMID:19621072

National Library of Medicine. (2014). *Greek medicine – The Hippocratic Oath*. Retrieved January 21, 2014 from http://www.nlm.nih.gov/hmd/greek/greek_oath.html

Ozdalga, E., Ozdalga, A., & Ahuja, N. (2012). The smartphone in medicine: A review of current and potential use among physicians and students. *Journal of Medical Internet Research*, *14*(5), e128. doi:10.2196/jmir.1994 PMID:23017375

Plint, A. C., Moher, D., Morrison, A., Schulz, K., Altman, D. G., Hill, C., & Gaboury, I. (2006). Does the CONSORT checklist improve the quality of reports of randomized controlled trials? A systematic review. *The Medical Journal of Australia*, *185*(5), 263–267. PMID:16948622

Research2Guidance. (2013). *Mobile Health market Report 2013-2017*. Retrieved January 21, 2014 from http://www.research2guidance.com/shop/index.php/mhealth-report-2

WHO. (1948). *Preamble to the constitution of the World Health Organization as adopted by the International Health Conference, New York, 19-22 June, 1946, signed on 22 July 1946 by the representatives of 61 states (official records of the World Health Organization, no. 2, p. 100) and entered into force on 7 April 1948*. WHO.

Wolf, J. A., Moreau, J. F., Akilov, O., Patton, T., English, J. C. III, Ho, J., & Ferris, L. K. (2013). Diagnostic inaccuracy of smartphone applications for melanoma detection. *JAMA Dermatology, 149*(4), 422–426. doi:10.1001/jamadermatol.2013.2382 PMID:23325302

KEY TERMS AND DEFINITIONS

App: A software application that is running on smartphones, tablet-pcs and other smart devices.

Health Care: Maintaining and restoration of health by preventing, diagnosing and treating disease.

Health: The state of complete physical, mental and social well-being and not merely the absence of disease or infirmity (WHO).

Medicine: The science of preventing, diagnosing, and treating disease and injury.

mHealth: The practice of medicine and public health supported by mobile devices.

Smartphone: A portable phone that inherits many computer functions.

Standards: A set of rules established by an authority for the measurement of quality.

Trustworthy Applications: Software that is functionally and technically reliable with valid content provided from reliable sources.

Chapter 8
Creating a Supportive Environment for Self-Management in Healthcare via Patient Electronic Tools

Sharazade Balouchi
Sewanee: The University of the South, USA

Ahmad Zbib
Heart and Stroke Foundation, Canada

Karim Keshavjee
InfoClin Inc, Canada & University of Victoria, Canada

Karim Vassanji
InfoClin Inc, Canada

Jastinder Toor
InfoClin Inc, Canada

ABSTRACT

Consumer electronic healthcare applications and tools, both Web-based and mobile apps, are increasingly available and used by citizens around the world. "eTools" denote the full range of electronic applications that consumers may use to assess, track, or treat their disease(s), including communicating with their healthcare provider. Consumer eTool use is prone to plateauing of use because it is one-sided (i.e., consumers use them without the assistance or advice of a healthcare provider). Patient eTools that allow patients to communicate with their healthcare providers, exchange data, and receive support and guidance between visits is a promising approach that could lead to more effective, sustained, and sustainable use of eTools. The key elements of a supportive environment for eTool use include 2-way data integration from patient home monitoring equipment to providers and from provider electronic medical records systems to patient eTools, mechanisms to support provider-patient communication between visits, the ability for providers to easily monitor incoming data from multiple patients, and for provider systems to leverage the team environment and delegate tasks to appropriate providers for education and follow-up. This is explored in this chapter.

DOI: 10.4018/978-1-4666-6150-9.ch008

INTRODUCTION

Patient-provider relationships rarely move beyond the confines of a doctor's office or hospital room. The typical patient-provider interaction is a time-honored tradition from the time of Hippocrates: a patient visits with his or her healthcare provider when experiencing symptoms or problems with his or her health. Based on this consultation and follow-up tests, the provider assesses the patient's condition and advises on the best method of treatment, which often includes prescribed medication, but also includes a variety of other modalities, such as physiotherapy, psychotherapy or non-pharmacological treatments. The patient proceeds by this method of treatment, or withdraws from it if he or she finds it ineffective or not feasible, until the next visit several months later. In between visits there is often no communication between the patient and the provider to discuss how the treatment is working. Although this approach does provide a great level of patient autonomy, it only works for low acuity diseases or when treatment regimes are relatively simple.

With the rapid growth in diagnostic and treatment modalities and preventive care approaches across a wide number of chronic diseases, it is increasingly difficult for patients to maintain their autonomy without additional supports. New technologies are trying to fill that gap, but may not provide the appropriate context and judgment patients need to maintain appropriate adherence to treatment recommendations over the long periods of time (sometimes decades) necessitated by today's preventive care protocols. For example, a patient with high cholesterol or high blood pressure may need to regularly monitor and treat his or her disease for 30, 40 or even 50 years to gain the benefits of stroke and heart attack prevention.

If medicine is to achieve economies of scale and capabilities, it is important that patients assume an active role in the management of their health because patients are more in tune with their own symptoms and healthcare providers are increas-ingly overworked. An approach that encourages patient involvement is self-management, which involves active collaboration between the patient and provider. Self-management is essential to long-term patient health, for it engages both the patient and provider to agree on the issues, establish goals, decide on priorities and agree on treatment plans (Schaefer et al 2009).

Electronic tools (eTools) are designed to assist patients with managing their diseases by identifying risk factors, monitoring symptoms, and facilitating communication with the patients' healthcare providers between visits (http://apps.nhs.uk/). eTools take many forms from personal health records to patient portals to mobile applications and social media. In particular, social media outlets and dedicated disease social networks have strong potential to enable the process of self-management since the effects and health outcomes from using social media appear positive (Merolli 2013).

A recent Pew Internet survey (2012) showed that over 70% of patients measure and track a health indicator for themselves or for a loved one. However, only 21% of patients use some form of technology to track their health; i.e., the remaining 49% track the metrics 'in their head'. This same rate appears in reports from the several years preceding 2012 as well, indicating a "pla-teaued" use of eTools in general. Plateaued use of specific health applications, as with many other apps, is quite common but poorly documented (Rudansky 2013). Nonetheless, it is an important metric for understanding the needs of users and providing tools that will work for them over an extended period of time. It also highlights the need for healthcare providers to reinforce the use of eTools, if they are to be effective in driving improved patient outcomes.

The marketplace distinguishes between two specific kinds of tools: *consumer* eTools – those applications that a person seeks out on his or her own to self-monitor health conditions – and *patient* eTools, which are designed for patients to use under the guidance of and through interaction with a healthcare provider. Consumer eTools do promote health awareness among patients but lack the patient-physician interaction necessary for long-term disease management. For example, consumer eTools are unlikely to integrate with the patient's electronic record maintained by their physician, thereby providing recommendations that may be at odds with what the patient's physician might recommend. Plateaued usage may be more likely in this setting because there is no reinforcing mechanism to encourage prolonged use. For this reason, this chapter focuses on how to create an environment where *patient* eTools can thrive. We analyze key barriers and enablers to incorporating them as part of a self-management program and make recommendations to healthcare providers on how to use patient eTools effectively. We believe that encouragement and accountability are two mechanisms that healthcare providers can use to support patients to continue using eTools for self-management and prevent plateauing of use. We also identify the clinical environment where eTools are most likely to succeed and examine the features that will make patient applications useful in the long run. Finally, we make recommendations to eTool developers on how to make their tools more effective for healthcare providers to use during their encounters with patients.

BACKGROUND AND LITERATURE REVIEW

Chronic diseases are the leading causes for 60% of deaths around the world, and the burden of chronic disease is predicted to rise over the next several decades. Self-management is critical in the case of chronic disease because lifestyle factors and medication adherence between healthcare provider visits are vital for the long-term health of patients. One definition of self-management is

"the systematic provision of supportive interventions by healthcare staff to increase patients' skills and confidence in managing their health problems, including regular assessment of progress and problems, goal setting, and problem-solving support… the key feature of these interventions is the aim of increasing patients' ability to deal with day-to-day consequences of their disease to maintain a satisfactory quality of life" (Trappenburg 2012). In fact, the recently adopted definition of health includes self-management as a key component (Huber 2011).

Because more people are seeking out health information on the web and via their mobile devices, the role of healthcare providers in supplying quality advice is more important than ever. There are many advantages to patients using the Internet and social media to learn about healthcare. Social media platforms allow users to share stories of sickness and health, which function as important sources of encouragement and empowerment. Social support from peers is a significant catalyst for behavior change. Brandt et al (2013) found that consumers interacting on a smoking cessation blog shared their personal stories, provided emotional support to each other and provided congratulatory messages, which served as encouragement to continue down a difficult path.

Users can also recommend doctors and healthcare facilities to one another. Recent studies reveal a surprisingly large amount of trust in social media content posted by other patients; 46% trust content posted by other patients, 55% trust content posted by hospitals, 56% by nurses and 60% by physicians (Ottenhoff 2012). There is also a positive correlation between provider use of social media and the quality of care delivered to a patient (Beck 2002, Manary 2013). The current clinical trends favor patient self-management as the most efficient approach in healthcare for treating chronic disease (Wagner 2002, Coleman 2009). In addition to experiencing better health outcomes, patients that are actively engaged in managing their diseases incur lower healthcare costs (Hibbard 2013).

Internet-based interventions are effective ways of engaging individuals that fall outside the range of conventional care, such as marginalized individuals that do not have access to primary care or those who may be unwilling to seek out traditional care. Online health programs can also be kept up-to-date with the latest treatment strategies and can capture demographic and usage data in large volumes to improve program content and efficacy. In this way, electronic health (eHealth) interventions can overcome challenges that traditional care cannot.

Web-based interventions are inherently personalized because users can freely browse and interact with content that is most relevant to them. Customized web-based algorithms already exist and have been successfully implemented in other industries, such as online advertising, and eHealth programs can use similar technology to personalize user content. The eTool registration page can imitate the face-to-face clinical information gathering process by having users input health-related parameters that tailor the eTool's content for a program more fitted to the user's health needs.

Moreover, the web has the added benefit of discussion and support forums where users can interact with others experiencing similar challenges; some programs are even moderated by experts, which ensures that the quality of health information is accurate in addition to supportive.

There is evidence that internet-based intervention is effective in treating mental health and addiction problems because users that fear stigmatization or struggle to prioritize self-care benefit from the anonymity of web-based interventions and the accessibility of information. Although the evidence shows that counseling and tailored self-help methods are effective methods, these avenues are underused and must be more accessible and up-to-date.

A study conducted by researchers at Evolution Health assessed the most active social network participants on two web-based smoking intervention sites and found that while most users posted infrequently, those who did post made regular contributions that strongly drive social network traffic. The study also revealed that the majority of users that posted to discussion boards were recent quitters, who ceased smoking for less than one year. The two eHealth social networks compared were the publicly run Canadian Cancer Society's Smokers' HelplineOnline and the privately run StopSmokingCenter.net. However, it is not clear what demographics frequent posters share; gender, age, and past smoking/quitting habits did not reveal significant differences. The key to effective social networks is to maintain a group of regular posters who offer direct help information, but there is very little research that explains the correlation between frequent posters and disengaged users (van Mierlo, et al. 2012).

Another study assessed how users engage with online weight loss tools. The results show that clinical characteristics can provide some indication into how a user interacts with an online health program. For example, there may be a correlation between gender and weight loss treatment strategies. Whereas for women the psychological influence of food may be a stronger factor in engaging with a weight loss tool, other factors may be more influential for men seeking weight loss tools. However, there is still very little research into how user demographics impact engagement with online intervention tools (Binks M, et al. 2012).

Simply providing health information is not enough to engage patients to change their health behaviors (Burns 2012). Some patients may feel overwhelmed and unprepared to manage their own health while others simply require more in-depth information to adequately care for themselves. A customized approach to healthcare that incorporates different health beliefs, goals, and motivations would improve clinical outcomes, lower costs, and heighten patient satisfaction.

Five key constructs appear to play an important role in enhancing and mediating patient self-management and improving patient outcomes. These constructs are real-world constructs that can be supported by eTools or can be detracted by poorly designed eTools. These constructs are: 1) Patient activation, as measured by the Patient Activation Measure (PAM); 2) patient-physician communications and patient preferences for communication styles and approaches; 3) patient behavior change models and 4) health literacy and 5) interoperability of data from provider electronic medical records (EMRs) to eTools and from remote monitoring devices to EMRs. An additional construct may be important in some cases, but is considered out of scope for this chapter discussion, namely the impact of mild to moderate cognitive impairment on use of eTools (Archer 2014). The impact of cognitive impairment on patient's understanding of their disease, disease process and self-management is very poorly understood. Although some consider cognitive impairment to be a special case of low health literacy, further research on the impact of cognitive impairment on disease and self-management are required before incorporating design recommendations into the next generation of eTools.

Hibbard et al (2013) and others (Hibbard 2008, Rask 2009, Skolasky 2011, Mosen 2007) have shown that patient activation, as measured by the Patient Activation Measure (PAM), is correlated with: healthier behaviors such as, physical activity and a diet higher in fruits and vegetables; more appropriate use of the healthcare system, including seeking regular care and not delaying care; more consumer-like behaviors such as making a list of questions for the doctor and researching doctor qualifications; more activity in self-management such as logging disease parameters and attending specialist visits; and better control of their disease, such as better control of blood pressure, HbA1c and fewer hospitalizations.

More importantly, patient activation has been found to be modifiable. Interventions that lead to changes in patient activation are not yet well-understood, but changes in patient activation from a low level to a higher level are associated with better health outcomes. As our understanding of the factors that lead to activation increases, it is likely that interventions will become more effective at changing health outcomes through personal agency. Early work with use of web-based interventions shows promise of being able to increase patient activation even in the absence of tailoring messages to the stage of the patient's level of activation (Solomon 2012). However, the authors caution against assuming that a short-term intervention is likely to have long-term, sustainable effects on patient activation.

Much has been written about patient-provider communication (Lam 2013, Farin 2012, de Jongh 2012). Farin et al (2011, 2012) have developed the KOPRA tool which measures communication preferences of patients with chronic disease. The KOPRA tool measures patient's communication preference along four dimensions: 1) effective and open communications, 2) patient participation and orientation, 3) emotionally supportive communication and 4) communication about personal circumstances. Interestingly, patients with different diseases prioritize different dimensions.

Older patients have different preferences from those of young people (older people are more comfortable with directive communications with less patient participation), and preferences appear to change over time or at different stages of a disease. When patients are particularly sick, they much prefer a directive approach rather than an open approach. Farin et al (2012) have also developed a provider communication style assessment questionnaire for patients. The so-called KOVA tool is an adaptation of the KOPRA tool but assesses whether providers' communication behaviors are in line with preferences. These two tools are good ways of assessing the congruence between provider communication behaviors and patient preferences.

Lam (2013) and de Jongh (2012) assess patient preference for specific communication media. Whether patients prefer to communicate by email, text messaging, social media or telephone can depend on age or disease. The effectiveness of communication also depends on disease and medium. eTools can be designed to assess patients' communication preferences in different situations and at different times in their lives to make sure that communications between patients and providers are the most effective ones. Ensuring appropriate communications with patients can be daunting when there are so many dimensions required which change for different diseases, severities of disease and ages of patients. These are exactly the types of situations where technologies, properly designed, can excel.

There are many behavior change models that have been studied over the last few years, including Prochaska's (1992) venerable transtheoretical model (TTM) of change, motivational interviewing (MI) and the health risk intervention (HRI) model (Prochaska 2008). The transtheoretical model has the longest history of research and has over 150 publications devoted to it. The model posits that people are at different stages of change at various times in their lives. The model describes 5 stages: 1) Individuals in the precontemplation stage engage in risky behaviors, but are not considering changing their behaviors. They typically do not have any facts about the risks of their behaviors or have tried to make changes unsuccessfully and have regressed back into the precontemplation stage; 2) Contemplators are those who are considering making a change. They are usually stuck weighing the benefits and costs of changing and are not yet convinced that they should change; 3) Preparers are individuals who have a plan to make a change (e.g., quit smoking, lose weight,

etc) because for them the benefits now outweigh the costs. Many have attempted a change in the past but have been unsuccessful. Although the Preparer has a plan, they may not have full commitment to the plan; 4) The Action stage is where the individual actually acts on their intent. They are doing what is required to make the change. If an individual has not sufficiently prepared for this stage, they are likely to revert back to their previous state; 5) Maintenance is the stage where the individual has successfully changed to a new set of behaviors for at least 6 months.

This model is well suited for development into eTools as the metrics are easily able to identify which stage a patient is in and can provide recommendations that are suited to the patient's stage. For example, while a patient who is in the Action stage may require encouragement and a reminder about the types of things that can lead to a relapse, a patient who is in the Precontemplation stage may need information about their disease and encouragement that behavior change is possible and sustainable. Chen et al (2012) report on a systematic review of eTools for smoking cessation. They concluded that eTools do have a small, but statistically significant impact on smoking cessation. Several other eTools for behavior change in a variety of health behaviors such as getting human papilloma virus vaccinations (Paiva 2014) and weight loss (Wee 2005) have been developed and tested.

A promising new area of behavior change is a method called adaptive elearning. As patients have increased access to technology and computers become more powerful, it is possible to create interactive tools that can assess a patient's knowledge and then provide them with the right information in the format that they like best and which is most effective at driving behavior change (Harris 2011). Although these authors reported poor results of this intervention that was found to be as costly as other current interventions, we speculate that costs are likely to come down and quality of the intervention is likely to go up over time. Adaptive elearning is likely here to stay.

Poor health literacy is well described as being associated with poor health and being disadvantaged when using the healthcare system. Patients with poor health literacy, which is estimated to be as high as 88% of patients over the age of 65, have a difficult time following treatment instructions, are more likely to make errors with their medications, have difficulty navigating the healthcare system, are more likely to be hospitalized and are more likely to incur higher costs (Health Literacy n.d).

eTools present a promising method to overcome poor health literacy. The ability to display pictures and graphs may help make numerical information more understandable. Showing patients pictures of their medications and displaying the time of day at which they are supposed to take them could be useful in communicating medication dosage information. Smith et al (2011) tried to automate a tool to improve the coherence of health text, building on a strong base of theoretical knowledge of how to write health related text in a manner that is easy to understand. Although they found that their approach was not scalable, it is only a matter of time before researchers crack the code on simplifying health text using automated algorithms.

Finally, eTools need to be able to get data from EMRs (Holbrook 2009) and share data with EMRs. Interoperability of data between healthcare provider systems and patient eTools is crucial for empowering patients to self-manage their diseases. Without interoperability, patients are blind in their use of eTools and their use is not sustainable.

Although the growing presence of sophisticated eTools that utilize complex notions of change in the realm of healthcare is engaging patients in the treatment of their own diseases and promoting health-consciousness, the drawbacks of a largely user-driven application are the lack of accountability, poor follow-up and lack of critical data that is usually in the hands of the provider.

The literature shows that over the long-term users disengage from using these applications. This could be attributed to several factors including the feeling of discouragement due to a lack of improvement in one's condition, the lack of feedback and validation needed to course correct or encourage one to stay on track, a lack of accountability for change other than to oneself, or a variety of other personal reasons such as busy schedules and life events taking priority.

Despite these barriers, recent surveys confirm a strong willingness by both physicians and patients to engage in the use of electronic tools, if it can provide better quality care. (Ottenhoff 2013, McGowan 2012). However, this is where the literature's role ends as there is very little written about the role of eTools in: 1) enhancing communication between healthcare providers and patients on an on-going basis; after all, it is unrealistic to expect patients with complex chronic diseases to self-manage for the 3-6 months between provider visits without some support or guidance from their care team; 2) enhancing the ability of the provider to track and monitor patient progress in between visits; currently there is no payment model for this type of service, other than a capitation funding model which may not explicitly require it and the tools to manage multiple data streams are still relatively primitive; 3) increasing patient accountability because somebody is monitoring progress on an on-going basis (Demiris 2008, Rosser 2009, van Gemert-Pijnen 2011).

GETTING PAST THE PLATEAU IN ETOOL USE

The Problem

The current patient-provider rapport does not effectively support communication between patients and providers between doctor visits – where the bulk of treatment takes place. As a patient undertakes the prescribed method of treatment, he or she can encounter complications such as experiencing side effects from a new medication, failing to see improvement in his or her condition after an adequate period of use of medication, or getting mixed messages about the safety or efficacy of the medication from family, friends and the Internet. As a result, patients may decide to stop taking a medication or stop following a course of treatment. This means that until the next doctor's visit (usually several months later) a patient is not treating his or her disease, during which time a patient's condition can worsen. The result is that doctors become frustrated and patients become discouraged because there is no structure in place to enable effective communication between the two parties in between visits.

At present, patient-provider communication tends to take the form of checklisting for medical information, which fails to incorporate the patient's personal and daily social demands, which can significantly impact the success of patient self-care. Quantitative measures are poor motivators for patient health behavior change because they don't hold significant relevance for patients in their daily lives. Often, the demand of self-care competes with many other demands in an individual's life, and it is important that providers take these social demands into account when working with patients to develop an effective treatment plan so that care is more manageable. Patients become discouraged and are less likely to take action when they do not feel that they can change their condition in a significant way. Treatment plans that incorporate patients' social demands are more manageable. It is also important to relate quantitative health indicators to how a patient is feeling in terms of pain, tiredness, etc. rather than simply as a physical result. (Farvolden et al. 2009)

Even with the support of eTools, patients tend to lose interest in health applications over time. While many people are initially willing to use health applications, they eventually become unmotivated and disengaged, which hinders disease management.

Controversies

The issue of how much support providers can give patients and the source of this support is controversial. Some tools that support self-management are purely patient-driven, while others are largely physician-controlled (e.g. tethered PHRs). Although self-management is not a new concept, it has not been widely adopted by providers. However, the trend is changing and some healthcare practices are now more willing to participate than others. In order to reduce the barrier for adoption of self-management in the care process, the important issue of how to provide enough support through an eTool must be addressed so that patients can succeed without critically disrupting the clinical workflow process and without overburdening already busy healthcare practitioners.

Barriers

Most eTools on the market today fall into the consumer eTool category. They are one-sided because the patient can download them without a prescription or recommendation from a healthcare provider and use them to manage their health autonomously without the guidance of their physician, who has access to valuable information that may not be available to the patient. It is also easier to develop eTools that don't require integration with EMRs as there are currently no universal standards for seamless integration into EMRs. The information that a patient may be missing include lab results, physiological readings and examination findings, a listing of previous diagnoses, alternative treatments and other best practice knowledge. Ultimately, this can cause inconsistencies between what patients are doing and what physicians might recommend. There are currently few systems in place to facilitate the sharing of information between the patient and the provider when a patient opts to use a consumer eTool.

Even most patient eTools today do not use best practices in helping patients and providers have postive, empowering interactions. eTools lack the customization that can be provided by staging patients in level of activation and stage of change. By assessing the level of activation and the stage of change, eTools can better identify where patients are in the self-management continuum and provide more customized and more effective interventions. eTools also lack the sophistication of understanding patient communication preferences with regard to their disease, not just their communication channel preferences. Finally, eTools lack the ability to present material at the appropriate level of health literacy for each patient that uses the eTool. Without better interoperability and sensitivity to a wider range of patients and their heterogenous needs, eTools will continue to miss the mark with encouraging self-management.

On the provider side, a key barrier is a lack of training. Many believe that self-management is more time consuming, yet there is no clear evidence that engaging patients is more time consuming than the typical care approach and in fact, encouraging self-management may in fact lead to better compliance and therefore better patient outcomes. Therefore, temporary incentives for

providers to adopt this method may be useful to overcome this misconception and barrier in the early stages of roll-out.

Providers also have few tools that allow them to manage data from multiple patients with multiple diseases; automated data collection from multiple eTools can easily overwhelm the current capacity of providers to manage incoming data. Lack of payment mechanisms to reimburse providers and lack of tools for reviewing, analyzing and responding to patient and remote device communications is yet another barrier preventing widespread adoption of these technologies.

Some critical barriers associated with adopting eTools into the primary care system include (Figure 1) concern for the privacy and security of patient personal information, lack of integration of eTools into the primary care workflow and lack of proof of their efficacy (Buijink 2012). Many information systems are not equipped to track patients throughout the care process. Furthermore, unlike the typical producer-consumer interaction that exists in a business transaction, the doctor-patient relationship involves greater risk because the stakes are so much higher. The threat of government regulation may also impede willingness to adopt and recommend eTools that

Figure 1. Barriers and enablers of eTool use

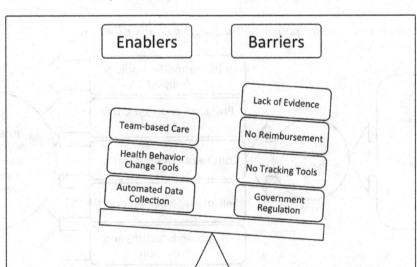

may end up, for example, being withdrawn from the market because of impending regulatory requirements (FDA 2011).

Enablers

Technological advances are facilitating the creation of more effective health tools. Automated data collection from a variety of devices is getting much easier and requires less effort from users, so patients are increasingly benefiting from applications without putting in very much work. Health behavior change tools and gamification of apps is another mechanism that keeps patients engaged with eTools longer. However, even gamified apps are soon abandoned if there are no strong external forces to help patients maintain use of their app for behavioral tracking and change over the long-term.

In addition to technological advances, other process and organizational enablers include team-based primary care, physician leadership within a culture of communication and quality improvement, support for patient self-management integrated into the primary care workflow, information technology support and an IT infrastructure that supports the use of eTools.

Although eTools are relatively new and it is still too early to be able to tell whether patients will use them for extended periods of time, patients do see their physicians for decades at a time and tend to be quite loyal to them. Basing a long-term intervention on known patterns of behavior (seeing a healthcare provider on a regular basis) is more likely to lead to success rather than relying on a relatively new technology to supplant existing relationships and ways of working.

Solutions and Recommendations

Based on interviews with key stakeholders (policy players, educational organizations and other organizations actively involved in designing, developing and deploying electronic channels of communication with healthcare providers), we identified several potential solutions.

An effective eTool will not only capture patient-collected data (e.g., home blood pressure readings, home blood sugar monitoring) but will also integrate with the provider's electronic medical record system (EMR) to collect relevant data for the management of the patient's condition (e.g., HbA1C for tracking diabetes, LDL for tracking high cholesterol, list of current medications, etc). The effective eTool will record a patient's healthcare goal, then track the patient's progress against that goal and send regular reports to providers so that they can support patients based on where they are in the treatment process. For example, an

Figure 2. Enabling environment for patient self-management and eTool use

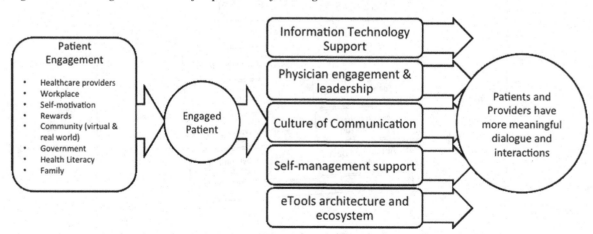

application might present a questionnaire shortly after a patient begins a new prescription. Through it, patients could voice concerns about side effects, new symptoms, and other treatment complications to their physicians in between visits. The application would send the questionnaire results to the provider, so they can gauge patient response to the treatment and provide feedback on how to proceed. eTools might also suggest questions for the patient to ask the provider.

Effective eTools also need to continue to use innovative best practices in enhancing patient self-management, including patient activation and patient behavior change. They also need to incorporate best practices in providing patients with communications in a manner that is congruent with their preferences and their expectations and in language that is easy to understand and implement.

Ultimately, patients benefit most from communicating with an advisor because technology alone cannot provide the accountability, encouragement and guidance that a human being can; therefore, healthcare management cannot be purely consumer-driven (Rock 2009, Rosser 2009). The self-management process must begin with a dialogue during which the provider recommends an eTool to the patient as a part of a self-management plan. Then, the provider requires some form of output or follow-up report from the eTool to serve as the focus for discussion at the next visit or as measure of efficacy in between visits. This focus on follow-up and on-going communication between visits creates the accountability that patients require to stay the course and continue using the app after the initial novelty has worn off. But before providers will adopt eTools, they must be effectively integrated into the primary care workflow.

The trend toward team-based care supports the integration of eTools into primary care workflows. The burden of follow-up need not fall on a single

provider because different providers on the team can each address issues that are relevant to their domain; e.g., the team pharmacist can address medication issues while the dietician can address nutrition issues. If provider EMRs allowed providers to tag patient issues according to team member competencies, then the appropriate provider could follow-up with patients to help them address their issue. Providers should be able to escalate or 'refer' a patient to another provider, if necessary.

Furthermore, provider-side applications will need to allow the provider to quickly separate the signals from the noise that is likely to come from eTools, allowing them to focus on the medical events that are most important and ignore the thousands of normal findings that might be reported about patient physiological measurements or medication compliance.

Although providers keep asking for evidence of efficacy, the reality is that until there is better understanding of which workflows are effective and which ones are not, it is unlikely that we will be able to garner the evidence that eTools are effective in the way that pharmaceutical agents are shown to be effective. The mechanism of action for an eTool is completely different from that of a pharmaceutical agent, so it is unlikely that we will have randomized controlled trial level evidence for eTool efficacy and effectiveness in the near term. Other than interacting with the eTool itself, eTools by themselves do not have a plausible mechanism for changing patient behaviors on a sustainable basis. Rather, what we will see is that assisting patients in self-management is effective because of the education, knowledge and behavior change support that is provided to them. eTools will only be a mechanism to measure progress between visits and to ensure consistency, replicability and mass customization of the self-management process across many patients.

FUTURE RESEARCH DIRECTIONS

Health behavior change is a rapidly evolving field. The inclusion of patient activation and health behavior change principles into eTools is also gaining ground (Pal 2013). The gamification of consumer and patient eTools is one facet of this evolving area, which is fuelled by the increasing ubiquity of smartphones that allow for rapid design of useful applications (Primack 2012),

eTools are a promising technology, but still in their infancy. Some key areas requiring further research include: 1) Impact of gamification and health behavior change methods on short- and long-term adherence to eTool use (Primack 2012). The role of gamification and other health behavior modification methods in the overall self-management paradigm needs to be better understood. 2) A better understanding of the elements of self-management that are effective for specific diseases and why they might be more effective for those diseases (Savage 2011, Li 2011, Effing 2007). It may be difficult to program effective interventions into eTool applications without a sound theoretical underpinning for patient self-management and a robust empirical base for proving the efficacy of interventions. 3) A better understanding of the mechanisms by which social and information forces exerted by providers, families, friends and social media can support or detract from patient wellness behaviors and patient well-being. Patients are bombarded by information from a variety of sources, many of which can be conflicting (Carpenter 2013). How they navigate those social and informational forces can have a big impact on medication compliance and follow through.

More information on tailored interventions is necessary to identify which strategies are the best for a given situation, in order to provide a framework under which dynamic approaches can be followed. Further research that could present the dynamic range of self-management programs supported by evidence of positive outcomes would support the transition towards self-management practices in primary care. For example, which kind of self-management intervention works best for which kind of patients and chronic diseases would be helpful in deciding which approach to take.

Developing multimodal eTools will be essential, and getting the most relevant information to patients will be critical in keeping the tools engaging and meaningful.

CONCLUSION

Patient self-management demands effective communication between patients and providers. Further, it requires a supportive and enabling environment for patient education and support. Social media is a powerful tool in this process because it can support or detract from provider efforts through social reinforcement or by presenting conflicting information. This points out that providers do not work in a vacuum and that providers cannot shape or control all the forces that patients need to navigate when taking care of themselves. Providers can only guide and support patients on how to navigate those forces if they themselves are aware of them and have effective mechanisms to overcome them.

Stand-alone, specialized tools may be effective for short-term use, and encourage patients to engage in monitoring their own health. But for eTools to be effective in the long run, they must be complemented by patient-provider communication within a broader environment and culture that supports patient self-management and is information technology- and information management-enabled to take advantage of new and evolving eTools and best practices.

An effective self-management program must customize its approach to treatment because a one-size-fits-all attitude does not account for individual patient experiences, desires, and concerns. Since patients cannot always meet with a doctor to discuss health issues, health applications can provide temporary support to a patient in between doctor visits. But electronic tools must move beyond the limitations of consumer applications before healthcare providers will adopt them. Furthermore, incorporating eTools does not eliminate the role of healthcare providers in the treatment process but, rather, promotes collaboration between patients and providers to achieve the best treatment strategies. This means engaging patients in the care process. Healthcare providers are key motivators for patient progress, and, as such, they should require some tangible output from eTools to keep patients engaged and accountable for self-management.

REFERENCES

Archer, N., Keshavjee, K., Demers, C., & Lee, R. (2014). Online self-management interventions for chronically ill patients: Cognitive impairment and technology issues. *International Journal of Medical Informatics, 83*(4), 264–272. doi:10.1016/j. ijmedinf.2014.01.005 PMID:24507762

Beck, R. S., Daughtridge, R., & Sloane, P. D. (2002). Physician-patient communication in the primary care office: A systematic review. *The Journal of the American Board of Family Practice, 15*(1), 25–38. PMID:11841136

Binks, M., van Mierlo, T., & Edwards, C.L. (2012). Relationships of the Psychological Influence of Food and Barriers to Lifestyle Change to Weight and Utilization of Online Weight Loss Tools. *The Open Medical Informatics Journal,* (6), 9-14.

Bodenheimer, T., Wagner, E. H., & Grumbach, K. (2002). Improving primary care for patients with chronic illness. *Journal of the American Medical Association, 288*(15), 1909–1914. doi:10.1001/jama.288.15.1909 PMID:12377092

Brandt, C. L., Dalum, P., Skov-Ettrup, L., & Tolstrup, J. S. (2013). After all–It doesn't kill you to quit smoking: An explorative analysis of the blog in a smoking cessation intervention. *Scandinavian Journal of Public Health, 41*(7), 655–661. doi:10.1177/1403494813489602 PMID:23696257

Buijink, A. W., Visser, B. J., & Marshall, L. (2013). Medical apps for smartphones: Lack of evidence undermines quality and safety. *Evidence-Based Medicine, 18*(3), 90–92. doi:10.1136/eb-2012-100885 PMID:22923708

Burns, J. (2012). The Next Frontier: Patient Engagement. *Managed Care.* Retrieved from http://www.managedcaremag.com/archives/1206/1206.engagement.html

Carpenter, D. M., Elstad, E. A., Blalock, S. J., & Devellis, R. F. (2014). Conflicting Medication Information: Prevalence, Sources, and Relationship to Medication Adherence. *Journal of Health Communication, 19*(1), 67–81. doi:10.1080/10810730.2013.798380 PMID:24015878

Chen, Y. F., Madan, J., Welton, N., Yahaya, I., Aveyard, P., & Bauld, L. et al. (2012). Effectiveness and cost-effectiveness of computer and other electronic aids for smoking cessation: A systematic review and network meta-analysis. *Health Technology Assessment, 16*(38). doi: doi:10.3310/hta16380 PMID:23046909

Coleman, K., Austin, B. T., Brach, C., & Wagner, E. H. (2009). Evidence on the Chronic Care Model in the new millennium. *Health Affairs, 28*(1), 75–85. doi:10.1377/hlthaff.28.1.75 PMID:19124857

de Jongh, T., Gurol-Urganci, I., Vodopivec-Jamsek, V., Car, J., & Atun, R. (2012). Mobile phone messaging for facilitating self-management of long-term illnesses. *Cochrane Database of Systematic Reviews, 12.* doi:10.1002/14651858. CD007459.pub2 PMID:23235644

Demiris, G., Afrin, L. B., Speedie, S., Courtney, K. L., Sondhi, M., Vimarlund, V., & Lynch, C. (2008). Patient-centered applications: Use of information technology to promote disease management and wellness. *Journal of the American Medical Informatics Association*, 15(1), 8–13. doi:10.1197/jamia.M2492 PMID:17947617

Effing, T., Monninkhof, E. M., van der Valk, P. D., van der Palen, J., van Herwaarden, C. L., & Partidge, M. R. et al. (2007). Self-management education for patients with chronic obstructive pulmonary disease. *Cochrane Database of Systematic Reviews*, 4. doi:10.1002/14651858. CD002990.pub2 PMID:17943778

Farin, E., Gramm, L., & Kosiol, D. (2011). Development of a questionnaire to assess communication preferences of patients with chronic illness. *Patient Education and Counseling*, 82(1), 81–88. doi:10.1016/j.pec.2010.02.011 PMID:20219317

Farin, E., Gramm, L., & Schmidt, E. (2012). Taking into account patients' communication preferences: Instrument development and results in chronic back pain patients. *Patient Education and Counseling*, 86(1), 41–48. doi:10.1016/j. pec.2011.04.012 PMID:21570795

Farvolden, P., Cunningham, J. A., van Mierlo, T., & Selby, P. (2009). Using E-health programs to overcome barriers to the effective treatment of mental health and addiction problems. *Journal of Technology in Human Services*, 27(1), 5–22. doi:10.1080/15228830802458889

Federal Drug Administration. (2011). *Draft Guidance for Industry and Food and Drug Administration Staff - Mobile Medical Applications*. Retrieved from http://x.co/1U9bc

Harris, J., Felix, L., Miners, A., Murray, E., Michie, S., & Ferguson, E. et al. (2011). Adaptive e-learning to improve dietary behavior: A systematic review and cost-effectiveness analysis. *Health Technology Assessment*, 15(37), 1–160. PMID:22030014

Health Literacy. (n.d.). Retrieved from http://healthliteracy.ca/en/professionals-and-service-providers.html

Hibbard, J., & Cunningham, P. J. (2008). How engaged are consumers in their health and health care, and why does it matter? *Research Briefs*, 8, 1–9. PMID:18946947

Hibbard, J. H., & Greene, J. (2013). What the evidence shows about patient activation: Better health outcomes and care experiences, fewer data on costs. *Health Affairs (Project Hope)*, 32(2), 207–214. doi:10.1377/hlthaff.2012.1061 PMID:23381511

Holbrook, A., Pullenayegum, E., Thabane, L., Troyan, S., Foster, G., & Keshavjee, K. et al. (2011). Shared electronic vascular risk decision support in primary care: Computerization of Medical Practices for the Enhancement of Therapeutic Effectiveness (COMPETE III) randomized trial. *Archives of Internal Medicine*, 171(19), 1736–1744. doi:10.1001/archinternmed.2011.471 PMID:22025430

Huber, M., Knottnerus, J. A., Green, L., Horst, H. V. D., Jadad, A. R., Kromhout, D., & Smid, H. (2011). How should we define health? *British Medical Journal*, 343(6). doi: doi:10.1136/bmj. d4163 PMID:21791490

Lam, R., Lin, V. S., Senelick, W. S., Tran, H. P., Moore, A. A., & Koretz, B. (2013). Older adult consumers' attitudes and preferences on electronic patient-physician messaging. *The American Journal of Managed Care, 19*(10), eSP7–eSP11. PMID:24511886

Li, T., Wu, H. M., Wang, F., Huang, C. Q., Yang, M., Dong, B. R., & Liu, G. J. (2011). Education programmes for people with diabetic kidney disease. *Cochrane Database of Systematic Reviews, 6*. doi:10.1002/14651858.CD007374.pub2 PMID:21678365

Manary, M. P., Boulding, W., Staelin, R., & Glickman, S. W. (2013). The patient experience and health outcomes. *The New England Journal of Medicine, 368*(3), 201–203. doi:10.1056/NEJMp1211775 PMID:23268647

McCallum, S. (2012). Gamification and serious games for personalized health. *Studies in Health Technology and Informatics*, 85–96. doi: doi:10.3233/978-1-61499-069-7-85 PMID:22942036

McGowan, B. S., Wasko, M., Vartabedian, B. S., Miller, R. S., Freiherr, D. D., & Abdolrasulnia, M. (2012). Understanding the factors that influence the adoption and meaningful use of social media by physicians to share medical information. *Journal of Medical Internet Research, 14*(5), e117. doi:10.2196/jmir.2138 PMID:23006336

Merolli, M., Gray, K., & Martin-Sanchez, F. (2013). Health Outcomes And Related Effects Of Using Social Media In Chronic Disease Management: A Literature Review And Analysis Of Affordances. *Journal of Biomedical Informatics, 46*(6), 957–969. doi:10.1016/j.jbi.2013.04.010 PMID:23702104

Mosen, D. M., Schmittdiel, J., Hibbard, J., Sobel, D., Remmers, C., & Bellows, J. (2007). Is patient activation associated with outcomes of care for adults with chronic conditions? *The Journal of Ambulatory Care Management, 30*(1), 21–29. doi:10.1097/00004479-200701000-00005 PMID:17170635

Ottenhoff, M. (2012). Infographic: Rising Use of Social and Mobile in Healthcare. *The Spark Report*. Retrieved from http://x.co/1U9fJ

Paiva, A. L., Lipschitz, J. M., Fernandez, A. C., Redding, C. A., & Prochaska, J. O. (2014). Evaluation of the acceptability and feasibility of a computer-tailored intervention to increase human papillomavirus vaccination among young adult women. *Journal of American College Health, 62*(1), 32–38. doi:10.1080/07448481.2013.843534 PMID:24313694

Pal, K., Eastwood, S. V., Michie, S., Farmer, A. J., Barnard, M. L., & Peacock, R. et al. (2013). Computer-based diabetes self-management interventions for adults with type 2 diabetes mellitus. *Cochrane Database of Systematic Reviews, 3*. doi:10.1002/14651858.CD008776.pub2 PMID:23543567

Pew Internet and American Life Project. (2012). *CHCF Health Survey Aug 7-Sep 6, 2012*. Retrieved from http://www.pewinternet.org/Reports/2013/Tracking-for-Health/Summary-of-Findings.aspx

Primack, B. A., Carroll, M. V., McNamara, M., Klem, M. L., King, B., & Rich, M. et al. (2012). Role of video games in improving health-related outcomes: A systematic review. *American Journal of Preventive Medicine, 42*(6), 630–638. doi:10.1016/j.amepre.2012.02.023 PMID:22608382

Prochaska, J. O., Butterworth, S., Redding, C. A., Burden, V., Perrin, N., & Leo, M. et al. (2008). Initial efficacy of MI, TTM tailoring and HRI's with multiple behaviors for employee health promotion. *Preventive Medicine, 46*(3), 226–231. doi:10.1016/j.ypmed.2007.11.007 PMID:18155287

Prochaska, J. O., DiClemente, C. C., & Norcross, J. C. (1992). In search of how people change: Applications to addictive behaviors. *The American Psychologist, 47*(9), 1102–1114. doi:10.1037/0003-066X.47.9.1102 PMID:1329589

Public Health Agency of Canada. (n.d.). Retrieved from http://www.phac-aspc.gc.ca/cd-mc/hl-ls/index-eng.php

Rask, K. J., Ziemer, D. C., Kohler, S. A., Hawley, J. N., Arinde, F. J., & Barnes, C. S. (2009). Patient activation is associated with healthy behaviors and ease in managing diabetes in an indigent population. *The Diabetes Educator, 35*(4), 622–630. doi:10.1177/0145721709335004 PMID:19419972

Rock, D. (2009). Managing with the Brain in Mind. *Strategy+ Business, 56*, 1-11.

Rosser, B. A., Vowles, K. E., Keogh, E., Eccleston, C., & Mountain, G. A. (2009). Technologically assisted behavior change: A systematic review of studies of novel technologies for the management of chronic illness. *Journal of Telemedicine and Telecare, 15*(7), 327–338. doi:10.1258/jtt.2009.090116 PMID:19815901

Rudansky, A. K. (2013, June 23). PayPal Founder's Fellowship Hatches Medication Reminder App. *Information Week Health Care.* Retrieved from http://x.co/1U6Xp

Savage, E., Beirne, P. V., Ni Chroinin, M., Duff, A., Fitzgerald, T., & Farrell, D. (2011). Self-management education for cystic fibrosis. *Cochrane Database of Systematic Reviews, 7.* doi:10.1002/14651858.CD007641.pub2 PMID:21735415

Schaefer, J., Miller, D., Goldstein, M., & Simmons, L. (2009). *Partnering in Self-Management Support: A Toolkit for Clinicians.* Institute for Healthcare Improvement. Retrieved from http://www.ihi.org/resources/Pages/Tools/SelfManagementToolkitforClinicians.aspx

Skolasky, R. L., Green, A. F., Scharfstein, D., Boult, C., Reider, L., & Wegener, S. T. (2011). Psychometric properties of the patient activation measure among multimorbid older adults. *Health Services Research, 46*(2), 457–478. doi:10.1111/j.1475-6773.2010.01210.x PMID:21091470

Smith, C. A., Hetzel, S., Dalrymple, P., & Keselman, A. (2011). Beyond readability: Investigating coherence of clinical text for consumers. *Journal of Medical Internet Research, 13*(4), e104. doi:10.2196/jmir.1842 PMID:22138127

Solomon, M., Wagner, S. L., & Goes, J. (2012). Effects of a web-based intervention for adults with chronic conditions on patient activation: online randomized controlled trial. *Journal of Medical Internet Research, 14*(1), e32. doi:10.2196/jmir.1924 PMID:22353433

Trappenburg, J., Jonkman, N., Jaarsma, T., van Os-Medendorp, H., Kort, H., & de Wit, N. et al. (2013). Self-management: one size does not fit all. *Patient Education and Counseling, 92*(1), 134–137. doi:10.1016/j.pec.2013.02.009 PMID:23499381 van Gemert-Pijnen, J. E., Nijland, N., van Limburg, M., Ossebaard, H. C., Kelders, S. M., Eysenbach, G., & Seydel, E. R. (2011). A holistic framework to improve the uptake and impact of eHealth technologies. *Journal of Medical Internet Research*, *13*(4), e111. doi:10.2196/jmir.1672 PMID:22155738

van Mierlo, T., Voci, S., Lee, S., Fournier, R., & Selby, P. (2012). Superusers in Social Networks for Smoking Cessation: Analysis of Demographic Characteristics and Posting Behavior from the Canadian Cancer Society's Smokers' Helpline Online and StopSmokingCenter.net. *Journal of Medical Internet Research*, *14*(3), e66. doi:10.2196/jmir.1854 PMID:22732103

Wee, C. C., Davis, R. B., & Phillips, R. S. (2005). Stage of readiness to control weight and adopt weight control behaviors in primary care. *Journal of General Internal Medicine*, *20*(5), 410–415. doi:10.1111/j.1525-1497.2005.0074.x PMID:15963162

ADDITIONAL READING

Berwick, D. (2010). *Connected for Health: using electronic health records to transform care delivery* (L. L. Liang, Ed.). Wiley.

KEY TERMS AND DEFINITIONS

Consumer: A person who uses goods and services voluntarily and of their own volition.

EMR: Software used by healthcare providers to document the care they provide. Usually used in real-time at the point of care.

eTool: A software application or website that is intended to help consumers or patients to monitor, track and/or treat a disease condition.

Gamification: Integration of game mechanics or game dynamics into software applications.

Patient: A person with a health condition who is in the care of a healthcare provider.

Team-Based Care: Interprofessional teams of healthcare providers who work together (virtually or in the real world) to provide care to patients in an integrated manner.

Section 3
Real Life Implementations and Cases

This section includes real implementation examples from the field of social media and mobile technologies in healthcare.

Chapter 9
Online Health Information:
Home Caregiver Population Driving Cyberspace Searches in the United States

Mary Schmeida
Kent State University, USA

Ramona McNeal
University of Northern Iowa, USA

ABSTRACT

Increasingly, the healthcare burden of an aging population in the United States is being "relieved" through family members caring for aging and ill loved ones at home. Today, families are turning to mobile technology to lessen their burden and to cope with the stress of caring for loved ones through activities ranging from healthcare information searches to social interactions with online health communities. The purpose of this chapter is to analyze factors predicting the characteristics and context of the U.S. home caregiver population. In addition, this chapter explores how mobile technologies are helping to mitigate some of the weight placed on the family caregiver. The authors explore these questions using multivariate regression analysis and individual level data from the Internet and American Life Project. The findings suggest that interaction with others in online support groups may be more important for the e-caregiver than other online activities.

INTRODUCTION

Mobile health (the use of wireless access for healthcare activities) has brought support to healthcare providers in the home environment across the United States. Mobile technology permits interface with health applications, government health information websites, healthcare providers, and social media such as health forums (Pew Research Center's Internet & American Life Project Mobile Health Survey, 2012a).

Parallel to mobile health is the growth of the family home caregiver role (Pew Research Center's Internet & American Life Project Family Caregivers Online, 2012b). The increased role of the family in caregiving is a phenomenon being experienced

DOI: 10.4018/978-1-4666-6150-9.ch009

in many industrialized countries because people are living longer, and consequently, have a greater chance of experiencing poorer health in their final years. This has resulted in a greater demand for long-term healthcare (Rhodes & Shaw, 1999; Organisation for Economic Co-operation and Development, 2009). Often, it is the family that provides the bulk of this care. For example, in Australia, the number of family members taking care of loved ones has been estimated to be five times more than full-time paid care providers. Similarly, in Canada it has been estimated that family is assuming 80-90% of family elder care (Stajduhar, Funk, Toye, Grande, Aoun, & Todd, 2010, p. 573).

Overtime, the care giving demands on family members is expected to increase. In the U.S., the adult population over 65 years is increasing at a rate faster than family who are able to care for them. It is projected that the number of individuals over 65 years will rise at a rate of 101% between 2000 and 2030, while the number of family members available to provide care will only increase at a rate of 25% during the same period (Mack & Thompson, 2001). By 2030, nearly 1 in 5 U.S. citizens is predicted to be 65 years or older (Murphy, 2005). The reliance on family to care for an increasing aging population does not come without a cost. Being a family caregiver is linked to a number of heath issues including depression, decline in physical health and increased mortality (Kiecolt-Glaser & Glaser, 2001; Schulz & Beach, 1999). The Internet has become an important resource for this unpaid labor force (Schmeida, 2005). Although several large studies help to define the characteristics of the average home caregiver in the U.S. (through the reporting of simple statistics such as percentages), few empirical studies exist that analyze these characteristics with certainty controlling/adjusting for factors using multivariate regression analysis. The objective of this chapter is to analyze an array of factors predicting the characteristics and context of the U.S. home caregiver population. In addition, this chapter explores how the Internet is

helping to mitigate some of the burden placed on the family caregiver and how mobile technology can be a supportive resource.

BACKGROUND

Mobile health is a form of telehealth that encompasses the use of electronic information and advanced communication technology (digital technologies) to support institutional healthcare services, consumer and provider education, health administration and health research (H.R. 2157, 2001). Technology gives the capability to connect different users, such as university hospitals with patients at home, and home healthcare givers with social health networks from different locations online (Center for Connected Health Policy, 2013). Healthcare consumers in sparsely populated regions can link to cutting edge urban healthcare services previously limited to urban residents, as well as apply for health insurance online. The goal of telehealth is to promote accessibility of public and private healthcare services in rural and urban areas, improve the quality of services, and promote efficiency by reducing service costs. It promises access to services, information, and social support to healthcare consumers and providers. The dramatic growth and importance of the Internet has led to evolvement of mobile technology and mobile health. Through the use of Internet connectivity, citizens can interface with health and medical information online, interact with healthcare providers via email, and participate in highly interactive social platforms.

Today's healthcare consumers are more sophisticated, demand better service quality, and are health information seekers who themselves are mobile. New generation technological devices include tablet computers and the multifunctional cell phones, which give consumers Internet access plus a phone. More healthcare consumers are now using the multifunctional cell phones, such as smartphones with downloadable health applications. Smartphone owners lead in looking for health advice at 52% versus 6% for non-smartphone owners, with health application downloading led by females, under age 50, better educated, and with a household earning over $75,000 per year (Pew, 2012a, p. 11). Current telehealth activities go beyond Internet consumerism to include social health interaction. These interactions take the form of social networking including online forums. Although the ability to connect with others with similar health issues is important to the online healthcare consumer, it has become particularly important to family caregivers who lead other groups in using social network sites (Pew, 2011). Healthcare social networking forums are growing and becoming a meeting place to exchange ideas, personal healthcare experiences and act as a support system to home caregivers (Pew, 2012a).

In addition to providing a meeting place for the online health community for sharing of experiences and emotional support, there are a multitude of online health activities that citizens are doing. These activities include reading reviews of healthcare providers and treatment options; attempting to diagnose a medical condition that they or a loved one is experiencing; and downloading applications that allow them to track their health. In the U.S., obtaining health insurance through the use of the Internet has become an important Internet service. A serious problem felt by many Americans is the inability to pay for health coverage. Historically, there has been a lack of health insurance among the poor, rural, children, and disabled population in the U.S. In 2009, it was estimated that the number of uninsured males was 27,463,000 and females at 23,211,000 (U.S. Census Bureau, 2012). These individuals typically do not have an option of getting insurance from their employer and do not qualify for Medicare or Medicaid. Medicare is the government health insurance program for people 65 years and older, disabled, and/ or with permanent kidney failure. Medicaid is the federal-state health insurance

program designed to assist the poor, such as low-income children, poor parents, pregnant women, the elderly, and disabled (Centers for Medicare & Medicaid Services, 2013). In 2010, the federal government attempted to reduce the number of uninsured through the Patient Protection and Affordable Care Act. Among the provisions of this act is the expansion of the Medicaid program by permitting young adults to stay on their parent's insurance plan until the age of 26 (Public Law 111-148). As an outreach effort to enroll the uninsured populations, the federal government and private sector have developed Internet websites. Medicare and Medicaid websites provide information on eligibility, enrollment forms, and provider information.

Home Caregiver Population Driving Cyberspace Searches in the United States

Family caregivers are among those individuals most likely to take advantage of the increased healthcare services provided online. According to the Pew Research Center's Internet & American Life Project (2012b), approximately 30% of adults in the United States provide care for another person, such as parent, spouse, child with a disability, or the chronically ill (p. 6). In addition to providing nursing care, the caregiver provides companionship, assists with household chores, and deals with bills and health insurance for the ill family member (AARP Public Policy Institute, 2011). While more American's are taking care of loved ones in their later stages of life, we do not have a clear picture of the home caregiver. Although several large studies help to define the characteristics of the average home caregiver in the U.S., few empirically analyze these characteristics with certainty controlling/ adjusting for factors using multivariate regression analysis. Demographic reporting show the average caregiver to be female, providing approximately 20 hours per week of uncompensated care to their mother

(AARP Public Policy Institute, 2011, p. 1), white, non-Hispanic, age 50-64 years, college graduate or more, married, and employed full-time (Pew, 2012b, p. 4 & 8; Tong, 2007).

Although the family caregiver is turning to the Internet for assistance, demographic factors play a role on the extent that the Internet is used for healthcare service support. The National Alliance for Caregiving (2009) reports online searches to be dominated by Asian American caregivers (66%), followed by Caucasian (54%), African Americans (44%), and Hispanics (50%). Additionally, only 30% of individuals over 65 years were found to use the Internet for caregiving support as compared to 56% for the younger cohort. Gender stands out in its importance in online healthcare searches and can be understood through the role that women play as caregivers in the United States. Even though demographic factors such as age, gender and race influence how much the home caregiver is relying on the Internet, the caregiver is outpacing others in online health information searches and across topic areas. Pew (2012a) found caregivers to lead non-caregivers in health or medical experiences/comments given on Internet news groups, websites or blogs (p. 14). Caregivers are more likely to follow personal health experiences of supports such as friends by using Internet websites such as Facebook (social networking website), LinkedIn (professional social network), or Google+ (online index of websites) (Pew, 2012b, p. 14). They lead non-caregivers in posting health provider reviews (Pew, 2012a, p. 16), in online health information social networking using Facebook and MySpace (20% versus 12%), consulting online reviews/rankings of medications (38% versus 18%), consulting healthcare providers (21% versus 13%), and healthcare institutions 20% versus 12% (Pew, 2012b, p. 15). In addition, home caregivers were more likely to use the Internet for health searches across all health topics surveyed, such as disease or medical condition (76% versus 61%), medical treatment (69% versus 50%), and information on hospitals, physicians, and health insurance (Pew,

2012b, p. 11). These findings are consistent with earlier research. Schmeida (2005) found that persons who are a primary or secondary caregiver to a household member are more likely to get online to search for information such as health insurance information.

PUBLIC POLICIES IN SUPPORT OF CAREGIVER NEEDS

Caregivers seem to have more hardships than their non-caregiver counterparts. Working age caregivers are more likely to face health concerns and disability. They are less likely to be employed outside the care giving environment, however, if employed they are more likely to miss work. Those unemployed face lack of employer-based health insurance (Commonwealth Fund, 2005). As a result, caregivers are more likely to experience hardship. Federal and state legislation have been passed to support the needs of the family home caregiver and lessen their hardship. For example, the federal Older Americans Act (P.L. 89-73, 1965; P.L. 110-246, 2008) provides funding for services, such as respite for family caregivers providing care to members 60 years and older. The Family and Medical Leave Act (103-3, 1993) permits working caregivers to take leave from work to assume care for family members with serious illness. Alzheimer's disease Demonstration Grants to States provides competitive grants that can assist states to help Alzheimer's patients, families, and caregivers with services such as respite for family caregivers (Public Law 78-410, 1991). The 2006 Lifespan Respite Care Act (P.L. 109-442, 2006) is a grant given to states administered by the U.S. Department of Health and Human Services Administration on Aging. It enables states to improve upon deficiencies of existing respite services and to oversee the implementation of new respite services to family caregivers. The states have also taken steps to lessen the burden of caring for loved ones. Almost 50% of the states have created Aging and Disability Resource Centers for residents to obtain information on state programs for the elderly. In addition, some states have programs aimed at improving the health of elderly citizens, such as West Virginia's statewide program to increase elderly physical activities with a walking regiment (Murphy, 2005).

Although both the federal and state governments have taken action to lessen the burden of the family caregiver, these policies may not be enough. Caregivers are increasingly turning to the Internet to augment government assistance. This trend raises a number of questions. Which family members are taking on the bulk of the caregiving duties? How is the Internet helping to mitigate some of the burden placed on the family caregiver? Can mobile technology enhance the capacity of the Internet assisting in the healthcare duties of loved ones?

EMPIRICAL MODEL: DATA AND METHODS

This study utilizes the *2012 Pew Health Tracking Survey* conducted for the Pew Internet & American Life Project, by the Princeton Survey Research Associates. The Pew Internet & American Life Project is part of the Pew Research Center, a nonpartisan, nonprofit group that conducts studies and provides information regarding factors that shape American society. Their surveys are random digit dial national telephone surveys limited to individuals 18 years or older and live in the continental United States. This study is based on a survey conducted for the Internet and American Life Project with a sample size (n) of 3,014 adults living in the US collected from August 7 to September 6, 2012.

Portrait of a Family Caregiver

This study begins with an examination of the demographic and geographical factors associated with an individual taking on the role of family caregiver using logistic regression analysis. Independent variables were selected based on findings from prior research. The dependent variable was constructed as a dummy variable using the following question: "In the past 12 months, have you provided unpaid care to an adult relative or friend 18 years or older to help them take care of themselves?" The variable is coded 1 if an individual responded yes and 0 otherwise.

Explanatory or independent variables include an *Income* measure on a 9-point scale where 1 indicates that family incomes range from $0 to $10,000 and 9 signifies a family income of $150,000 or more. *Education* is measured using a 7-point scale, ranging from eighth-grade education or less to post-graduate training/ professional training, which includes Masters/ Ph.D., law and medical school. Based on prior research (Pew, 2012b) it is expected that both income and education to be positively associated with the role of family caregiver. *Gender* is measured using a binary variable coded 1 for female and 0 for male. The literature (AARP Public Policy Institute, 2011; Pew, 2012b; Tong, 2007) overwhelmingly suggests that women are more likely to take on the caregiver role. This same research suggests that caregivers are more likely to be middle aged and caring for a parent. Since this suggests the relationship between becoming a family caregiver and age is quadratic, both age and age squared are included in the model.

To control for race and ethnicity, dummy variables are included for *African Americans*, *Asian Americans*, and *Latinos* with *non-Hispanic Whites* as the reference group. Based on current literature (Pew, 2012b) it is expected that the family caregiver will have a greater likelihood of being a non-Hispanic White. Dummy variables for the *Midwest, Northeast and West* regions are included to control for regional differences. The South is designated as the reference group because states in the South contain the greatest percentage of the U.S. aging population. In 2004, 36% of the population over 55 lived in the South (Murphy, 2004). Since research on healthcare access (Schmeida & McNeal, 2007) finds a persistent gap in urban/ rural areas, two dummy variables were included for the respondent's community type (*Suburban and Urban*) with rural as the reference group. Residents living in rural areas are expected to be more likely to take on the role of family caregiver compared to those living in suburban and urban areas because of limited access to health care delivery sites. To control for *Marital Status* a dummy variable is included coded 1 if the respondent was married or living with a partner and 0 otherwise. Finally, dummy variables for *Employed Fulltime* and *Employed Part-Time* are added to control for employment status. Prior research (Pew, 2012b) suggests full time employed individuals and married individuals are more likely to take on the caregiver role.

E-Caregiver

Since this study also explores how the Internet may help to mitigate some of the burden placed on the family caregiver, additional models are calculated to determine if Internet use by caregivers varies from that of non-caregivers. Control variables are selected based on findings from prior research on barriers to Internet usage and e-caregiver activities. Although there are many ways the Internet could potentially assist the online health information seeker, we chose two questions to consider. The first is: "In the last 12 months, have you downloaded forms online or applied for health insurance online, including private insurance, Medicare, or Medicaid?" This question is chosen because of the growing inability to pay for health coverage, a serious issue experienced by many Americans today. Since both caregivers and non-caregivers are likely to take part in this online activity, it is a useful question for examining whether caregivers are more likely to use the Internet for healthcare assistance. The second question is: "In the past 12 months, have you read someone else's commentary or experiences about health or medical issues online?" This question was selected to help gauge how important online forums are to the well being of caregivers when compared to non-caregivers. Both variables are coded 1 if the individual took part in the online healthcare activity and 0 otherwise.

As with the previous model (Table 1), demographic and geographical measures will be used as control variables but their inclusion is based on a different literature. Instead of considering indicators of access to healthcare and the literature on caregivers, this section considers the literature on Internet access and technological skill. It is unrealistic to assume that all caregivers will use the Internet equally when providing assistance to a family member or friend. The ability to do so can be limited by access to the Internet and the ability to use it. According to the latest National Telecommunication and Information Administration (NTIA) study (2011, p. 5), the percentage of U.S. citizens with Internet access is rising with 68.2% of households having broadband access at home, and 72% of citizens having Internet access at some location such as school, work or library. There are still however, individuals without Internet access. They are primarily elderly, less affluent, less educated, minorities (Hispanic and African American), living with a disability, unemployed, and those who reside in rural areas (NTIA, 2011, p. 28).

Access to the Internet does not guarantee usage. Other factors help determine how much the Internet is used and why. Among the factors found to influence whether an individual goes online and the extent to which it is used is technical skills. According to Mossberger, Tolbert & Stansbury (2003), technological skills can be thought of in two ways. The first (technical competencies) encompasses knowing how to use hardware and software. The second category (information literacy) indicates the ability to determine what information to get from the Internet to perform a specific task. Adams, Stubbs & Woods (2005)

Table 1. Portrait of a family caregiver, 2012

Variables	Family Caregiver b(se)	p>|z|
Environmental Variables		
Suburban	**-.296(.123)**	**.017**
Urban	**-.298(.130)**	**.022**
Midwest	-.070(.120)	.599
Northeast	-.208(.131)	.111
West	-.093(.114)	.420
Individual Level Variables		
Age	**.048(.014)**	**.001**
Age Squared	**-.000(.000)**	**.001**
Female	.116(.088)	.187
Latino	-.094(.135)	.488
Black	**.210(.122)**	**.086**
Asian	-.247(.267)	.357
Education	.016(.026)	.588
Income	**.049(.022)**	**.029**
Married	**.172(.097)**	**.074**
Work Full Time Work Part Time	-.080(.108) **.347(.147)**	.454 **.019**
Constant Pseudo R2	**-1.711(.248)** .0181	**.000**
LR Chi² (16)	56.98	.000
N	2379	

Sources: *2012 Pew Health Tracking Survey.* Logistic regression estimates with standard errors in parentheses. Reported probabilities are based on two-tailed tests. Statistically significant coefficients at .10 or less in bold.

also argue that psychological factors such as motivation are important to the development of technical skills and Internet usage.

Among the measures included in these regression models on Internet access and technological skills are *Income, Age* and *Education*. Based on the literature (NTIA, 2011; Mossberger, Tolbert & Stansbury, 2003) it is expected that *Income* and *Education* to be positively associated with Internet searches while *Age* would be negatively associated. There is conflicting research (Schmeida & McNeal, 2007; Schmeida & McNeal, 2013), which finds for at least one online healthcare activity (searching for Medicare and Medicaid informa-

tion) the less affluent are more likely to take part in this activity. This conflicting research can be explained by Adams, Stubbs & Woods (2005), who find that factors such as motivation or need can be important in predicting Internet use. Since the Medicaid program was designed to help the poor, it is not unusual that the less affluent would be more likely to use the Internet to find information on this topic. A dummy variable was also included for *Female*. Although the literature doesn't point to a difference in Internet use by gender, it is expected that females will be more likely to use the Internet for healthcare activities. This follows the literature (AARP Public Policy Institute, 2011

Pew, 2012b; Tong, 2007), which overwhelming finds that women assume the role of caregiver in the United States more often.

To control for race and ethnicity, dummy variables were included for *African American*, *Asian American*, and *Latino* with *Non-Hispanic White* as the reference group. Based on Internet access and technology skills literature, it is assumed that Asian Americans are most likely to take part in Internet activities, followed by non-Hispanic Whites. This assumption is supported by the National Alliance for Caregiving (2009) that found online health searches to be dominated by Asian American caregivers (66%), followed by Caucasian (54%), African Americans (44%), and Hispanics (50%). A dummy variable was included for *Mobile Technology* coded 1 if they answered yes to the question, "do you access the internet on a cell phone, tablet or other mobile handheld device, at least occasionally?" and coded 0 otherwise. This control was included because studies (Selwyn, 2004; Mossberger, Tolbert, & McNeal, 2007) found when Internet access is more convenient and quicker, it leads to greater usage and improved technology skills. These findings suggest that mobile technology users may be more likely to use the Internet for healthcare activities.

Since research on Internet access (NTIA, 2011) finds a persistent gap in urban/rural areas, two dummy variables were included for the respondent's geographic area (*Suburban* and *Urban*) with rural as the reference group. Residents living in suburban and urban areas are expected to be more likely to conduct Internet searches compared to those living in rural areas. Dummy variables for the *Midwest, Northeast and West* regions were included to control for regional differences, with the South designated as the reference group because West and Miller (2006) found that the South region had the lowest levels of Internet connectivity. Finally, measurements were added for *Health Status* of the respondent, *Care for an Adult*, and *Care for a Child*. The variable *Health Status* is a 4-point scale where the respondent

rated her/his own health from poor to excellent. *Care for an Adult* was constructed as a dummy variable using the following question: "In the past 12 months, have you provided unpaid care to an adult relative or friend 18 years or older to help them take care of themselves?" It is coded 1 if an individual responded yes and 0 otherwise. *Care for a Child* was constructed as a dummy variable using the question: "In the past 12 months, have you provided unpaid care to any child under the age of 18 because of a medical, behavioral, or other condition or disability?" It is coded 1 if an individual responded yes and 0 otherwise. These three variables were included because they represent perceived need.

FINDINGS AND DISCUSSION

Portrait of a Family Caregiver

In Table 1, the dependent variable is coded so that higher scores are associated with increased likelihood of caring for an elderly family member or friend. Since the dependent variable is binary, the model is estimated using logistic regression. The findings below do not entirely correspond to prior research on demographic studies of family caregivers in the United States, but this is expected. Most of these earlier studies reported simple statistics such as percentage and did not analyze these characteristics using a statistical method that would control for the impact of other factors. Among the findings that did agree with earlier research are those for age, income, marital status and community type. These findings suggest that individuals most likely to care for an older loved one are middle aged, more affluent, married or living with a partner and in a rural region.

While some findings are consistent with previous research, others are not. Even though Southern states have a greater proportion of elderly citizens, there were no statistical differences found based on region. Perhaps this suggests that, unlike community type, there are no differences in access to health care delivery sites across regions. Similarly, neither education nor gender was found related to the role of caregiver. This is inconsistent with previous findings (AARP Public Policy Institute, 2011; Pew, 2012b; Tong, 2007), that find the more educated and females are more likely to take on the role of caregiver. There are two possible explanations for these findings. The first is the "graying" of America. As a larger percentage of the U.S. population turns 65 or older, those who might not have normally taken on the role of caregiver find themselves assuming roles traditionally taken by females. A second possibility is that the measure for the dependent variable may be too "blunt" of an instrument. It only asked the respondent if they had provided care in the last 12 months; it did not measure how long the respondent provided care and to what extent. We might find greater differences in care based on individual factors, if the dependent variable was more specific. In contrast to previous research and reports (Pew, 2012b; National Alliance for Caregiving, 2009), the findings indicate that those employed part-time and African Americans were most likely to be caregivers. This suggests that caregivers may not be able to work full time outside the caregiver role. Also, blacks may have a greater need to assume the role due to fewer resources to hire outside help or long-term facility placement. Although this earlier study found that those employed full time were more likely to be caregivers, this finding is more intuitive. Working fulltime and acting as a caregiver would be extremely difficult. Among the findings that did agree with earlier research are those for age, income, marital status and community type.

E-Caregiver

In Table 2, the dependent variables are coded so that higher scores are associated with increased likelihood of taking part in the individual online healthcare activity. Since the dependent variables are binary, models are estimated using logistic regression. While the findings for individual level variables were consistent across the two online activities, there are considerable differences based on environmental variables. For both dependent variables, education and income were positively related to engaging in the online health activity. This is consistent with the literature on both Internet access and technological skill (NTIA, 2011; Mossberger, Tolbert & Stansbury, 2003). The finding that income is positively associated with online health activity conflicts with research (Schmeida & McNeal, 2007; Schmeida & McNeal, 2013) that show for at least one online healthcare activity (searching for Medicare and Medicaid insurance information) the less affluent are more likely to take part in this activity. This conflicting research can be explained by technological skills. Both the activities explored in this study required greater information literacy, downloading, and filling out insurance forms online. All of these activities would involve greater technical competencies than just searching for health information.

Online health activities were also found more likely to be done by the young and women. The findings regarding age are consistent with previous research on Internet access and technological skills. This literature does not provide help in predicting the influence of gender on online activities. Early research (prior to 2000) found that Internet users were more likely to be male but current research generally agreed that differences in gender had disappeared (NTIA, 2011). The finding that women are more likely to take part in online healthcare activities is consistent with the literature on caregiver. In addition, this outcome adds support to the concern that the dependent variable in Table 1 may not be sufficiently precise. The results in Table 1 indicate that gender is not a significant predictor of family caregiver, which is inconsistent with the findings in Table 2 that shows gender to be statistically significant.

Race/ ethnicity factors are not associated with the dependent variable in either model. These findings conflict with those (NTIA, 2011) that indicate

Table 2. E-Caregiver activities, 2012

Variables	Download Insurance Forms		Read Other's Health Experience Online	
	b(se)	p>|z|	b(se)	p>|z|
Environmental Variables				
Suburban	**.405(.226)**	**.073**	.213(.194)	.851
Urban	.201(.239)	.399	.141(.166)	.394
Midwest	-.200(.206)	.330	**.247(.150)**	**.100**
Northeast	**-.371(.217)**	**.087**	.077(.158)	.627
West	.143(.175)	.415	**.309(.138)**	**.025**
Individual Level Variables				
Age	**-.010(.005)**	**.034**	**- .026(.004)**	**.000**
Female	**.247(.142)**	**.082**	**.238(.108)**	**.028**
Latino	.044(.212)	.835	-.018(.161)	.913
Black	-.225(.213)	.292	-.203(.157)	.198
Asian	-.638(.445)	.152	-.015(.275)	.956
Education	**.201(.042)**	**.000**	**.179(.032)**	**.000**
Income	**.060(.035)**	**.081**	**.066(.026)**	**.011**
Mobile Technology	**.708(.181)**	**.000**	**.611(.131)**	**.000**
Care for Adult	**.459(.143)**	**.001**	**.676(.109)**	**.000**
Care for Child	**.523(.201)**	**.009**	**.576(.165)**	**.000**
Health Status	**-.212(.097)**	**.030**	-.108(.076)	.147
Constant **Pseudo R2**	-3.351(.487) .0878	**.000**	-1.945(.360) .1193	**.000**
LR Chi² (16)	139.98	.000	300.57	.000
N	2376		2376	

Sources: *2012 Pew Health Tracking Survey* Logistic regression estimates with standard errors in parentheses. Reported probabilities are based on two-tailed tests. Statistically significant coefficients at .10 or less in bold.

race/ ethnic minorities (African Americans and Hispanics) are less likely to have Internet access. They are however, consistent with Mossberger, Tolbert, & Gilbert (2006) who found variations in Internet usage by race/ ethnicity are the result of concentrated poverty and racial segregation. They found that once factors such as education attainment and median family income are controlled for, the appearance of differences in Internet usage based on race/ ethnicity disappear. This outcome is also consistent with earlier research (Schmeida & McNeal, 2007; Schmeida & McNeal, 2013)

that found no relationship between race/ ethnicity and the online healthcare activity of searching for Medicare and Medicaid information online.

There is limited support for the argument that geographic differences including region and community type (urban, suburban and rural) can influence online healthcare activities. Regarding the dependent variable *Reading Other's Health Experience Online,* residents of the West and Midwest were found to be more likely to take part in this activity, which corresponds with West and Miller (2006) who found the South to have the lowest levels of Internet connectivity. However, the finding that resident's of the Northeast are less likely to download and fill out insurance forms does not. Finally, the only result that corresponds to the prediction that those living in urban and suburban areas would be more likely to take part in online healthcare activities is that suburban residents were more likely to download and fill out insurance forms online.

Measurements were added for *Health Status* of the respondent, *Care for an Adult* and *Care for a Child* with the belief that family caregivers and individuals with poorer health would have greater need to seek online healthcare assistance. The findings from both models supported these predictions. In Table 2 both models, family caregivers were positively associated with the dependent variable and individuals who rated their own health more poorly were more likely to download and fill out insurance forms online. Finally, following Selwyn (2004), and Mossberger, Tolbert, & McNeal (2007) we added a control for mobile technology use. These studies (based on broadband) found that when Internet access is more convenient and quicker, it leads to greater usage and improved technology skills. For both models, individuals with mobile technology were more likely to take part in online healthcare activities. This adds support to the earlier research on broadband access.

Monte Carlo Simulations

As a final method for examining the effect of caregiver status and mobile technology, the percentage of individuals who took part in each online healthcare activity from Table 2 is presented in Table 3 and 4. While the findings in Table 2 indicate a positive effect of caregiver status and mobile technology on online healthcare activities, it is not likely that each factor would equally impact these activities. To illustrate the extent to which each factor can increase online health activities, the coefficients reported in Table 2 were converted to predicted probabilities of taking part in each online healthcare activity (King, Tomz, & Wittenberg, 2000). The simulations compare the probability of taking part in each activity for individuals who have taken on different levels of family care giving and those who "do" and "do not" have mobile technology. Probability simulations were calculated holding the variable age at its mean and income, health status and education at their median values. Gender was set at female, race at non-Hispanic white, region at Midwest, and community type at suburban and urban. Expected probabilities were calculated for different levels of family healthcare giving, by statistically varying the variable "use of mobile technology" that was set at "does not use mobile technology" or "do use mobile technology."

Table 3. Mobile technology and the expected probability of reading about other's health experiences online (2012)

Predicted Probability of Reading About Other's Health Experiences Online	Not a Family Caregiver	Caregiver for Child	Caregiver for Adult	Caregiver for both Child and Adult
No Mobile Technology	13.8% (.030)	22.2% (.050)	23.9% (.047)	35.6% (.065)
Yes Mobile Technology	22.8% (.044)	34.2% (.064)	36.4% (.058)	50.2% (.069)
Difference (yes-no)	9.0%	12.0%	12.5%	14.6%

Note: Standard deviations are in parentheses. To simulate different levels of mobile technology usage, usage was set at "does use mobile technology" and "does not use mobile technology." Value for age was set at the mean. Values for income, education and level of health were set at their median. Gender was set at female, race at non-Hispanic white, region at Midwest, and community type at urban and suburban. Estimations were produced using Clarify: Software for Interpreting and Presenting Statistical Results, by Michael Tomz, Jason Wittenberg, and Gary King (2000).

Table 4. Mobile technology and the expected probability of downloading insurance forms or applying for insurance online (2012)

Predicted Probability of Downloading Insurance Forms or Applying for Insurance Online	Not a Family Caregiver	Caregiver for Child	Caregiver for Adult	Caregiver for both Child and Adult
No Mobile Technology	6.5% (.022)	10.7% (.039)	9.9% (.033)	15.9% (.054)
Yes Mobile Technology	12.1% (.037)	19.2% (.056)	17.9% (.053)	27.1% (.075)
Difference (yes-no)	5.6%	8.5%	8.0%	11.2%

Note: Standard deviations are in parentheses. To simulate different levels of mobile technology usage, usage was set at "does use mobile technology" and "does not use mobile technology." Value for age was set at the mean. Values for income, education and level of health were set at their median. Gender was set at female, race at non-Hispanic white, region at Midwest, and community type at urban and suburban. Estimations were produced using Clarify: Software for Interpreting and Presenting Statistical Results, by Michael Tomz, Jason Wittenberg, and Gary King (2000).

READING ABOUT OTHER'S HEALTH EXPERIENCES ONLINE

Table 3 presents the predicted probabilities for the dependent question, "In the past 12 months, have you read someone else's commentary or experiences about health or medical issues online?" The findings provide a clearer picture of the impact the three variables (mobile technology, care for an adult, and care for a child) have on the likelihood that an individual will seek out information regarding other's experiences with a particular health issue. The probability of taking part in this activity increases between 9% and 14.6% when comparing individuals who "do" and "do not" use mobile technology. After holding other factors constant, the effects of mobile technology results in an increased probability of taking part in this activity of 9% for individuals who haven't taken on the role of caregiver, and 12% for those who are taking care of a child. It also represents an approximate 12.5% increased probability for those providing care to an adult, and a 14.6% high probability for those providing care to both a child and adult. The findings suggest that the role of caregiver has a greater impact than mobile technology in this online health activity. For individuals without mobile technology, those who provide care to both adults and children are

35.6% - 13.8% or 21.8% more likely to take part in this activity. The impact of the role of caregiver is even larger for those individuals with mobile technology. For individuals with mobile technology, those who provide care to both adults and children are 50.2% - 22.8% or 27.4% more likely to take part in this activity.

DOWNLOADING INSURANCE FORMS OR APPLYING FOR INSURANCE ONLINE

Table 4 presents the predicted probabilities for the dependent question, "In the last 12 months, have you downloaded forms online or applied for health insurance online, including private insurance, government Medicare or Medicaid?" The findings provide a clearer picture of the impact that the three variables (mobile technology, care for an adult, and care for a child) have on the likelihood that an individual will download insurance forms online or apply for insurance online. The probability of taking part in this activity increases between 5.6% and 11.2%, when comparing individuals who "do" and "do not" use mobile technology. After holding other factors constant, the effects of mobile technology results in an increased probability of taking part in this activity of 5.6% for individuals who haven't taken on the role of caregiver, and 8.5% for those who are taking care of a child. It also represents an approximate 8% increased probability for those providing care to an adult, and an 11.2% high probability for those providing care to both a child and adult. The findings suggest that the role of caregiver has a similar impact to that of mobile technology for this online health activity. For individuals without mobile technology, those who provide care to both adults and children are 15.9% - 6.5% or 9.4% more likely to take part in this activity. The impact of the role of caregiver is even larger for those individuals with mobile technology. For individuals with mobile technology, those who provide care to both adults and children are 27.1% - 12.1% or 15% more likely to take part in this activity.

Although Tables 3 and 4 support the findings from Table 2 showing the variables mobile technology, caregiver for child, and caregiver for adult increase the likelihood of engaging in online healthcare activities, the impact is not the same across activities. All three independent variables had a greater impact on the dependent variable, *Reading about Other's Health Experiences*. In addition, for this variable the role of caregiver resulted in a greater likelihood of taking part in this activity than using mobile technology. The effect of all three variables was smaller for the *Online Insurance* dependent variable and all three variables had a similar impact. These differences may be attributable to the current economic climate, particularly with the number of individuals relying on Medicaid continuing to rise (Vestal, 2012). Individuals across various demographic groups may find the necessity to take part in this activity whether or not they are a caregiver.

Solutions and Recommendations

Home caregivers face the potential for physical, financial and emotional stress. Spouses and adult children commonly report emotional stress while spouses also report more physical strain and finan-

cial strain. Caregiving has been found to worsen pre-existing health problems and caregivers are more likely to have health problems than non-caregiver counterparts (Administration on Aging, 2011; Commonwealth Fund, 2005). In the U.S., caregivers have responsibilities to elderly parents, spouses, and children. The need for elder support is not expected to diminish anytime soon. With the younger population growing fewer, elder generation living longer, and the demand for elder care growing, government responsibility to the aged generation is expected to accelerate. Title III of The Older Americans Act of 1965 has authorized the Administration on Aging to implement programs in support of the needs of caregivers. Support is provided for information, supplemental services, respite, training or education (Administration on Aging, 2011, p. 3). These services can both extend the amount of time that the aged can remain in their homes and lessen the burden for the caregiver. As significant as these measures are, this study also points to the importance of mobile health. The availability of online forums is serving a critical role to relieve caregiver stress and to provide them with emotional support. Our research findings point to a growing need for government support of programs facilitating better Internet service to the population that is a portrait of the family healthcare giver, specifically the middle aged, more affluent, married (or living with a partner) and in a rural region. Since rural America has traditionally lagged behind urbanites in Internet access/ use, pushing government programs to facilitate the spread of Internet service supporting mobile technology to these underserved regions is a priority.

FUTURE RESEARCH DIRECTIONS

In examining the role of the e-caregiver, this chapter relied on secondary data analysis or data collected by another entity. There are advantages and disadvantages associated with all forms of data analysis. One disadvantage associated with secondary data analysis is that the data was collected for a specific purpose and may not be ideally suited for other research. In general, these datasets have been well suited for this study. Nevertheless, there are a few instances where different wording of several questions may have improved upon this study. Of particular concern are the instruments for *Care for a Child* and *Care for an Adult*. The questions available in this survey for these measures were, "In the past 12 months, have you provided unpaid care to an adult relative or friend 18 years or older to help them take care of themselves?" and "In the past 12 months, have you provided unpaid care to any child under the age of 18 because of a medical, behavioral, or other condition or disability?" These questions may both be too "blunt" of an instrument. For future studies it may be better to develop questions that measure to what extent the respondent provided care and how long.

Another issue to consider for future research is that this study relies on a cross-sectional design that depicts individual action at one point in time. Both the dependent and independent variables are being measured at roughly the same time. This makes it more difficult to establish time order, therefore weakening internal validity. While this study suggests that certain demographic factors are important in determining who takes on the role of caregiver, it is more difficult to make the argument that there is a causal effect. The same argument could be made for the findings regarding the importance of both the role of caregiver and access to mobile technology in the likelihood that an individual will take part in a particular online health activity. Finally, the use of a cross-sectional design suggests factors may only be relevant during this time period. The results of a longitudinal study, on the other hand, might find that these variables are only significantly related to this topic during a specific time period. Such a study could find that, in the long run, other factors play a more important role. There are several

trends that future research will need to consider when exploring this topic. The first is the "graying" of America. Currently, 1 in 8 Americans are 65 years or older. Between 2010 and 2050, the population of Americans 65 years and older is expected to double from 40.2 million (2010) to 88.5 million for year 2050 (U.S. Census Bureau, 2010). The second is the rapid adoption of mobile technology for online health activities. Pew (2012a) found that in 2010 approximately 17% of cell phone owners had used their phones for health searches. By 2012, the number had risen to 31%. It is expected that mobile technology will continue to play an increasing role in individual healthcare in the future.

CONCLUSION

This chapter began by noting several overlapping trends: the expansion of mobile health, the "graying" of America and the increased role of family in the care of aging family members and loved ones. These two trends are placing stress on the current health system and placing an increasing burden on the family. Studies (Kiecolt-Glasser & Glaser, 2001; Schulz & Beach, 1999) find the role of family caregiver is associated with a number of heath related issues including depression, decline in physical health and increased mortality. To examine whether the first trend (expansion of mobile health) holds promise for alleviating some of the weight on family members, we initially began by looking at factors that predicted who is taking on the job of caregiver. Next, this research examined two questions that measure extent to which an individual uses mobile health. The first was, "In the last 12 months, have you downloaded forms online or applied for health insurance online, including private insurance, Medicare, or Medicaid?" This question was chosen because both caregivers and non-caregivers are likely to take part in this online activity; it is a useful question for examining whether caregivers are more likely to use the Internet for healthcare assistance. The second question is, "In the past 12 months, have you read someone else's commentary or experiences about health or medical issues online?" This question was selected to help gauge how important online forums are to the well-being of caregivers. Much of the help that the Internet provides to the caregiver is in the form of information, but the online forums serve a different function – to relieve stress and provide emotional support.

This study found that individuals most likely to take on the role of caregiver live in rural areas, are middle aged, African American, married, work part time and are more affluent. This portrait of a family caregiver points to a combination of need and capacity. Those living in rural areas and African Americans may have less access to health care facilities suggesting that they are assuming the role out of necessity. Married and middle-aged caregivers points to those who are part of the "sandwich" generation. They represent a segment of the population who are both grappling with elderly parents needing assistance and simultaneously raising children, or helping with grandchildren. Finally, those working part time and are more affluent may have greater resources that allow them to take on this role.

While this study finds that certain segments of society are more likely to take on the role of caregiver, they do not all equally make use of the Internet for health assistance. These individuals are most likely to take part in online health activities including those who were more affluent, younger, better educated, have mobile technology, female, have health issues of their own, and have taken on the role of caregiver. These findings point to a combination of need, Internet access and possession of technological skills. Those individuals who most likely have technological skills and Internet access are younger, better educated and affluent. At the same time, those most in need of Internet health resources are those who have taken on the role of caregiver, are suffering from health problems and female. Although this study did not

find a gender difference in the role of caregiver, many (AARP Public Policy Institute, 2011; Pew, 2012b; Tong, 2007) have found that women are more likely to be caregivers. It is possible that while both genders are now taking on the role of caregiver, women are still more extensively involved in this activity. The measures used for caregiver in this study were not precise enough to determine the extent to which an individual may assume this role. The finding that those with mobile technology are more likely to take part in online health activities points to the role of technology itself. Earlier studies on broadband (Selwyn, 2004; Mossberger, Tolbert, & McNeal, 2007) found that when Internet access is more convenient and quicker, it leads to greater usage and improved technology skills. Mobile technology may have a similar effect.

Finally, this study used Monte Carlo simulations to explore the extent to which the role of care giving and the use of mobile technology can influence online health activities. For the variable *Online Insurance Activities*, being a caregiver increased the likelihood of taking part in these activities between 5.6% and 11.2% and while using mobile technology increased it between 9.4% and 15%. With regard to *Reading About Other's Experiences*, being a caregiver increased the likelihood of taking part in these activities between 9% and 14.6% and while using mobile technology increased it between 21.8% and 27.4%. Mobile technology and the role of caregiver had less of an impact on online insurance activities. This suggests, partly, that many Americans from the general population are engaging in this activity. On the other hand, the findings indicate that online health forums help to provide emotional support that may be particularly important to the individual who has taken on the role of caregiver. Worth noting is that mobile technology significantly increases the likelihood that a caretaker will take part in these forums which supports earlier work on broadband (Selwyn, 2004; Mossberger, Tolbert, & McNeal, 2007) that found when Internet access is more convenient and quicker, it leads to greater usage and improved Internet skills.

Overall, our research impacts the study of mobile health and social networking technology in several ways. First, it reminds us of the growing importance of family caregiver. In many industrialized countries they are becoming the "stress joint" holding the healthcare system together. Yet, they can easily be overlooked by researchers examining healthcare trends. Since the family caregiver as part of the U.S. healthcare delivery system is critical, their significance requires research attention from the analytic community. Second, this study finds both mobile health and social networking sites to play a nontrivial role in the mental health of family caregivers. This suggests the importance of focusing on how these new technologies can be used to further the accessibility to online support groups. Social networking is vital to caregivers without a spouse or significant other, serving as a therapeutic support system to "regroup" from caring functions, much important for mental-health and balance of life. Through Internet connectivity, the caregiver can interface with highly interactive social platforms, and find solace with other caregivers online. Finally, this research reinforces policy initiatives that facilitate better Internet services to citizens relying on cyberspace to connect with public and private-sector services, such as online health insurance forms, online libraries for health and medical information, among other supportive resources.

REFERENCES

AARP Public Policy Institute. (2011). *Valuing the invaluable: 2011 update the growing contributions and costs of family caregiving*. Retrieved July 13, 2012, from http://www.aarp.org/relationships/caregiving/info-07-2011/valuing-the-invaluable.html

Adams, N., Stubbs, V., & Woods, V. (2005). Psychological barriers to Internet usage among older adults in the U.K. *Medical Informatics and the Internet in Medicine*, *30*(1), 3–17. doi:10.1080/14639230500066876 PMID:16036626

Administration on Aging. (2011). Supporting family caregivers through Title III of the OAA (Research Brief No. 5). Retrieved July 12, 2013, from http://www.aoa.gov/AoARoot/Program_Results/docs/2011/AoA5_SupportFamilyCaregvrs.pdf

Center for Connected Health Policy. (2013). *What is telehealth?* Retrieved July 27, 2013, from http://cchpca.org/

Centers for Medicare & Medicaid Services. (2013). *Medicare program - general information*. Retrieved July 12, 2013, from http://www.cms.gov/

Commonwealth Fund. (2005). *Issue brief: A look at working-age caregivers' roles, health concerns, and need for support*. Retrieved November 2, 2010, from http://www.commonwealthfunorg

H. R. 2157. (2001). *Rural Health Care Improvement Act of 2001*. 107th Congress. 1st Session.

Kiecolt-Glaser, J., & Glaser, R. (2001). Stress and immunity: age enhances the risks. *Current Directions in Psychological Science*, *10*(1), 18–21. doi:10.1111/1467-8721.00105

King, G., Tomz, M., & Wittenberg, J. (2000). Making the most of statistical analysis: Improving interpretation and presentation. *American Journal of Political Science*, *44*(2), 347–361. doi:10.2307/2669316

Mack, K., & Thompson, L. (2001). *Data: Profiles, family caregivers of older persons: Adult children*. Georgetown University, The Center on an Aging Society.

Mossberger, K., Tolbert, C., & Gilbert, M. (2006). Race, concentrated poverty and information technology. *Urban Affairs Review, 41*(5), 583–620. doi:10.1177/1078087405283511

Mossberger, K., Tolbert, C., & McNeal, R. (2007). *Digital citizenship: The internet, society and participation.* Cambridge, MA: MIT Press.

Mossberger, K., Tolbert, C., & Stansbury, M. (2003). *Virtual inequality: Beyond the digital divide.* Washington, DC: Georgetown Press.

Murphy, K. (2005, June 30). *Aging surge poses challenge for states.* Retrieved June 3, 2013, from http://www.pewstates.org/projects/stateline/headlines/aging-surge-poses-challenge-for-states-85899389790

National Alliance for Caregiving. (2009). *Caregiving in the U.S. 2009.* Retrieved June 8, 2013, from http://www.caregiving.org/data/Caregiving_in_the_US_2009_full_report.pdf

National Telecommunications and Information Administration. (2011). *Digital nation: Expanding internet usage.* Retrieved March 15, 2012, from http://www.ntia.doc.gov/files/ntia/publications/ntia_internet_use_report_february_2011.pdf

Organisation for Economic Co-operation and Development (OECD). (2009). *The long-term care workforce: Overview and strategies to adapt supply to a growing demand.* Paris: OCED.

Pew Research Center's Internet & American Life Project. (2011, May 12). *The social life of health information, 2011.* Retrieved April 8, 2012, from http://www.pewinternet.org/Reports/2011/Social-Life-of-Health-Info.aspx

Pew Research Center's Internet & American Life Project. (2012a). *Mobile health 2012.* Retrieved March 9, 2013, from http://www.pewinternet.org/Reports/2012/Mobile-Health.aspx

Pew Research Center's Internet & American Life Project. (2012b). *Family caregivers online.* Retrieved February 10, 2013, from http://www.pewinternet.org/Reports/2012/Caregivers-online.aspx

Public Law 103-3. (1993). *Family and Medical Leave Act.*

Public Law 109-442. (2006). *Lifespan Respite Care Act.*

Public Law 110-246. (2008). *The Older Americans Act.*

Public Law (111-148). (2010). *Patient Protection and Affordable Care Act.*

Public Law 78-410. (1991). *Public Health Service Act.*

Public Law 89-73. (1965). *Older Americans Act.*

Rhodes, P., & Shaw, S. (1999). Informal care and terminal illness. *Health & Social Care in the Community, 7*(1), 39–50. doi:10.1046/j.1365-2524.1999.00147.x PMID:11560621

Schmeida, M. (2005). *Telehealth innovation in the American states.* Ann Arbor, MI: ProQuest.

Schmeida, M., & McNeal, R. (2007). The telehealth divide: disparities to searching public health information online. *Journal of Health Care for the Poor and Underserved, 18*(3), 637–647. doi:10.1353/hpu.2007.0068 PMID:17675719

Schmeida, M., & McNeal, R. (2013). Bridging the inequality gap to searching Medicare and Medicaid information online: An empirical analysis of e-government success 2002 through 2010. In J. Ramon Gil-Garcia (Ed.), *E-government success around the world: Cases, empirical studies, and practical recommendations.* Hershey, PA: IGI Global. doi:10.4018/978-1-4666-4173-0.ch004

Schulz, R., & Beach, S. (1999). Caregiving as a risk factor for mortality: The caregiver health effect study. *Journal of the American Medical Association*, 282(23), 2215–2219. doi:10.1001/jama.282.23.2215 PMID:10605972

Selwyn, N. (2004). Reconsidering political and popular understandings of the digital divide. *New Media & Society*, 6(3), 341–362. doi:10.1177/1461444804042519

Stajduhar, K., Funk, L., Toye, C., Grande, G., Aoun, S., & Todd, C. (2010). Part I: Home-based family caregiving at the end of life: A comprehensive review of quantitative research (1998-2008). *Palliative Medicine*, 24(6), 573–593. doi:10.1177/0269216310371412 PMID:20562171

Tong, R. (2007). Gender-based disparities east/west: Rethinking the burden of care in the United States and Taiwan. *Bioethics*, 21(9), 488–499. doi:10.1111/j.1467-8519.2007.00594.x PMID:17927625

U.S. Census Bureau. (2010, May). *The next four decades, the older population in the United States: 2010 to 2050*. Retrieved July 24, 2013, from http://www.census.gov/prod/2010pubs/p25-1138.pdf

U.S. Census Bureau. (2012). *The 2012 statistical abstract, the national databook*. Retrieved July 29, 2013, from http://www.census.gov/compendia/statab/cats/health_nutrition.html

Vestal, C. (2012). *Medicaid: a year of excruciating decisions*. Retrieved May 17, 2012, from www.stateline.org/live/prntable/story?contentId=624072

West, D., & Miller, E. (2006). The digital divide in public e-health: Barriers to accessibility and privacy in state health department web sites. *Journal of Health Care for the Poor and Underserved*, 17(3), 652–667. doi:10.1353/hpu.2006.0115 PMID:16960328

ADDITIONAL READING

Bell, B., Reddy, P., & Rainie, L. (2004). Rural areas and the Internet: rural Americans' Internet use has grown but they continue to lag behind others. Retrieved November 18, 2008, from http://www.pewinternet.org/pdfs/PIP_Rural_Report.pdf.

Brooks, E., Turvey, C., & Augusterfer, E. (2013). Provider barriers to telemental health: obstacles overcome, obstacles remaining. *Telemedicine Journal and e-Health*, 19(6), 433–437. doi:10.1089/tmj.2013.0068 PMID:23590176

Dugdale, A., Daly, A., Papandrea, F., & Maley, M. (2005). Accessing e-government: Challenges for citizens and organizations. *International Review of Administrative Sciences*, 71(1), 109–118. doi:10.1177/0020852305051687

Fujioka, Y., & Stewart, E. (2013). How do physicians discuss e-health with patients? The relationship of physicians' e-health beliefs to physician mediation styles. Do physicians discuss e-health with patients? *Health Communication*, 28(4), 317–328. doi:10.1080/10410236.2012.682971 PMID:22716050

Hage, E., Roo, J., van Offenbeek, M., & Boonstra, A. (2013). Implementation factors and their effect on e-health service adoption in rural communities: a systematic literature review. *BMC Health Services Research*, 13(1), 1–16. doi:10.1186/1472-6963-13-19 PMID:23311452

Hargittai, E., & Hinnant, A. (2008). Digital inequalities: Differences in young adults' use of the Internet. *Communication Research*, 35(5), 602–621. doi:10.1177/0093650208321782

Hitt, W., Low, G., Bird, T., & Ott, R. (2013). Telemedical cervical cancer screening to bridge Medicaid service care gap for rural women. *Telemedicine Journal and e-Health*, 19(5), 403–408. doi:10.1089/tmj.2012.0148 PMID:23600410

Huniche, L., Dinesen, B., Nielsen, C., Grann, O., & Toft, E. (2013). Patients' use of self-monitored readings for managing everyday life with COPD: a qualitative study. *Telemedicine Journal and e-Health, 19*(5), 396–402. doi:10.1089/tmj.2012.0135 PMID:23531094

Jacobus, C., & Lichtenstein, E. Cybernet Medical. (June, 2006). Telehealth outcomes. Retrieved March 25, 2007, from www.cybernetmedical.com/%22www.cybernetmedical.comwww.cybernetmedical.com

Jaglal, S., Haroun, V., Salbach, N., Hawker, G., Voth, J., & Lou, W. et al. (2013). Increasing access to chronic disease self-management programs in rural and remote communities using telehealth. *Telemedicine Journal and e-Health, 19*(6), 467–473. doi:10.1089/tmj.2012.0197 PMID:23570277

Kernaghan, K. (2005). Moving toward the virtual state: Integrating services and service channels for citizen-centered delivery. *International Review of Administrative Sciences, 71*(1), 119–131. doi:10.1177/0020852305051688

Koh, H., Brach, C., Harris, L., & Parchman, M. (2013). A proposed health literate care model would constitute a systems approach to improving patients' engagement in care. *Health Affairs, 32*(2), 357–367. doi:10.1377/hlthaff.2012.1205 PMID:23381529

McNeal, R., Hale, K., & Dotterweich, L. (2008). Citizen-government interaction and the internet: expectations and accomplishments in contact, quality and trust. *Journal of Information Technology & Politics, 5*(2), 213–229. doi:10.1080/19331680802298298

Mosier, J., & Sakles, J. (2013). Telebation: next generation telemedicine in remote airway management using current wireless technologies. *Telemedicine Journal and e-Health, 19*(2), 95–98. doi:10.1089/tmj.2012.0093 PMID:23215736

Office for the Advancement of Telehealth. (2001). 2001 Tele-medicine Report to Congress. http://telehealth.hrsa/gov

Paschou, M., Sakkopoulos, E., & Tsakalidis, A. (2013). easyHealthApps: e-health apps dynamic generation for smartphones & tablets. *Journal of Medical Systems, 37*(3), 1–12. doi:10.1007/s10916-013-9951-6 PMID:23666429

Sawyer, S., & Tapia, A. (2005). The sociotechnical nature of mobile computing work: evidence from a study of policing in the United States. *International Journal of Technology and Human Interaction, 1*(3), 1–14. doi:10.4018/jthi.2005070101

Stajduhar, K., Funk, L., & Outcalt, L. (2013). Family caregiver learning—how family caregivers learn to provide care at the end of life: A qualitative secondary analysis of four datasets. *Palliative Medicine, 27*(7), 657–664. doi:10.1177/0269216313487765 PMID:23695826

Stanley, L. D. (2003). Beyond access: psychosocial barrier to computer literacy. *The Information Society, 19*(5), 407–416. doi:10.1080/715720560

Steele, R., & Lo, A. (2013). Telehealth and ubiquitous computing for bandwidth-constrained rural and remote areas. *Personal and Ubiquitous Computing, 17*(3), 533–543. doi:10.1007/s00779-012-0506-5

Stover, S. (1999). *Rural internet connectivity*. Rural Policy Research Institute. Retrieved June 21, 2000, from http://www.rupi.org.

Stovers, S., Chapman, G., & Walters, J. (2004). Beyond community networking and CTCs: Access, development, and public policy. *Telecommunications Policy, 28*(7-8), 465–485. doi:10.1016/j.telpol.2004.05.008

Van Dijk, J., & Hacker, K. (2003). The digital divide as a complex and dynamic phenomenon. *The Information Society, 19*(4), 315–326. doi:10.1080/01972240309487

Vilaplana, J., Solsona, F., Abella, F., Filgueira, R., & Rius, J. (2013). The cloud paradigm applied to e-health. *BMC Medical Informatics and Decision Making*, *13*(3), 1–10. PMID:23496912

Waterson, P., Glenn, Y., & Eason, G. (2012). Preparing the ground for the 'paperless hospital': A case study of medical records management in a U.K. outpatient service department. *International Journal of Medical Informatics*, *81*(2), 114–129. doi:10.1016/j.ijmedinf.2011.10.011 PMID:22088601

KEY TERMS AND DEFINITIONS

Caregiver: An individual who provides nursing care and/ or companionship, assistance for another person, such as parent, spouse, child with a disability or chronically ill.

Facebook: Online social network service.

Information Literacy: The ability to determine which information found on the Internet is appropriate for a specific task.

LinkedIn: Social networking website for professional people.

Medicaid: Public health insurance program sponsored by the U.S. government for the impoverished of all age groups, for the blind, disabled, and medically needy considered impoverished. It is the second largest U.S. public health insurance program.

Medicare: Public health insurance program sponsored by the U.S. government for persons under 65 years of age with a certain disability, age 65 or older, and all age groups with End-Stage Renal Disease. It is the largest U.S. public health insurance program.

Mobile Caregiver: The use of advanced communication technology, such as the Internet or multifunctional cell phone for meeting caregiver function(s).

Technical Competency: Necessary skills to use hardware and software, such as typing and using a mouse.

Chapter 10
Nurses Using Social Media and Mobile Technology for Continuing Professional Development:
Case Studies from Australia

Carey Mather
University of Tasmania, Australia

Elizabeth Cummings
University of Tasmania, Australia

ABSTRACT

Continuing professional development is mandatory for all healthcare professionals in Australia. This chapter explores how the expectations of the regulatory and professional organisations of nursing and midwifery can be integrated within the profession by enrolled and registered nurses and midwives to meet the requirements and maintain their registrations. Using actual case studies as a basis, the chapter demonstrates how continuing professional development can be delivered as mobile or m-learning using social media or mobile technologies within this health profession. This chapter focuses on case studies from the Australian healthcare sector; however, it appears that similar issues arise in other countries and so the challenges and solutions described in the case studies can inform practice in other countries. It concludes by discussing the potential for continuing professional development m-learning into the future.

INTRODUCTION

Health professionals use a complex network of communication strategies to share important information within professions and multidisciplinary teams to improve patient or client outcomes and ensure high quality care is safely delivered. Building on the ubiquitous use of a variety of communication strategies can transform how continuing professional development (CPD) is delivered and accessed. By extending communication beyond the borders of the workplace it is

DOI: 10.4018/978-1-4666-6150-9.ch010

possible to improve access and enable a flexibility that is unprecedented. Regulatory authorities have provided direction and scope regarding what CPD is and how it can be achieved.

Social media and the use of mobile technologies is the way of the future for CPD of health professionals. CPD is mandatory for the 580,000 health professionals registered by the Australian Health Practitioner Regulation Agency (AHPRA). Annual evidence of compliance with the CPD Standard for each health profession is required to ensure competence is maintained. CPD is essential for health professionals to be contemporary in their knowledge and use best practice to ensure high quality and safe care. Additionally, it provides opportunities for practitioners to be exposed to innovation within their field. There are other less tangible benefits that include opportunities for interdisciplinary collaboration and networking with colleagues.

CONTINUING PROFESSIONAL DEVELOPMENT

In Australia, AHPRA regulates the practice of 15 health professional bodies, all members of which are required to undertake CPD on an annual basis. Each profession has its own standards, codes, guidelines and policies that describe the requirements necessary to meet AHPRA requirements for maintaining registration within the profession (AHPRA, 2013).

The Nursing and Midwifery Board of Australia (NMBA) is the professional body for nurses and midwives and they define continuing professional development or CPD as:

...the means by which members of the profession maintain, improve and broaden their knowledge, expertise and competence, and develop personal and professional qualities required through their professional lives. (NMBA, 2013, p1)

The NMBA CPD Registration Standard prescribes that there must be documented evidence of a minimum number of hours of CPD undertaken each year or per triennium, in areas relevant to the health professional (NMBA, 2013). It describes acceptable CPD activities that may be undertaken. CPD may include formal courses, conferences, or online learning. Self-directed programs that are planned and developed by individuals are acceptable provided they include reflection. Nurses are required to keep written documentation and verified evidence of compliance within a personal portfolio (NMBA, 2013).

The NMBA CPD Registration Standard supports a range of activities that can be undertaken as e-learning, using social media or mobile technologies (NMBA, 2013). The development of a range of digital technologies and the growth of social media ensure mobile technologies are well positioned over time to replace traditional learning and teaching models of CPD. Development and delivery of CPD opportunities to health professionals is only limited by imagination about the utility of social media and mobile technology as a strategy for achieving CPD requirements.

CPD is embedded within each of the Australian Nursing and Midwifery Council (ANMC, now NMBA) competency domains (ANMC, 2006). It is encapsulated in critical thinking and analysis (Domain 3, Element 4) that states nurses will "participate in ongoing professional development of self and others" (ANMC, 2006: p4).

Health informatics and health technology competency is now included in Standard 4 about program content of the Australian Nursing and Midwifery Council (ANMAC) Standards (ANMAC, 2012). ANMAC is the independent accrediting authority responsible for monitoring education providers and nursing and midwifery programs of study leading to registration or professional endorsement in Australia. There are accreditation assessment standards that must be attained to be authorised to develop curricula and assess student performance (ANMAC, 2012).

Information communication technology (ICT) competency is now embedded in each of the nine standards. They were written with the expectation that stakeholders will facilitate and provide the means to support the development of ICT literacy of student nurses. Additionally, ICT competency standards for Australia are currently being developed (Borycki, Foster, Sahama, Frisch, & Kushniruk, 2013; Staggers, Gassert, & Curran, 2002). The inclusion of health informatics and health technology has major implications for delivery of CPD using social media and mobile technologies with the current enrolled and registered nurse and midwifery workforce. CPD using m-learning approaches will need to focus on developing appropriate knowledge and skills of the current workforce in using this technology. Whereas the focus for new graduates will be ensuring they understand the legal and ethical implications of embedding these emerging technologies into their career and professional development.

Whilst the requirement for CPD is mandatory for all Australian healthcare professionals, this chapter is limited to discussion of the possibilities for enrolled and registered nurses, and midwives – referred to as healthcare professionals. It explores how the expectations of the regulatory and professional organisations of nursing and midwifery can be integrated within the profession by enrolled and registered nurses and midwives to meet the requirements and maintain their registrations. Furthermore, this chapter discusses the background to the current situation and using case studies from Australia will demonstrate how CPD can be delivered as m-learning using social media or mobile technologies within this health profession. It appears that similar issues arise in other countries and so the challenges and solutions of using social media and mobile technologies within health care settings may be transferrable.

TERMINOLOGY CONSIDERATIONS

There is a lack of standard definitions for describing terminology in informatics that enables easy discussion about using social media and mobile technology for CPD (Georgiev, Georgieva, & Smrikarov, 2004; Ruiz, Mintzer, & Leipzig, 2006). For the purpose of this chapter information communication technology is used to describe all branches of informatics and digital media. Subgroupings of health informatics also known as e-health and refers to clinical and health service delivery hardware, middleware and software. Health technology refers to web-based software and mobile applications to diagnose, monitor, treat or educate end-users. Kaplan and Haenlein (2010; 60) define Social media as "a group of internet-based applications that build on ideological and technological foundations of Web 2.0. and that allow the creation and exchange of User Generated Content". This definition encompasses a range of applications that include Facebook, YouTube, Flickr, Twitter and Instagram. New applications are constantly being created that include varying levels of social presence, media richness, self presentation and self-disclosure (Kaplan and Haenlein 2010). These classifications impact on the way social media is viewed in the literature. This description satisfactorily defines social media in this chapter.

M-health is a sub-grouping of e-health that relates to any mobile technology or computing used to interface with any stakeholder group involved with digital health service delivery or care (WHO, 2011). E-learning encompasses pedagogical frameworks that use the digital mediums for delivery and interaction. M-learning refers specifically to learning and teaching interaction that uses mobile hand-held devices such as electronic notebooks, tablets or smartphones (Traxler, 2007).

The use of the term connected health to describe digitally mediated healthcare by Wicklund (2013) has merit. Over time there will no longer be the need to distinguish ICT in health from mobile technology used to as a platform to learn in this environment.

The current lack of standard definitions to describe social media and mobile technologies requires further exploration. Consideration of the terms used and standardisation of terminology would improve communication and clarify meaning for researchers, health service providers, educators and other end-users of this emerging technology.

AUSTRALIAN POLICY DEVELOPMENT

There has been a significant increase in the development and use of ICT in healthcare at individual and systems levels (Abbott & Coenen, 2008; Smedley, 2005; While & Dewsberry, 2011). The rapid change in healthcare delivery and communication models has implications for different healthcare settings. A number of challenges and potential solutions in relation to meeting the needs of stakeholders within the healthcare sector in Australia have been outlined in the Australian National E-Health Strategy (Australian Health Ministers' Conference, 2008). An ICT skilled health workforce was identified as a key resource required to drive change and the adoption of technological solutions.

There is a requirement for the higher education sector and professional bodies to encourage and support their students and health professionals in gaining high quality educational experiences that support this changing environment (Bembridge, Levett-Jones, & Yeun-Sim Jeong, 2011; MacKay & Harding, 2009). Therefore, the development and provision of educational programs that meet and extend the demand and transference of ICT skills in the Australian workplace is imperative.

Additionally, digital platforms provide flexibility and e-learning CPD opportunities that were unavailable before the advent of the Australian Government's 'Digital Education Revolution' (DEEWR, 2008).

The introduction of the Australian Government's 'Digital Education Revolution' policy (2008) is particularly relevant to e-learning, CPD and the use of social media and mobile technologies (DEEWR, 2008). The policy reorientated secondary school students for post-secondary education and training, by routinely introducing them to digital media technologies (DEEWR, 2008; White, 2008). Literature regarding the use of digital technology in tertiary institutions, especially universities, suggests introducing students to the technology prior to attending the experiential environment (ALTC, 2008; Kenny, Neste-Kenny, Park, Burton, & Meiers, 2009; Mather, 2012b). By enabling the current nursing workforce to develop knowledge and skills in the use of social media and mobile technologies it is possible to foster collaboration and create opportunities to integrate student knowledge, skills and expectations to promote collegiality. Furthermore, offering m-learning CPD opportunities that are accessible within the clinical workplace can be used as a vehicle to model and engender life-long learning required by the profession (ACN, 2013a).

The capacity for health professionals to use digital platforms for CPD is mixed. There are a number of factors that currently impede or improve the likelihood of engagement of health professional use of mobile technologies for CPD (Mather, Marlow, & Cummings, 2013a). Reducing or minimising the barriers to using mobile platforms has the potential to globalise the health professions and create unprecedented inter-professional collaboration and CPD opportunities. By harnessing the capacity of digital technologies for CPD has the ability to accelerate the implementation of the national digital E-health strategy, meet the aims of ANMAC and support the aims and philosophy of the ANMC competency standards.

If the tertiary nursing education curriculum is to remain responsive to the changing clinical workplace environment and meet the needs of current and future nurses there is a need to develop, monitor and evaluate the usefulness of these emerging technologies within the clinical nursing environment. Furthermore, CPD opportunities must match current needs and plan for future requirements of nurses who work in a variety of urban and rural settings within Australia.

SPECIFIC CPD REQUIREMENTS FOR NURSES

The Nursing and Midwifery Board of Australia (NMBA, 2013) mandates that nurses and midwives registered in Australia will participate in at least 20 hours of CPD per year in each category. The NMBA CPD Registration Standard also prescribes that one hour of active learning will equal one hour of CPD. The CPD must be relevant to the nurse's context of practice. The standard also provides detailed information about the documentation required to enable it to be used as evidence. There is recommendation of the use of a portfolio for capturing elements required for completion of the CPD cycle (NMBA, 2013).

As clinical informatics becomes widespread within nursing environments there is an expectation that nurses are already, or will become familiar with e-health and m-health technologies as they are developed and implemented in the workplace. The personally controlled electronic health record (PCEHR) is an example of the Australian e-health strategy initiative (DoHA, 2013) that requires clinicians and consumers to have a functional understanding of computer and internet use. Nurses are expected to be advocates and assist potential registrants in becoming part of this user-centric mobile technology assisted initiative.

CPD in relation to the use of digital technologies is paramount to support clinicians in developing the necessary technical skills to undertake their role and function as nurses. Developing digitally supported CPD meets both the process and content requirements to be competent in decision-making regarding the use of digital technology. Digital technology, especially mobile platforms are easily accessible and can be used to meet CPD registration requirements. While accessing digital technology to complete CPD is not new, using mobile technology to deliver m-learning CPD through this media channel will become more popular. It will be multimedia supported, easily accessible, with flexible modes of delivery in real-time at workplaces.

IMPACT ON CPD OPPORTUNITIES

Workforce Considerations

Currently, CPD may be initiated by an individual health professional, facilitated by a supervisor or provided by an institution and undertaken or delivered at different levels (Lorenzo & Ittelson, 2005; Mason, Pegler, & Weller, 2004). Ownership of CPD can be invested with individuals, supervisors or companies (Lorenzo & Ittelson, 2005). However, within this framework there are workplace factors that impede CPD using traditional delivery models. These limitations include shift work, part-time employment, recreation leave, staffing skill mix and patient or client workload that make consistent, flexible or easy delivery of learning and teaching to support CPD difficult in the workplace (Mather, 2011, 2012b; Mather & Marlow, 2012). Additionally, geographic isolation can compound equity of access to CPD opportunities (Mather & Marlow, 2012). The advent of digital technologies and the growth of m-learning technologies is an attractive alternative for the development of e-learning CPD opportunities.

The expansion of CPD opportunities using social media and mobile technologies provides opportunities for health professionals bridge gaps of health technology knowledge and skills in the workplace. Use of social media and mobile technologies could enable health professionals to learn in situ, without the need for face-to-face tuition. Instruction on how to use new equipment or software could be undertaken remotely. Health professionals could obtain instructions from a supervisor as required, while learning how to master new skills or behaviour or gain feedback about performance (Kuiz et al., 2006). Additionally, the availability for browsing multimedia information for learning or being reminded about a topic could occur quickly and easily if access was provided by an organisation. Point and shoot collection of objects and artefacts could facilitate access to expert advice or opinion rapidly on a global scale. Observation or recording of activities could be undertaken for discussion, reflection or peer review after completion (Ruiz et al., 2006; While & Dewsberry, 2011). Mobile technology offers learners the opportunity to have control over the content, pace of learning and enable them to individualise their learning objectives. There is also potential for collaborative learning with health professionals from the same and different fields. Encouragement to collaborate to meet CPD requirements could be facilitated by organisations by supporting access to mobile devices and provision of easy access to data delivery (Kenny et al., 2009; Ruiz et al., 2006).

Generational Cohort Considerations

Brunetto, Farr-Wharton and Shacklock (2012) describe generational cohort differences that may influence the use of the digital media strategies for CPD. The average age of registered nurses in Australia, as with many countries, is increasing to the extent that in 2011 the average age was 44.4 years and 22% of all nurses were aged over 55 years (HWA, 2013a). Experienced registered nurses are more likely to be Baby Boomers or Generation X clinicians. These generations are acknowledged to be less likely to use digital technology for communication (Brunetto et al.,

2012; Windham, 2005) which may limit their uptake of e-learning opportunities. Mather et al. (2013b) identified that registered nurses need to be educationally prepared in ICT skills to be able to confidently engage in sharing information that would facilitate CPD.

Nelsey and Brownie (2012) describe the values and needs of Baby Boomers, X and Y generations that represent a large component of the nursing workforce (HWA, 2013a). Career aspirations of these groups are important when considering CPD opportunities and how social media or mobile technology could be adopted and integrated into their learning culture. Baby Boomers value learning and training opportunities while Generation X enjoy working independently and have a tendency to be self-reliant. Generation Y pursue life-long learning and are technologically advanced (Nelsey & Brownie, 2012).

Oblinger (2003), Oblinger and Oblinger (2005) and Skiba and Barton (2006) defined the age range of the 'digital native' or millennial generation described by Prensky (2001) as born between 1980 and the mid 1990s and are known as the Net generation or Millenials (Epstein & Howes, 2006). Millenials are accustomed to active, rather than passive, learning, preferring flexible and multi-faceted approaches than previous generations (ALTC, 2008). They tend to prefer online learning rather than the formal classroom approach but they need an interactive multimedia and multi-faceted approach to online educational delivery (Dede, 2005; Windham, 2005). Millenials are comfortable using computers for social networking and web interfacing, but that does not translate into them having the appropriate ICT skills required for use in the workplace (ALTC, 2008; Mather, 2012a). Additionally, this generation of nurses want information immediately and will seek answers through their computers or mobile phones rather than use other sources of media such as newspapers (Windham, 2005). These nurses are considered to be able to engage effectively and more widely through social networking and global communication services, than earlier generations. For them the notion of 'friendship' extends further than the geographical boundaries of where they live. The Internet opens networks beyond any local or national boundary, and enables a connectedness that was not available to previous generations of nurses (Dede, 2005).

Australian workplaces are increasingly an intergenerational mix of health professionals so it can be advantageous to harness the characteristics of generational cohorts to enhance or strengthen opportunities for undertaking CPD that uses m-learning technology in the workplace. This approach also provides secondary advantages that include improving collegiality, team work and mentoring within healthcare settings (Nelsey & Brownie, 2012).

Educational Considerations

Use of traditional models of punctuated access to learning opportunities to meet CPD can stifle the opportunities provided by real-time learning. Mobile computing offers multimedia access in real-time (Kenny et al., 2009; Kovachev, Aksakali, & Klamma, 2012; Lupton, 2012; Ruiz et al., 2006). Self-directed learning can be completed on the job as desired, rather than being completed later, away from the workplace. While it is not possible to complete more structured modules or courses during usual daily activities, by using mobile technologies, it is possible to collect and collate artefacts or learning objects as evidence that can be reviewed or reflected on once the shift is completed (Van der Rijt & Hoffman, 2013). Strategic use of mobile devices or software and applications will require re-orientation of learning behaviour and habits to change the culture of how CPD is undertaken. How and what evidence is accumulated has the opportunity to create a constant and consistent updating of knowledge and skills which can augment reflective processes that is a key behaviour required for e-learning to be effective (Kenny et al., 2009; Phillips, Kennedy, &

McNaught, 2012). This change in behaviour has the opportunity to revolutionise the workplace, create learning organisations (Senge, 1990) that are globally connected to best practice and expert opinion.

Technology Considerations

The availability of m-learning opportunities for CPD using social media and mobile technologies will continue to increase in parallel with the commercialisation of this technology. There will be a burgeoning increase in access to platforms to meet user demand. The main barrier to continued growth will be missing regulations regarding security, privacy and ownership of data issues (Treuer & Jenson, 2003). Similarly, issues of copyright, authenticity and access still need to be addressed and incorporated into any standards that are developed (ALTC, 2008; Treuer & Jenson, 2003). Potential users may lack the confidence, understanding or knowledge and skills to embark on using these platforms through fear of making mistakes that breach professional or workplace policies and guidelines (Mather, Marlow, & Cummings, 2013b). Additionally, some users may have concerns about data security and privacy issues associated with data storage and retrieval (ALTC, 2008). Lack of standardisation of terminology to describe use of these technologies, may also create issues that could impede uptake of m-learning by health professionals (Burgess, Bruns, & Hjort, 2013).

Access to mobile data services that provide sufficient bandwidth to support multimedia resources, sharing and storage of files need to be considered (Mather, 2011). Delivery support for m-learning may be problematic in some settings where healthcare facility policies and guidelines or geographic isolation may render access to data difficult (Mather et al., 2013b).

At an individual level, m-learning for CPD requires clinicians to have access to a mobile device, data support services, formal m-learning modules or a self-directed plan. The current choice of operating system, device, screen size, data storage, memory and battery life impact on the access to the type of m-learning users will choose. Furthermore as multimedia content delivery and creation becomes more complex so will the pressure for being competent with management of mobile learning interfaces. End users, such as health professionals, will be required to understand how keyboard, touch screen, stylus use and speech recognition assisted software operates as well as an understanding of the importance of data security.

Funding Considerations

The cost of investment to develop the infrastructure to support mobile technology is well recognised (Pagan, Higgs, & Cunningham, 2008). Pagan, Higgs and Cunningham (2008) reported that 3% of total Australian healthcare costs, or about $1-2 billion annually was spent on ICT. These estimates exclude expenditure specifically related to learning and teaching in the tertiary sector. The report stated that software based technologies will need to be developed to assist healthcare providers with understanding complex systems including educating and skilling medical professionals individually and in teams (Pagan et al., 2008).

Prior to embarking on m-learning CPD health professionals will need to consider the cost of any chosen mobile device, data support services, formal m-learning modules or a self-directed plan. They will need to consider their choice of operating system, screen size of the device, amount of data storage, memory and battery life that will impact on the access to the type of m-learning they can utilise. Furthermore, users will need to consider whether they are required to purchase a pre-paid or a data management contract from a commercial provider or whether their organisation will allow them to use the organisational data delivery provider.

THE NEXUS OF DIGITAL TECHNOLOGY AND EDUCATION TO SUPPORT CPD OPPORTUNITIES

Currently digital technology is used as a platform to offer a range of online CPD opportunities. Professional bodies such as the Australian Federation of Nurses (ANF) and the Australian College of Nursing (ACN) offer CPD portals to their members (ACN, 2013a; ANF, 2013). Commercial companies and education providers also offer a range of stand-alone digital educational opportunities for purchase that are endorsed by the ACN as meeting the CPD requirements (ACN, 2013b). Regardless of the supplier of e-learning to nurses, the majority of the digital CPD available is delivered as self-paced online modules that may include asynchronous discussion and submission of online assessments (ACN, 2013a; ANF, 2013). There are also national initiatives such as the Health Workforce Australia NHET-Sim program that utilises both face to face and online modules for completion of the program (HWA, 2013b). The majority of these fee-paying programs are yet to be adapted for tablet or smart phone use. Additionally these forms of CPD do not utilise social media or mobile technologies that could provide a level of connection that has previously been untapped.

Recently there has been an emergence of digital media research (Burgess et al., 2013), including a number of studies of undergraduate students (Kocoglu, 2008; MacKay & Harding, 2009; Mather, 2011, 2012b; Twomey, 2004) or health professional behaviour (Mather et al., 2013a, 2013b). Studies directly relating to the use of m-learning for CPD within a healthcare context are scant. The following case studies provide insights into the strengths and limitations of delivering m-learning for CPD in the clinical setting. The first relates to the implementation of e-portfolios to the experiential environment (Mather, 2011). The second describes the use of a social media platform to disseminate and share information (Mather et al., 2013a). The final case study demonstrates how the use of more than one m-learning platform can create a collaborative and connected learning community (Mather et al., 2013a).

Case Study 1. Use of Mobile Technology: E-Portfolios

One key factor in CPD is maintaining evidence of competence. Collation of evidence to meet the ANMC competency standards (ANMC, 2006) recognised by AHPRA can be facilitated through the use of an e-portfolio. Mobile technologies support a range of e-portfolio software that can be used as a repository and for documenting self-directed CPD (NMBA, 2013). Case study 1 demonstrates how the implementation and experience of e-portfolios as a user-centric mobile technology can be used to support learning outcomes.

E-portfolios are a function of the 'knowledge economy' with relevance across all industry sectors (ALTC, 2008). The technology is considered useful as increasing nurses' skills and competencies in ICT thereby better preparing them for the workplace to be more work ready at registration (Wade, Abrami, & Sclater, 2005). Used effectively e-portfolios can be an excellent tool for creating meaning and relevance to nurses exploring their professional interests and potential while in practice (ALTC, 2008). Capturing personal and professional development in an easily accessible format can enable individuals to make stronger links between their own aspirations and the within professional opportunities available (ALTC, 2008) A critical element for implementing the use of an e-portfolio is relevance throughout the learning and professional development of an individual and their portability, flexibility and adaptability that make them a usable tool in the workplace (Madden, 2007). An evaluation of the implementation

of an e-portfolio into the experiential environment of a foundation unit of a Bachelor of Nursing program in Australia was undertaken during 2010. The study provided valuable insights and uncovered assumptions about user understanding about ICT use.

This study was conducted across four campuses in two states of Australia. Students were allocated to approximately 250 placement agencies that included a range of healthcare environments. These were tertiary and district acute care services in hospitals, residential aged care facilities, multi-purpose health centres, general practice surgeries and community based health service settings. Organisations took one or up to 60 students depending on its size and the capacity to provide high quality supervision experience for students.

Prior to implementation of the technology there was the development of a range of learner support artefacts including face-to-face tutorials, web conferencing, media vignettes, narrated slide presentations, a user manual and fact sheets. Technical support was also provided prior and during the implementation phase.

Online surveys completed by students resulted in a response rate of 60% (311/511). Pre-implementation findings indicated that approximately half the students had not used a portfolio before. It was found that 82% of students used social media even though only 15% of respondents indicated they used file sharing sites such as Flickr, YouTube, Tumblr or Picasa. Eight percent of participants had their own website and only 2% had used an e-portfolio before.

The post-use findings indicated that 66% of students strongly agreed or agreed they liked the e-portfolio blog tool for reflection and 78% strongly agreed or agreed or the use of blogs enabled them to feel connected with peers. Furthermore, 65% of respondents strongly agreed or agreed that e-portfolios supported integration of knowledge and skills. Qualitative responses from students also indicated that more training in the use of the technology was required. Others indicated that security of data was cause for concern.

The findings of the evaluation indicated the assumption that students could utilise learning and teaching software was flawed. Furthermore the notion that students had a base-line understanding of computing and software terminology was ill-founded. Although the use of computers is ubiquitous in the environment it became apparent that although students used digital media for a variety of uses, it did not translate into understanding about the purpose of an e-portfolio.

This case study also demonstrated that lead-time and appropriate technical support were paramount for enabling appropriate use of the software within the clinical environment. Additionally, the development of applications suitable for tablet and smartphones have been developed since this study was completed (Mather, 2012b). Adapta-

tion of e-portfolios with mobile technology has improved access and the development of native applications will enhance usability.

The implications from this study for using m-learning for CPD include ensuring that health professionals have the opportunity to become familiar with the device and software to be used for delivery of the m-learning CPD. An e-portfolio is a recommended method for collection and collation of evidence. Therefore it is imperative that current practitioners gain understanding and access to this platform to support their CPD journey. The collection and storage of artefacts and objects in this repository will further increase the possibilities for collaboration and sharing of multimedia information. As millennial generation professionals embark on CPD, they will build on their digital knowledge and skills to create content that will be disseminated and shared using mobile technologies. It will be imperative that this generation of

Figure 1. Mobile technology supports the use of an e-portfolio for mobile learning

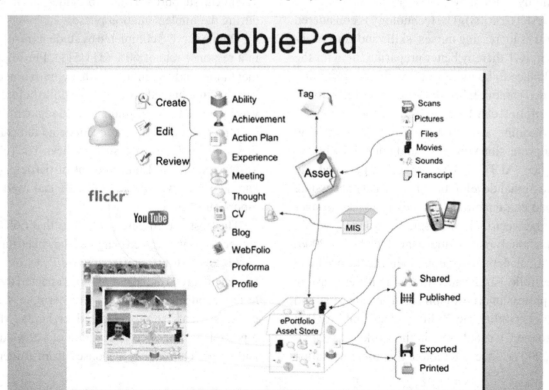

nurses are provided with a sound understanding of privacy and security issues surrounding any content captured or developed using mobile technology (Van der Rijt & Hoffman, 2013). As m-learning for CPD diffuses into the workplace repurposing artefacts and objects for peer learning will also be enabled. Health professionals will be able to demonstrate their commitment to maintaining their registration by documentation of their CPD plan, storage of artefacts and objects and inclusion of their learning through using a reflective practice within their e-portfolio.

Case Study 2. Use of Social Media: Micro Blogging

Self-directed learning is an acceptable method of CPD (NMBA, 2013). An evaluation of the implementation of using micro blogging for m-learning about clinical supervision for health professionals as self-directed CPD was undertaken during 2012. Initially 12 clinicians who undertook clinical supervision of students were identified and were offered the opportunity to attend workshops aimed at up-skilling and building confidence in the use of ICT. These clinically based practitioners were orientated to mobile technology and supplied with a tablet computer. They undertook workshops to learn how to use the micro blogging social media platform known as Twitter.

Twitter was chosen as it was free, easy to set up and use. Importantly this form of connection was limited to information transfer of 140 characters per interaction making it useful as a text message on any smartphone. These short messages were advantageous to users in rural areas where internet connectivity could be unreliable or slow (Mather & Marlow, 2012). Clinicians could choose to have messages directly pushed to their mobile telephone or accessed at an appropriate time via their hand held device or by computer. Depending on the settings, this software enabled the development of public or private communities and users could

search or follow topics, individuals or organisations of interest. Participants could choose whether they wanted to contribute or ignore any conversations or tweets. They could also disseminate information by sending or retweeting messages to others. The @PEPCommunity account was managed using a social media management tool known as Hootesuite. This software enabled scheduling dissemination of information of interest to clinical supervisors.

The micro blog data tweeted by participants was limited to sharing information about clinical supervision. The digital strategy focused on improving connectedness and increasing communication flow among group members. Discussion relating to personal data was not a focus of the strategy and no personal or sensitive data or information about patients, clients or health professionals was shared using this software platform.

The security of these data relied on the privacy controls provided and updated by the owners of the digital communication platform. However, participants could customise their own accounts to control the level of visibility that suited their needs. Participants from this University or its partner organizations were expected to adhere to the social media guidelines that outlined appropriate use and consequences of breaching confidentiality (RCNA, 2011; University of Tasmania, 2010).

Baseline data about current digital media use by clinicians was obtained by online questionnaire. These clinicians became key change agents for disseminating information about this digital communication strategy in their clinical environments. Additionally, two personal capture vignettes and four fact sheets about the digital communication strategy and how to join were developed and hosted on the clinical supervision webpage within the University website. Technical support was provided by an ICT consultant throughout the study. It was intended that these clinicians would promote cultural change by modelling the communication strategy in the

Figure 2. @PEPCommunity microblog showing information feed or 'tweets'

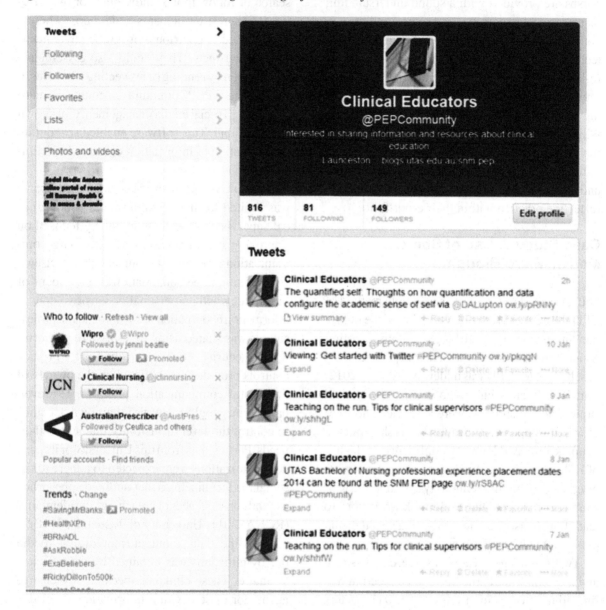

clinical environment. The digital media survey attracted 29 respondents and although numbers were low, it provided useful feedback about the clinicians that were prepared to be involved with the study. Over 66% of participants indicated they were aged over 46 years. Furthermore, 72% of respondents indicated they were from regional or rural areas. The remaining participants (24%)

were from urban environments. The majority of respondents (93%) indicated they had used the internet for more than 5 years.

During the study the micro blog @PEPCommunity account attracted 103 members or followers. The group consisted of 25 nurses known to be associated with the University and 18 other nurses. There were 16 academics involved of which 11 were identified as nurse academics. The remainder of participants were medical and allied health personnel involved with higher education or health organisations (n=27). There were 6 participants that were unidentified. TweetReach software indicated that the account content posted reached an average of 5000 accounts and 10 000 impressions per week. Of the 447 micro blogs posted or tweeted the content was evenly distributed between learning and teaching; students; practice tips; education; social media and clinical supervision.

Qualitative feedback about using this methodology was mixed. The majority of respondents indicated they liked receiving information from the micro blog few felt competent or comfortable with commenting or providing information. There were a small group (n=4) that were familiar with using Twitter. At interview they were enthusiastic about the potential reach of the platform. One respondent indicated it provided a connectedness

to the University that was previously lacking. This respondent indicated they followed up the information posted on the micro blog and retweeted information to their own networks.

Case Study 3. Use of Social Media and Mobile Technology to Support a Community of Practice for Peer Learning

As previously stated, self-directed learning is an acceptable method for accumulation of CPD hours (NMBA, 2013). An evaluation of the use of a blog and micro blogging to support and disseminate contemporary clinical supervision information as self-directed CPD was undertaken during 2012. It also provided a conduit to promote connectedness among this group of health professionals. The development of this Web 2.0 enhanced digital media strategy was to support the development of a community of practice of clinical supervisors.

Figure 3. Summary of micro blog key words by Vizify (Source: https://www.vizify.com/clinical-educators)

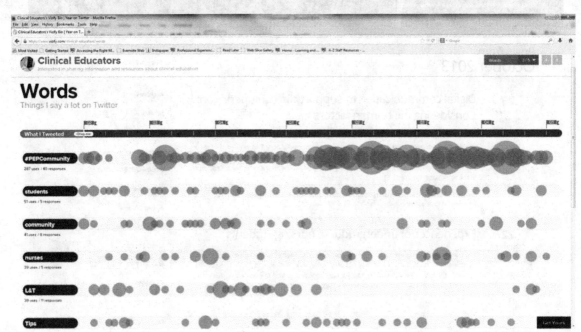

It was implemented to strengthen partnerships by information sharing and access to resources between the University, organizations, facilities and registered nurses who supervise students. The use of an asynchronous or synchronous digital methodology enabled feedback or information sharing to occur at the users' convenience.

The Professional Experience Placement blog was hosted by the University web service and Google Analytics were used to track visits to the blog content. Clinical supervisors were provided with a weekly précis of contemporary clinical supervision information via the blog. These updates matched the cycle of students attending the experiential environment during their course. Blogs were approximately 300-400 words each

and provided contemporary information about clinical supervision. Topics spanned the role, function and student-supervisor interface. It included scholarly discussion about orientation; preparedness; belongingness; or giving and receiving feedback. There was capacity to provide comment on the blogs and it also displayed a web link to the micro blog. Now, rather than relying on receiving information via their organization, registered nurses had the opportunity to choose to receive the information directly from the University through engaging with the blog or micro blog activity. Additionally, it enabled registered nurses to have access to information such as key dates that previously may have been sent to managers at organizations rather than the clinicians

Figure 4. Blog showing information posted about clinical supervision

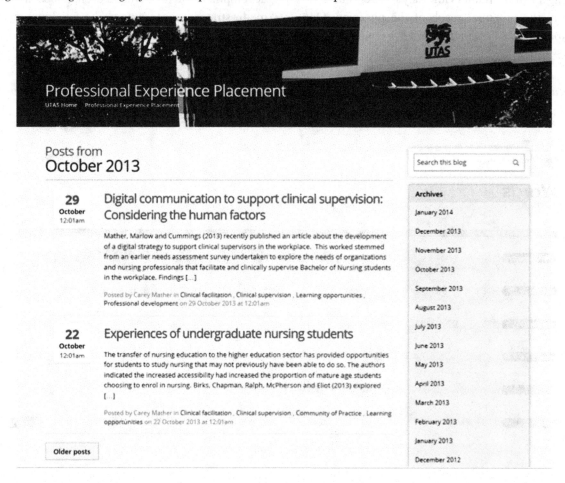

responsible for nurses. Registered nurses were able to access updates about changes within the BN curriculum that may impact on learning and teaching of students (Mather et al., 2013b).

During the first 12 months of the implementation of the blog, 67 blogs were published. Each new blog was announced on the micro blog, with a resulting spike in views recorded in the 24 hours after the broadcast. The blog page attracted an average of 60 page views per week; with an average viewing time of three minutes per visit. Visitors to the blog were global, however, the majority (70%) originated in Australia. Other regular visitors registered from Canada, United Kingdom, India, Philippines, Vietnam, Spain and Malaysia. Access to the micro blog was also available via a widget link on the blog web page.

Eighteen face-to-face interviews were conducted to elicit qualitative information about the development of the community of practice using

Web 2.0 technology. Findings from this evaluation highlighted a number of structural barriers for CPD that will need to be addressed prior to the large scale inception of CPD within the workplace. It was found that clinicians at some sites were unable to access the internet while at work. Hospital policy precluded the use of mobile technology during work time. Staff at other facilities reported that using mobile technology while working with patients or clients was considered poor role modelling and was discouraged as it demonstrated a lack of social presence in the workplace (Condon, 2013). Further discussion with regarding the issue uncovered a perception by a few of the community of practice members that some of their peers did not understand the capacity of the technology. Colleagues were unaware they could learn about clinical conditions or receive feedback and suggestions about patient or client care from peers or an expert external to

Figure 5. Google analytics captured information about blog use

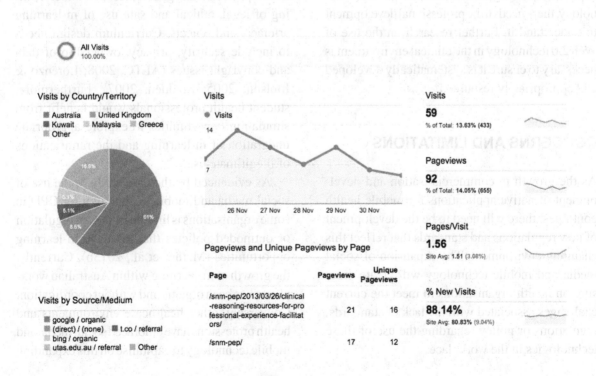

the organisation, while in the workplace. Some practitioners identified they lacked confidence in how to respond using the software platform while other practitioners reported they were satisfied with 'lurking' or being passive members of the group. They did not perceive they needed to post comments or messages to feel part of the group. There was a core group of participants that found the community of practice was beneficial for their learning. One respondent indicated they waited for the blog to be published each week. It was the only CPD they undertook regularly. They stated that as it was relevant to their role and function it was all they needed to remain contemporary in their practice as a nurse.

To increase equity of access to m-learning opportunities to augment and facilitate CPD opportunities, a change in organisational policy regarding Web 2.0 technology is required. Additionally, a cultural shift by health professionals in the perception of the uses of this technology needs to occur to enable legitimisation of its use for CPD in the workplace or in real-time. Ironically, to develop understanding about the capacity and capability of using social media and mobile technology, there needs to be professional development to understand it. Further research on the use of Web 2.0 technology in the clinical environment is necessary to ensure it is systematically developed and appropriately resourced.

CONCERNS AND LIMITATIONS

As the growth in commercialisation and development of native applications for mobile health continues, there will need to be the development of new regulations and standards that reflect this changing environment. The expansion of social media and mobile technology will create pressure on health organisations to meet the current challenges associated with the lack of standards, regulations or policy regarding the use of these technologies in the workplace.

In response there is a need for technology planning, enabling education, and fostering cultural change of health professionals, and empowerment of their staff to enable those organizations that do allow the personal use of m-learning supported devices, to be easily accessible and reliable. There needs to be parallel development of social etiquette and conduct within organisations that promote the potential of developing learning organisations. Educational institutions, professional bodies, CPD providers and health professionals need to become involved and fully conversant with policy development regarding security, privacy, ownership of data and copyright issues. All stakeholders have an important role in guiding current and future health professionals on effective and responsible use of social media and mobile technology use in the workplace, with control, access and standards for use being a major challenge (Lorenzo & Ittelson, 2005; Treuer & Jenson, 2003). It is therefore incumbent on educational institutions to introduce foundation information in their courses about ethical and legal issues surrounding this technology. They are vested with ensuring that health professionals gain a thorough understanding of legal, ethical and safe use of m-learning artefacts and objects. Curriculum design needs to include security, privacy, ownership of data and copyright issues (ALTC, 2008; Lorenzo & Ittelson, 2005; Madden, 2007). Furthermore, student health professionals would benefit from simulation opportunities to explore appropriate integration of m-learning and the ramifications of illegitimate use.

As evidenced by the case study 3, the use of social media and mobile technology for CPD in some organisations is limited by lack of regulation or outmoded policies that dissuade m-learning opportunities (Mather et al., 2013b). Currently, the growth of m-learning within Australian workplaces has been organic and without coordination. Conversely, other healthcare environments and health professions have embraced social media and mobile technology to capitalise on this expanding area of communication and interest in participatory healthcare by patients or clients (iHealthBeat, 2011; Ramsay Health Care, 2012). Case study 3 demonstrates there are opportunities for interested groups to develop discourse regarding a global or national approach to self-directed CPD opportunities using Web 2.0 technology. Once social media and m-learning is embedded as an accepted form of CPD there will be opportunities to develop novel and innovative approaches for a more structured approach for CPD that can attract formal recognition as acceptable m-learning in situ, in the workplace in real-time.

There are challenges that have been identified for preparing health professionals in developing understanding and skills in social media and mobile technology use. These factors included cost, maintenance and lack of training (Russin & Davis, 1990). An ageing workforce may initially impede the pace of integration of m-learning into the workplace. However, for the successful introduction of m-learning platforms, nurses must first acquire the necessary information, communication and technology program skills. One of the inherent dangers of embedding social media and mobile technology into the workplace for m-learning is that the technological novelty of the product could overshadow the purpose its introduction, resulting in the learning opportunities being subsumed by the technology itself (Kenny et al., 2009; Woodward & Nanlohy, 2004). Furthermore, as the pace for contemporary information increases and new information is rapidly available there will be a need for health professionals to filter information, and also demonstrate maintenance of currency in their area of specialisation.

FORMAL AND INFORMAL METHODS OF CPD

There are opportunities to undertake massive open online courses (MOOCs) (WDREC, 2013). These modules may be undertaken as web-based activities or can be adapted for mobile computing. Similarly there has been rapid development of mobile educational gaming opportunities (DiPietro, Ferdig, Boyer, & Black, 2007; Sánchez & Olivares, 2011). Completion of these formal courses or objects can be used as evidence to demonstrate CPD. This formal approach enables demonstration of evidence to meet the annual requirements for CPD.

Informal self-directed CPD may initially be more difficult to set-up, however there are advantages to using local context opportunities to learn in situ. Development of the knowledge and skills to develop a learning plan, documentation and recording evidence of learning will facilitate health professionals to create artefacts and objects using a range of Web 2.0 technologies will require commitment by health professionals. The use of point and shoot learning using mobile device embedded cameras will enable artefact creation. The generation of content to facilitate learning artefacts that can be shared and repurposed to maximise their use will become more popular. This informal strategy to promote learning opportunities that can be used for obtaining CPD hours may become more acceptable as mobile technology becomes more embedded in the workplace.

THE FUTURE OF M-LEARNING IN CPD

The nature and scope of the potential reach of human interface technology is being explored, however, there is much work to be undertaken if they are to become widely used or accepted (Davis, 2009). Growth and commercialisation within these digital technology fields is occurring more rapidly than incumbent 'mature' or Baby Boomer educators from the health sciences or education fields can innovate within the curriculum before further advances render it is superseded (Kurzweil, 2001; Moore, 1965; Skiba & Barton, 2006).

Simulation has been used to teach a range of skills such as beginning nurse communication and skills competency, at undergraduate and graduate levels (Nehring & Lashley, 2009). The scope of using mobile hosted human interface technology applications is broad. For example augmented reality technology can be used to support fundamental anatomy and physiology and complex skill development in the simulation skills laboratory or the experiential environment (Rolland, Wright, & Kancherla, 1996; Sherstyuk, Vincent, & Berg, 2008; Vilkoniene, 2009). As the development of applications that support augmented reality increase, so will the number of healthcare professionals who benefit from the learning and teaching opportunities the mobile augmented reality technology can provide (Mather, 2010). This technology can be used as an adjunct to traditional CPD and to enhance accepted technologies such as mannequin simulation or in situ learning in the practice environment (Mather, 2010). There is an urgency for educational providers to respond creatively in the development of m-learning artefacts and objects to engage current and future health professionals with m-learning opportunities that challenge and inspire them to remain contemporary and competent in their chosen fields (Kenny et al., 2009; Skiba & Barton, 2006).

Ausburn and Ausburn (2004) discuss the use of human interface technology within the industrial, technical instruction education environment. They critique the capabilities, limitations and effectiveness of human interface technology maintaining it is an important emerging technology where competence with complex technical skills is required. They state the technology has the capacity to re-orientate the m-learning environment (Ausburn & Ausburn, 2004). Human interface technology can enable healthcare professionals to gain an understanding of complex concepts and develop competence in cognitive and behavioural attributes that are desirable in their chosen profession (Ausburn & Ausburn, 2004; Georgiev et al., 2004; Ruiz et al., 2006).

By CPD becoming more embedded within the workplace, in situ learning in real-time will become faster and more collaborative. The creation of self-directed content that is shared between colleagues or interested others will be possible (Kenny et al., 2009). Increased opportunity for increased connectivity between nurses with similar interests will enable the use of social media to develop and sustain communities of practice. The rapid evolution of ideas and concepts will become more commonplace and feedback from experts and peers about performance support and knowledge will become possible (Mather et al., 2013a). Content creation and sharing between interested practitioners will encourage diffusion of information and innovations (Rogers, 1995; Sanson-Fisher, 2004). Collation of evidence, owned by the user, stored in e-repositories external to workplace and allowing access or sharing with colleagues and peers as necessary will be popular. Repurposing of artefacts and objects as learning tools among members will be widespread as m-learning for CPD will become more accessible and flexible.

CONCLUSION

In conclusion, social media and mobile technology will become embedded in healthcare and become part of what will be known as connected health, rather than remain with the fragmented terminology currently used to differentiate between the fields (Wicklund, 2013).

Recent Australian policy development regarding accountability and responsibility of health professionals to maintain their registration by demonstration of evidence of competency has provided opportunities to reorientate the CPD landscape. In conjunction with these changes has been the rapid expansion of social media and mobile technology that is now becoming embedded within healthcare. There are currently gaps in the knowledge and skills of health professionals to maximise the integration of this technology, to include CPD in the workplace. The lag in the development of standards, policies and guidelines related to legal and ethical issues, may be an advantage as there remains sufficient time to explore opportunities to reorientate CPD using this technology. Human interface technology, including wearable computing sensors and accelerometers, will be developed and will be used for feedback and provide mobile performance support (Lupton, 2012).

The introduction of mobile technology based CPD could promote life-long learning opportunities at the beginning of a nurse's career. Over time it will promote a cultural shift in how CPD is viewed and undertaken. The development and adaptation of mobile applications to facilitate reflective practice and enable the collation of a repository for storage of artefacts as evidence to demonstrate competency will become more refined. There will be further integration of CPD in real-time, rather than as an asynchronous entity conducted outside the workplace. M-learning using social media and mobile technology will become ubiquitous in the workplace.

Connected health is possible through the success of market penetration of mobile technology within healthcare and will exert pressure on healthcare professionals to adopt and keep up with the changing trends of digital technology use both within and external to the workplace. During the next 5 years it is predicted that commercialisation of e-health and m-health tools will become embedded within the healthcare settings (Walsh, 2013). To meet the demand for competent use of this technology, CPD providers will rapidly adapt to deliver e-learning opportunities through a range of mobile technology including tablet and smartphone applications rather than web-based software. To maintain competency in the workplace health professionals will need to embrace new ways of undertaking CPD. Learning in situ, in real-time with the assistance of augmented reality applications will be possible.

The possibilities of m-learning using social media and mobile technologies for CPD are bounded only by the limits of current technology and the pace of acceptance by health professionals and regulatory bodies as a legitimate strategy for learning.

REFERENCES

Abbott, P., & Coenen, A. (2008). Globalisation and advances in information and communication technologies: The impact of nursing and health. *Nursing Outlook, 56*(5), 238–246, 246.e2. doi:10.1016/j.outlook.2008.06.009 PMID:18922277

ACN. (2013a). *Continuing Professional Development*. Retrieved 23 July 2013, from http://www.nursing.edu.au/CPDh

ACN. (2013b). *External CPD providers*. Retrieved 23 July, from http://www.nursing.edu.au/CPDh

AHPRA. (2013). *Australian Health Practitioner Regulation Agency Registration Standards*. Retrieved 24 July 2013, from http://www.ahpra.gov.au/Registration/Registration-Standards.aspx

ALTC. (2008). *e-Portfolio use by university students in Australia: Informing excellence in policy and practice*. Australian E-Portfolio Project final Report. Retrieved 20 July 2011, from http://www.altc.edu.au/resources?text=Australian+E-Portfolio+Project

ANF. (2013). *Continuing Professional Education*. Retrieved 25 July 2013, from http://anf.org.au/pages/cpe

ANMAC. (2012). *Australian Nursing and Midwifery Accreditation Council Registered Nurse Accreditation Standards*. Retrieved 23 July 2013, from http://www.anmac.org.au/sites/default/files/documents/ANMAC_RN_Accreditation_Standards_2012.pdf

ANMC. (2006). *Australian Nursing and Midwifery Competency Standards for Nurses and Midwives*. Retrieved 26 February 2011, from http://www.nursingmidwiferyboard.gov.au/Codes-and-Guidelines.aspx

Ausburn, L., & Ausburn, F. (2004). Desktop Virtual Reality: A Powerful New Technology for Teaching and Research in Industrial Teacher Education. *Journal of Industrial Teacher Education, 41*(4), 33–58.

Australian Health Ministers' Conference. (2008). *National E-Health Strategy*. Author.

Bembridge, E., Levett-Jones, T., & Yeun-Sim Jeong, S. (2011). The transferability of information and communication technology skills from university to the workplace: A qualitative descriptive study. *Nurse Education Today, 31*(3), 245–252. doi:10.1016/j.nedt.2010.10.020 PMID:21093125

Borycki, E., Foster, J., Sahama, T., Frisch, N., & Kushniruk, A. (2013). Developing national level informatics competencies for undergraduate nurses: Methodological approaches from Australia and Canada. *Studies in Health Technology and Informatics, 183*, 345–349. PMID:23388312

Brunetto, Y., Farr-Wharton, R., & Shacklock, K. (2012). Communication, Training, wellbeing and commitment across generations. *Nursing Outlook, 60*(1), 7–15. doi:10.1016/j.outlook.2011.04.004 PMID:21703652

Burgess, J., Bruns, A., & Hjort, L. (2013). Emerging methods for digital research: An introduction. *Journal of Broadcasting & Electronic Media, 57*(1), 1–3. doi:10.1080/08838151.2012.761706

Condon, B. (2013). The present state of presence in technology. *Nursing Science Quarterly, 26*(1), 24–28. doi:10.1177/0894318412466738 PMID:23247344

Davis, R. (2009). Exploring Possibilities: Virtual Reality in Nursing Research. *Research and Theory for Nursing Practice: An International Journal, 23*(2), 133–147. doi:10.1891/1541-6577.23.2.133 PMID:19558028

Dede, C. (2005). *Planning for Neomillennial Learning Styles: Implications for Investments in Technology and Faculty*. Retrieved 30 July 2013, from www.educause.edu/educatingthenetgen

DEEWR. (2008). *Digital education revolution: Overview*. Retrieved 20 June 2013, from http://www.digitaleducationrevolution.gov.au/about.htm

DiPietro, M., Ferdig, R. E., Boyer, J., & Black, E. W. (2007). Towards a Framework for Understanding Electronic Educational Gaming. *Journal of Educational Multimedia and Hypermedia, 16*(3), 225–248.

DoHA. (2013). *Welcome to eHealth.gov.au*. Retrieved 25 July, from http://www.ehealth.gov.au/internet/ehealth/publishing.nsf/Content/home

Epstein, M., & Howes, P. (2006, September-October). The Millennial Generation: Recruiting, Retaining and Managing. *Today's CPA,* 66-75.

Georgiev, T., Georgieva, E., & Smrikarov, A. (2004). *M-Learning - A New Stage of E- Learning*. Paper presented at the ComSysTech'2004. New York, NY.

HWA. (2013a). Nurses in focus. *Australia's Health Workforce Series*. Retrieved 23 July 2013, from https://www.hwa.gov.au/sites/uploads/Nurses-in-Focus-FINAL.pdf

HWA. (2013b). NHETsim. *Training the Healthcare simulation community*. Retrieved 23 July, from http://www.nhet-sim.edu.au/

iHealthBeat. (2011). Mayo Clinic launches social networking site on health care issues. *iHealthBeat, 15*. Retrieved 17 August 2011, from http://www.ihealthbeat.org/articles/2011/7/15/mayo-clinic-launches-social-networking-site-on-health-care-issues.aspx

Kaplan, A. M., & Haenlein, M. (2010). Users of the world, unite! The challenges and opportunities of social media. *Business Horizons, 53*(1), 59–68. doi:10.1016/j.bushor.2009.09.003

Kenny, R., Neste-Kenny, J., Park, C., Burton, P., & Meiers, J. (2009). Mobile learning in Nursing practice education: Applying Koole's FRAME model. *Journal of Distance Education, 23*(3), 75–96.

Kocoglu, Z. (2008). Turkish EFL student teachers' perceptions on the role of Electronic portfolios in their professional development. *The Turkish Online Journal of Educational Technology, 7*, Article 8,

Kovachev, D., Aksakali, G., & Klamma, R. (2012). *A real-time collaboration-enabled Mobile Augmented Reality system with semantic multimedia*. Paper presented at the Collaborative Computing: Networking, Applications and Worksharing (CollaborateCom), 8th International Conference. Pittsburgh, PA. doi:10.4108/icst.collaboratecom.2012.25043610.4108/icst.collaboratecom.2012.250436

Kurzweil, R. (2001). Law of Accelerating returns. *KurzweilAI.net*. Retrieved 23 July 2013, from http://www.kurzweilai.net/articles/art0134.html?printable=1

Lorenzo, G., & Ittelson, G. (2005). An overview of e-portfolios. *Educause Learning Initiative*. Retrieved 14 February 2010, from www.educause.edu

Lupton, D. (2012). M-health and health promotion: The digital cyborg and surveillance society. *Social Theory & Health, 10*(3), 229–244. doi:10.1057/sth.2012.6

MacKay, B., & Harding, T. (2009). M-support: Keeping in touch on placement in primary health care settings. *Nursing Praxis in New Zealand Inc, 25*(2), 30–40. PMID:19928649

Madden, T. (2007). *Supporting student e-Portfolios: A physical sciences practice guide*. Hull, UK: Higher Education Academy Physical Sciences Centre.

Mason, R., Pegler, C., & Weller, M. (2004). E-portfolios: An assessment tool for online courses. *British Journal of Educational Technology, 35*(6), 717–727. doi:10.1111/j.1467-8535.2004.00429.x

Mather, C. A. (2010). *Human interface technology: Enhancing tertiary nursing education to ensure workplace readiness*. Paper presented at the International Technology, Education and Development Conference. New York, NY.

Mather, C. A. (2011). *E-portfolios: Lessons from an interdisciplinary collaboration: The School of nursing and Midwifery experience abstract*. Paper presented at the EDULEARN11 (3rd International Conference on Education and New Learning Technologies). Barcelona, Spain.

Mather, C. A. (2012a). An Interdisciplinary evaluation of an e-portfolio: WIL at the University of Tasmania. In C. Simmons, W. Sher, A. Williams, & T. Levett-Jones (Eds.), *Workready. E-portfolios to support professional placements in nursing and construction management degrees in Australia* (pp. 73–88). Sydney: Office for Learning and Teaching.

Mather, C. A. (2012b). *Embedding an e-portfolio into a work Integrated learning environment: The School of Nursing and Midwifery experience.* Paper presented at the EDULEARN12 (4th International Conference on Education and New Learning Technologies). Barcelona, Spain.

Mather, C. A., & Marlow, A. (2012). Audio teleconferencing: Creative use of a forgotten innovation. *Contemporary Nurse, 41*(2), 177–183. doi:10.5172/conu.2012.41.2.177 PMID:22800383

Mather, C. A., Marlow, A., & Cummings, E. (2013a). Digital communication to support clinical supervision: Considering the human factors. *Studies in Health Technology and Informatics, 194*, 160–165. PMID:23941949

Mather, C. A., Marlow, A., & Cummings, E. (2013b). *Web 2.0 strategies to enhance support of clinical supervisors of undergraduate nursing students: An Australian experience.* Paper presented at the EDULEARN13 (5th International Conference on Education and New Learning Technologies). New York, NY.

Moore, G. (1965). Cramming more components into integrated circuits. *Electronics, 38*(8), 114.

Nehring, W., & Lashley, F. (2009). Nursing Simulation: A Review of the Past 40 Years. *Simulation & Gaming, 40*(4), 528–552. doi:10.1177/1046878109332282

Nelsey, L., & Brownie, S. (2012). Effective leadership, teamwork and mentoring – Essential elements in promoting generational cohesion in the nursing workforce and retaining nurses. *Collegian (Royal College of Nursing, Australia), 19*(4), 197–202. doi:10.1016/j.colegn.2012.03.002 PMID:23362605

NMBA. (2013). *Nursing and Midwifery Continuing Professional Development Registration Standard.* Retrieved 23 July 2013, from http://www.nursingmidwiferyboard.gov.au/Registration-Standards.aspx

Oblinger, D. (2003). Boomers, Gen-Xers and Millenials: Understanding the New Students. *Educause Review.* Retrieved 14 February 2010, from www.educause.edu/educatingthenetgen

Oblinger, D., & Oblinger, J. (2005). *Educating the Net Generation.* Retrieved 23 December 2009, from http://www.educause.edu/educatingthenetgen

Pagan, J., Higgs, P., & Cunningham, S. (2008). *Getting Creative in Healthcare: The contribution of creative activities to Australian Healthcare.* Retrieved 23 july 2013, from http://eprints.qut.edu.au/14757/

Phillips, R., Kennedy, G., & McNaught, C. (2012). The role of theory in learning technology evaluation research. *Australasian Journal of Educational Technology, 28*(7), 1103–1118.

Prensky, M. (2001). Digital Natives, Digital Immigrants On the Horizon. MCB University Press, 9(5).

Ramsay Health Care. (2012). *Ramsay Health Care's Social Media Policy.* Retrieved 6 May 2013, from http://www.youtube.com/watch?v=f-xo0237n6U

RCNA. (2011). *RCNA Social Media Guidelines for Nurses.* Canberra, Australia: Royal College of Nursing Australia.

Rogers, E. (1995). *Diffusion of Innovations* (5th ed.). New York: Free Press.

Rolland, J., Wright, D., & Kancherla, A. (1996). Towards a Novel Augmented-Reality Tool to Visualise Dynamic 3-D Anatomy. In J. Westwood, S. Westwood, L. Felländer-Tsai, R. Haluck, R. Robb, S. Senger, & K. Vosburgh (Eds.), *Medicine Meets Virtual Reality: Global healthcare grid* (pp. 337–348). Washington, DC: IOS Press.

Ruiz, J., Mintzer, M., & Leipzig, R. (2006). The impact of E-learning in medical education. *Academic Medicine*, *81*(3), 207–212. doi:10.1097/00001888-200603000-00002 PMID:16501260

Russin, M., & Davis, J. (1990). Continuing education electronic bulletin board system: Provider readiness and interest. *Journal of Continuing Education in Nursing*, *21*(1), 23–27. PMID:2106537

Sánchez, J., & Olivares, R. (2011). Problem solving and collaboration using mobile serious games. *Computers & Education*, *57*(3), 1943–1952. doi:10.1016/j.compedu.2011.04.012

Sanson-Fisher, R. (2004). Diffusion of innovation theory for clinical change. *The Medical Journal of Australia*, *180*, S55–S56. PMID:15012582

Senge, P. M. (1990). *The Fifth Discipline*. New York: Doubleday/Currency.

Sherstyuk, A., Vincent, D., & Berg, B. (2008). *Creating Mixed Reality Manikins for Medical Education*. Paper presented at the Artificial Reality and Telexistance (ICAT, 2008). Yokohoma, Japan.

Skiba, D., & Barton, A. (2006). Adapting your Teaching to Accommodate the Net Generation of Learners. *The Online Journal of Issues in Nursing*, *11*(2), Manuscript 4.

Smedley, A. (2005). The importance of informatics competencies in Nursing: An Australian Perspective. *Computers, Informatics, Nursing. CIN*, *23*(2), 106–110. PMID:15772512

Staggers, N., Gassert, C., & Curran, C. (2002). A Delphi study to determine Informatics competencies for nurses at four levels of practice. *Nursing Research*, *51*(6), 383–390. doi:10.1097/00006199-200211000-00006 PMID:12464758

Traxler, J. (2007). Defining, discussing and evaluating mobile learning: The moving Finger writes and having writ. *International Review of Research in Open and Distance Learning*, *8*(2), 67–75.

Treuer, P., & Jenson, J. (2003). Electronic Portfolios Need Standards to Thrive: The proliferation of e-portfolio applications requires compatible software and design standards to support lifelong learning. *EDUCAUSE Quarterly*, *2*, 34–42.

Twomey, A. (2004). Web-based teaching in nursing: Lessons from the literature. *Nurse Education Today*, *24*(6), 452–458. doi:10.1016/j.nedt.2004.04.010 PMID:15312954

University of Tasmania. (2010). *Social Media Guidelines*. Retrieved 15 January 2013, from http://www.utas.edu.au/__data/assets/pdf_file/0007/82843/Social-Media-Guidelines.pdf

Van der Rijt, R., & Hoffman, S. (2013). Ethical considerations of clinical photography in an area of emerging technology and smartphones. *Journal of Medical Ethics*. PMID:23800451

Vilkoniene, M. (2009). Influence of augmented reality technology upon pupils' knowledge about human digestive system: The results of the experiment. *US-China Education Review*, *6*(1), 36–43.

Wade, A., Abrami, P., & Sclater, J. (2005). An Electronic Portfolio to Support Learning. *Canadian Journal of Learning and Technology*, *31*(3).

Walsh, B. (2013). *mHealth market poised for explosive growth*. Retrieved 25 July, from http://www.clinical-innovation.com/topics/mobile-tele-health/mhealth-market-poised-explosive-growth

WDREC. (2013). *Understanding Dementia Free online course*. Retrieved 23 July 2013, from http://www.utas.edu.au/wicking/wca/mooc

While, A., & Dewsberry, G. (2011). Nursing and information and communication technology (ICT), A discussion of trends and future directions. *International Journal of Nursing Studies, 48*(10), 1302–1310. doi:10.1016/j.ijnurstu.2011.02.020 PMID:21474135

White, G. (2008). *Digital learning: An Australian research agenda*. Retrieved 24 July 2013, from www.acer.edu.au/documents/TLL_DigitalLearn-ingResearch.doc

WHO. (2011). *mHealth: New Horizons for health through mobile technologies: Second survey on ehealth*. Retrieved 23 July 2013, from http://www.who.int/goe/publications/goe_mhealth_web.pdf

Wicklund, R. (2013). When mhealth and telehealth become just healthcare. *Government Health IT*. Retrieved 26 July 2013, from http://www.gov-healthit.com/news/when-mhealth-and-telehealth-become-just-healthcare

Windham, C. (2005). The Student's Perspective. *Educating the Net Generation, Educause*. Retrieved 14 February 2010, from www.educause.edu/educatingthenetgen

Woodward, H., & Nanlohy, P. (2004). Digital portfolios: Fact or fashion? *Assessment & Evaluation in Higher Education, 29*(2), 228–238. doi:10.1080/0260293042000188492

ADDITIONAL READING

Abbott, P., & Coenen, A. (2008). Globalisation and advances in information and communication technologies: The impact of nursing and health. *Nursing Outlook, 56*(5), 238–246, 246.e2. doi:10.1016/j.outlook.2008.06.009 PMID:18922277

Bembridge, E., Levett-Jones, T., & Yeun-Sim Jeong, S. (2011). The transferability of information and communication technology skills from university to the workplace: A qualitative descriptive study. *Nurse Education Today, 31*(3), 245–252. doi:10.1016/j.nedt.2010.10.020 PMID:21093125

Borycki, E., Foster, J., Sahama, T., Frisch, N., & Kushniruk, A. (2013). Developing national level informatics competencies for undergraduate nurses: methodological approaches from Australia and Canada. *Studies in Health Technology and Informatics, 183*, 345–349. PMID:23388312

Brunetto, Y., Farr-Wharton, R., & Shacklock, K. (2012). Communication, Training, wellbeing and commitment across generations. *Nursing Outlook, 60*(1), 7–15. doi:10.1016/j.outlook.2011.04.004 PMID:21703652

Condon, B. (2013). The present state of presence in technology. *Nursing Science Quarterly, 26*(1), 24–28. doi:10.1177/0894318412466738 PMID:23247344

Davis, R. (2009). Exploring Possibilities: Virtual Reality in Nursing Research. *Research and Theory for Nursing Practice: An International Journal, 23*(2), 133–147. doi:10.1891/1541-6577.23.2.133 PMID:19558028

Dede, C. (2005). Planning for Neomillennial Learning Styles: Implications for Investments in Technology and Faculty Retrieved 30 July 2013, from www.educause.edu/educatingthenetgen

Duncan, I., Yarwood-Ross, L., & Haigh, C. (2013). YouTube as a source of clinical skills education. Nurse Education Today. In Press Available online 14 January 2013.

Farr-Wharton, R., Brunetto, Y., & Shacklock, K. (2012). The use of intuition nurse-supervisor relationships and the impact on empowerment and affective commitment. *Journal of Advanced Nursing*, 68(6), 1391–1401. doi:10.1111/j.1365-2648.2011.05852.x PMID:22032539

Househ, M. (2013). The use of Social media in healthcare: organisational, clinical and patient perspectives. *Studies in Health Technology and Informatics*, 183, 244–248. PMID:23388291

Kaplan, A. M., & Haenlein, M. (2010). Users of the world, unite! The challenges and opportunities of social media. *Business Horizons*, 53(1), 59–68. doi:10.1016/j.bushor.2009.09.003

Kenny, R., Neste-Kenny, J., Park, C., Burton, P., & Meiers, J. (2009). Mobile learning in Nursing practice education: Applying Koole's FRAME model. *Journal of Distance Education*, 23(3), 75–96.

Lupton, D. (2012). M-health and health promotion: The digital cyborg and surveillance society. *Social Theory & Health*, 10(3), 229–244. doi:10.1057/sth.2012.6

MacKay, B., & Harding, T. (2009). M-support: Keeping in touch on placement in primary health care settings. *Nursing Praxis in New Zealand Inc*, 25(2), 30–40. PMID:19928649

Mather, C. A., & Marlow, A. (2012). Audio teleconferencing: Creative use of a forgotten innovation. *Contemporary Nurse*, 41(2), 177–183. doi:10.5172/conu.2012.41.2.177 PMID:22800383

Mather, C. A., Marlow, A., & Cummings, E. (2013). Web 2.0 strategies to enhance support of clinical supervisors of undergraduate nursing students: An Australian experience. Paper presented at the EDULEARN13 (5th International Conference on Education and New Learning Technologies).

McLean, R., Richards, B. H., & Wardman, J. (2007). The effect of Web 2.0 on the future of medical practice and education: Darwinian evolution or folksonomic revolution. *The Medical Journal of Australia*, 187, 174–177. PMID:17680746

Periera, R., Baranauskas, M. C., & da Silva, S. R. P. (2010). A discussion on social software: Concepts, building blocks and challenges. *International Journal for Informatics*, 3(4), 382–391.

Phillips, R., Kennedy, G., & McNaught, C. (2012). The role of theory in learning technology evaluation research. *Australasian Journal of Educational Technology*, 28(7), 1103–1118.

Salminen, L., Stolt, M., Saarikoski, M., Suikkala, A., Vaartio, H., & Leino-Kilpi, H. (2010). Future challenges for nursing education - A European perspective. *Nurse Education Today*, 30(3), 233–238. doi:10.1016/j.nedt.2009.11.004 PMID:20005606

Sharples, M., Taylor, J., & Vavoula, G. (2005). *Towards a theory of Mobile learning* Paper presented at the mLearn 2005, Cape Town, South Africa.

Sherstyuk, A., Vincent, D., & Berg, B. (2008, December 01-03). Creating Mixed Reality Manikins for Medical Education. Paper presented at the Artificial Reality and Telexistance (ICAT, 2008), Yokohoma, Japan.

Skiba, D., & Barton, A. (2006). Adapting your Teaching to Accommodate the Net Generation of Learners. *The Online Journal of Issues in Nursing*, 11(2), Manuscript 4.

Smedley, A. (2005). The importance of informatics competencies in Nursing: An Australian Perspective. Computers, Informatics, Nursing. *CIN, 23*(2), 106–110. PMID:15772512

Strickland, K., Adamson, E., McInally, W., Tiittanen, H., & Metcalfe, S. (2013, Oct). Developing global citizenship online: An authentic alternative to overseas clinical placement. *Nurse Education Today, 33*(10), 1160–1165. doi:10.1016/j.nedt.2012.11.016 PMID:23260621

Traxler, J. (2007). Defining, discussing and evaluating mobile learning: The moving Finger writes and having writ. *International Review of Research in Open and Distance Learning, 8*(2), 67–75.

Treuer, P., & Jenson, J. (2003). Electronic Portfolios Need Standards to Thrive: The proliferation of e-portfolio applications requires compatible software and design standards to support lifelong learning. *EDUCAUSE Quarterly, 2*, 34–42.

Van der Rijt, R., & Hoffman, S. (2013). Ethical considerations of clinical photography in an area of emerging technology and smartphones. Journal of Medical Ethics, Published Online First 25 June 2013

WHO. (2011). mHealth: New Horizons for health through mobile technologies: second survey on ehealth [Electronic Version]. Retrieved 23 July 2013, from http://www.who.int/goe/publications/goe_mhealth_web.pdf

Wicklund, R. (2013). When mhealth and telehealth become just healthcare [Electronic Version]. Government Health IT. Retrieved 26 July 2013, from http://www.govhealthit.com/news/when-mhealth-and-telehealth-become-just-healthcare

Wilson, R., Ranse, J., Cashin, A., & McNamara, P. (2013). Nurses and Twitter: The Good, the bad and the reluctant. Collegian, Early Online 1 November 2013.

KEY TERMS AND DEFINITIONS

Health Technology Competency: As for technology competency but with a specific focus on the health industry.

M-Health: Relates to any mobile technology or computing used to interface with any stakeholder group involved with digital health service delivery or care.

Micro Blogging: Allows subscribers to use a web service to broadcast short posts to other subscribers.

M-Learning: Refers specifically to learning and teaching interaction that uses mobile handheld devices such as electronic notebooks, tablets or smartphones.

Technology Competency: Observable and measurable factors representing the knowledge and skills in relation to the use of technology that are required for performing and supporting the underlying required work processes.

Chapter 11
An Android Mobile-Based Environmental Health Information Source for Malaysian Context

Lau Tiu Chung
Swinburne University of Technology – Sarawak, Malaysia

Lau Bee Theng
Swinburne University of Technology – Sarawak, Malaysia

H. Lee Seldon
Multimedia University, Malaysia

ABSTRACT

An anticipated research activity in healthcare is the involvement of populations and social media to identify health problems, including environmental ones. In this chapter, the authors propose an Android mobile-based system for collection and targeted distribution of the latest alerts and real-time environmental factors to the Malaysian population. This mobile system is designed to facilitate and encourage research into environmental health quality issues by providing a comprehensive tracking and monitoring tool correlated to social media networks. This system is embedded with Google Maps and Geocoding services to visualize the location and environmental health reports from the aggregated social media news feeds; the output is also shared across the social media networks.

INTRODUCTION

Social media networks help in creating big impact and public awareness toward environmental health tracking and monitoring. Tracking disease through online activity has been done before; Google found that search terms were good indicators of flu activity in 2008 and 2009 (Lowensohn, 2008; Google, 2012). Later Google introduced public estimation for flu activity through Google flu tracking system. Unlike basic internet searches from traditional search engines like Google or

DOI: 10.4018/978-1-4666-6150-9.ch011

Yahoo, social media networks seem to have introduced crowd-sharing and posting information across the given platforms. "Traditional" search requests are generally motivated only by a desire to learn more about given subject, such as infectious disease and healthcare topics, but social media networks seem to be motivated by the desire to gain more popularity by doing what one's friends do. For example, if haze is forming near one's living location, the person can easily make a short written post on Facebook or Twitter, so the short written post can ideally "go viral" and be exposed to others in the social media network. In other words, social media networks inherently explore more contexts to the individual's situation surrounding them. For someone who reads and writes a lot about the environment, Twitter and Facebook provide a great way to keep track of what others in the same field are working on.

Social media network is nowadays inseparable from Mobile. With smart phone usage projected to grow exponentially across the region, and with mobile data speeds increasing, and with the roll-out of wireless internet services and social media networks improving their mobile offering, social networking is becoming more mobile-oriented by nature (Firefly, 2012). There is no denying that the growth of social networking cannot be separated from increasing mobility, and will only be fuelled further by the advance of the smart phone in consumer's lives. So does the growth of the smart phone and increased mobility signify a new phase or dimension for social media? These situations imply and drive mobile users' behavior towards the way they receive environmental health information.

In this research, the establishment of an Android mobile-based environmental health information system associated with social media networks will play a key role in helping to provide the information needed to ideally improve public health. This paper presents several study areas such as environmental health tracking, the use of social media networks in tracking diseases, the social media network in RSS, and the use of mobile health technologies in Malaysia. Besides, it also includes the proposed solutions such as multi-tier architecture that used in developing Android mobile applications, word level n-gram approach used to match social media text inputs against a dictionary of known patterns, integrated environmental health ontological model in Malaysian context adopted in Android mobile-based environmental health information system, and the evaluation of system accuracy testing results.

BACKGROUND

In the past, many environmental health issues were not delivered to the public efficiently. The print and television press often did not headline environmental news. The mobile technologies revolution in the late 1990s mostly served the purpose of providing voice communication over the phone. People were passive consumers of news reports about environmental health hazards, seldom ones which could affect their own health.

In the early 2000s several studies of environmental health tracking tools were established with a main goal: to protect communities by providing federal, state, and local agencies with information they could use to plan, apply and evaluate environmental health actions (California Environmental Health Investigation Branch, 2012; Center for Disease Control and Prevention, 2010; European Environment Agency, 2011; Freifeld & Brownstein, 2007; Wisconsin Department of Health Services, 2011). While existing environmental health surveillance systems have been proven to serve as an effective mode for spreading health information to their respective users, the idea of "borderless" information dissemination should be also considered.

The Rise of Environmental Health Tracking

Environmental health tracking is the on-going, systematic collection, integration, analysis, interpretation, and dissemination of data from monitoring of environmental hazards and health effects (California Environmental Health Investigation Branch, 2012; Center for Disease Control and Prevention, 2012; HealthMap, 2012; New York Department of Health, 2009).The component parts of environmental health tracking are hazard identification and mapping, exposure assessment and quantification, development of biomonitoring, systematic review of health outcomes and disease surveillance, horizon scanning, and development of environment and health indicators (Health Protection Agency, 2012).

Environmental health tracking serves to protect the health of people by monitoring environmental contaminants and their related diseases, study the impact of these contaminants on human health, and inform the public about how to best protect their health from harmful pollutants (California Environmental Health Investigation Branch, 2012). It is interesting to know that checking the weather forecast every morning may help one with more than just deciding which clothes to wear; it may help one to prepare for how one feels that day, health wise. Weather forecasts may show a high level of humidity which may lead to headache or acne in certain people if they do not prepare themselves in advance. In this particular research context, environmental health tracking is a type of surveillance that endeavours to bring together specific health and environmental monitoring data in Malaysia from a number of different online media news.

The Use of Social Media Networks in Tracking Diseases

Social media has been widely used to predict some desirable results such as weekend box office takings for movies and elections (Taylor, 2013). However, a social media network in tracking disease raised curiosity and attention in public and health officials. Many serious researchers are becoming more interested in the reliability of social media in delivering quality health messages to the public (Avnet, 2013). According to Schmidt (2012), traditional flu surveillance by the Center for Disease Control and prevention (CDC) relies on outpatient reporting and virological test results supplied by laboratories nationwide. However, the system confirms outbreaks within about two weeks after they begin, but social media can flag more immediate concerns and actions. Tweets with location information may allow officials to plot points on a map to detect a trend, then alert providers to gear up for a possible outbreak (Bautista, 2013). Besides, the use of Twitter to track levels of disease activity and public concern in the U.S. during the Influenza A H1N1 pandemic in 2009 by several researchers has demonstrated that Twitter traffic can be used not only descriptively, i.e. to track users' interests and concerns related to H1N1 influenza, but also to estimate disease activity in real time, i.e., one to two weeks faster than current practice allows. According to Taylor (2013), 250,000 social media users in U.S said they got the flu. To make use of Twitter as a source of collecting environmental health data can be very impressive due to volume and speed. One interesting statistic is that 87.9% of Malaysians has internet access via Facebook (Factbroser.com, 2012), Another fact is that Malaysia's mobile penetration is more than 100%, compared to 59% for internet and 41% for social media (Factbroser.com, 2012).

Social Media Network in RSS

Social media networks are becoming great tools for tapping into news and conversations about issues critical to the environment, both from public health and healthcare agencies (Chunara, Andrews, & Brownstein, 2012). Recently it has been suggested that the existing real-time platforms such as Facebook (Facebook, 2012) and Twitter (Twitter, 2012) can be used as main sources to improve public health. Social media is a great choice of data input because of the simple structure of their reports – RSS feed. Every news feed may consist of the following details:

1. **The Title:** It describes the main topic of the news report.
2. **The Published Date:** It describes the date when the news is released.
3. **URL:** It describes where the online report is located on the web server.
4. **Description:** It describes the content of the news report.
5. **Address:** It describes either the news report published location or incident reported location.

RSS feed eases data collection as one can track down the user post through Twitter/Facebook user account timeline. There are two ways to access Twitter RSS feeds: through user id or user name. Both create the same outcome, in XML format. For example, a Twitter user name can be written in https://Twitter.com/statuses/user_timeline/healthmap.rssor while a Twitter user id can be written in https://Twitter.com/statuses/user_timeline/20149254.rss (Woodfin, 2011). Figure 1 shows an example of twitter user name while Figure 2 shows an example of twitter user ID.

Figure 1 and Figure 2 show twitter's information format that is encoded in plain view or can be described as XML document. XML contains markup symbols to describe the contents of a page that allow processing by RSS feed reader. Many application programming interfaces (APIs) such as Twitter and Facebook have been developed to aid RSS feed reader with processing XML data. The rise of "Web 2.0" technologies (O'Reilly, 2005) including the proliferation of Really Simple Syndication (RSS) (Cayzer, 2004) and Asynchronous JavaScript and XML (AJAX) (Garrett, 2005) make the process of data collection simple. All these RSS feeds, regardless from Twitter or Facebook, are structured in XML. With given the RSS feed, it allows many automated mechanisms such as RSS readers to retrieve the information from the given site URL.

The Use of Mobile Health Technologies in Malaysia

According to Vodafone (2012), cost-effective and easy-to-deploy mobile devices, with their ability

Figure 1. Twitter user name

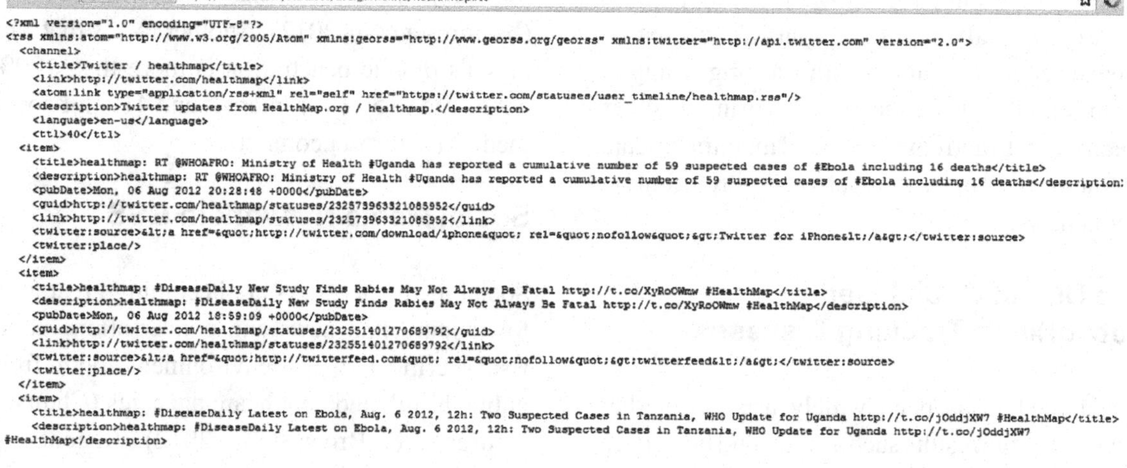
Twitter, Inc. [US] https://twitter.com/statuses/user_timeline/healthmap.rss


```
<?xml version="1.0" encoding="UTF-8"?>
<rss xmlns:atom="http://www.w3.org/2005/Atom" xmlns:georss="http://www.georss.org/georss" xmlns:twitter="http://api.twitter.com" version="2.0">
  <channel>
    <title>Twitter / healthmap</title>
    <link>http://twitter.com/healthmap</link>
    <atom:link type="application/rss+xml" rel="self" href="https://twitter.com/statuses/user_timeline/healthmap.rss"/>
    <description>Twitter updates from HealthMap.org / healthmap.</description>
    <language>en-us</language>
    <ttl>40</ttl>
  <item>
    <title>healthmap: RT @WHOAFRO: Ministry of Health #Uganda has reported a cumulative number of 59 suspected cases of #Ebola including 16 deaths</title>
    <description>healthmap: RT @WHOAFRO: Ministry of Health #Uganda has reported a cumulative number of 59 suspected cases of #Ebola including 16 deaths</description:
    <pubDate>Mon, 06 Aug 2012 20:28:48 +0000</pubDate>
    <guid>http://twitter.com/healthmap/statuses/232573963321085952</guid>
    <link>http://twitter.com/healthmap/statuses/232573963321085952</link>
    <twitter:source>&lt;a href=&quot;http://twitter.com/download/iphone&quot; rel=&quot;nofollow&quot;&gt;Twitter for iPhone&lt;/a&gt;</twitter:source>
    <twitter:place/>
  </item>
  <item>
    <title>healthmap: #DiseaseDaily New Study Finds Rabies May Not Always Be Fatal http://t.co/XyRoOWmw #HealthMap</title>
    <description>healthmap: #DiseaseDaily New Study Finds Rabies May Not Always Be Fatal http://t.co/XyRoOWmw #HealthMap</description>
    <pubDate>Mon, 06 Aug 2012 18:59:09 +0000</pubDate>
    <guid>http://twitter.com/healthmap/statuses/232551401270689792</guid>
    <link>http://twitter.com/healthmap/statuses/232551401270689792</link>
    <twitter:source>&lt;a href=&quot;http://twitterfeed.com&quot; rel=&quot;nofollow&quot;&gt;twitterfeed&lt;/a&gt;</twitter:source>
    <twitter:place/>
  </item>
  <item>
    <title>healthmap: #DiseaseDaily Latest on Ebola, Aug. 6 2012, 12h: Two Suspected Cases in Tanzania, WHO Update for Uganda http://t.co/jOddjXW7 #HealthMap</title>
    <description>healthmap: #DiseaseDaily Latest on Ebola, Aug. 6 2012, 12h: Two Suspected Cases in Tanzania, WHO Update for Uganda http://t.co/jOddjXW7
#HealthMap</description>
```

Figure 2. Twitter user ID

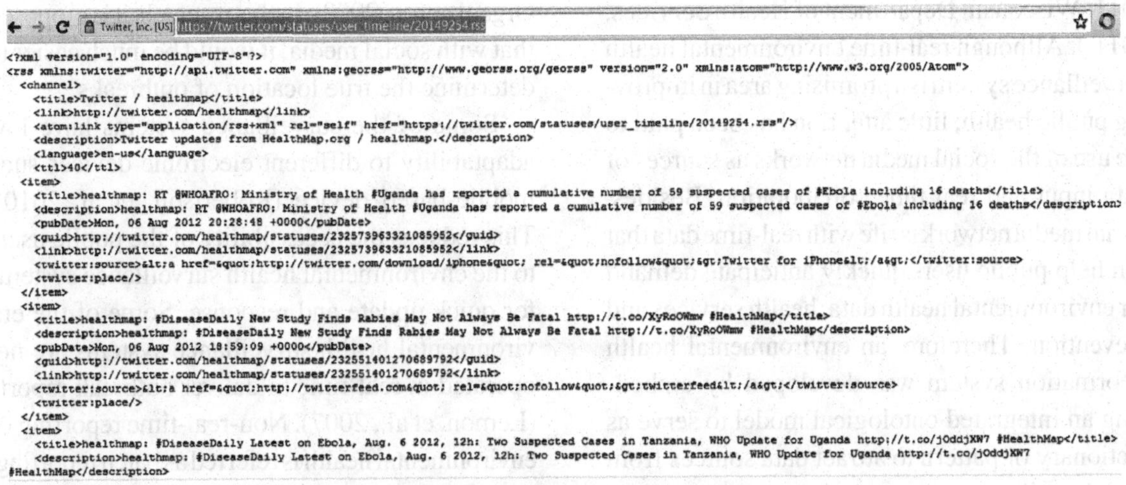


```
<?xml version="1.0" encoding="UTF-8"?>
<rss xmlns:twitter="http://api.twitter.com" xmlns:georss="http://www.georss.org/georss" version="2.0" xmlns:atom="http://www.w3.org/2005/Atom">
  <channel>
    <title>Twitter / healthmap</title>
    <link>http://twitter.com/healthmap</link>
    <atom:link type="application/rss+xml" rel="self" href="https://twitter.com/statuses/user_timeline/20149254.rss"/>
    <description>Twitter updates from HealthMap.org / healthmap.</description>
    <language>en-us</language>
    <ttl>40</ttl>
  <item>
    <title>healthmap: RT @WHOAFRO: Ministry of Health #Uganda has reported a cumulative number of 59 suspected cases of #Ebola including 16 deaths</title>
    <description>healthmap: RT @WHOAFRO: Ministry of Health #Uganda has reported a cumulative number of 59 suspected cases of #Ebola including 16 deaths</description>
    <pubDate>Mon, 06 Aug 2012 20:28:48 +0000</pubDate>
    <guid>http://twitter.com/healthmap/statuses/232573963321085952</guid>
    <link>http://twitter.com/healthmap/statuses/232573963321085952</link>
    <twitter:source>&lt;a href=&quot;http://twitter.com/download/iphone&quot; rel=&quot;nofollow&quot;&gt;Twitter for iPhone&lt;/a&gt;</twitter:source>
    <twitter:place/>
  </item>
  <item>
    <title>healthmap: #DiseaseDaily New Study Finds Rabies May Not Always Be Fatal http://t.co/XyRoOWmw #HealthMap</title>
    <description>healthmap: #DiseaseDaily New Study Finds Rabies May Not Always Be Fatal http://t.co/XyRoOWmw #HealthMap</description>
    <pubDate>Mon, 06 Aug 2012 18:59:09 +0000</pubDate>
    <guid>http://twitter.com/healthmap/statuses/232551401270689792</guid>
    <link>http://twitter.com/healthmap/statuses/232551401270689792</link>
    <twitter:source>&lt;a href=&quot;http://twitterfeed.com&quot; rel=&quot;nofollow&quot;&gt;twitterfeed&lt;/a&gt;</twitter:source>
    <twitter:place/>
  </item>
  <item>
    <title>healthmap: #DiseaseDaily Latest on Ebola, Aug. 6 2012, 12h: Two Suspected Cases in Tanzania, WHO Update for Uganda http://t.co/jOddjXN7 #HealthMap</title>
    <description>healthmap: #DiseaseDaily Latest on Ebola, Aug. 6 2012, 12h: Two Suspected Cases in Tanzania, WHO Update for Uganda http://t.co/jOddjXN7
#HealthMap</description>
```


to quickly capture and transmit data on disease incidence, can be decisive in the prevention and containment of outbreaks. With the right information and effective monitoring of both social media networks and environmental health issues, mobile health technologies are supporting effective environmental health tracking and enabling the identification of health trends. This literally allows governments and health authorities to allocate resources more effectively and, if required, adapt the programme and policies in place to manage emergency.

In Malaysia the internet digital divide limited the reach of computerized health behavior interventions for lower socioeconomic groups for years, if not decades. In contrast, mobile phone use has been rapidly and widely adopted among virtually all demographic groups. Malaysia has 34 million mobile subscribers and 17.5 million internet users (Factbrowser.com, 2012) in a population of about 27 million. Mobile health technologies are not unfamiliar in Malaysia as people begin to appreciate having health information at their fingertip. Malaysian Ministry of Health initiated myHealth application which provides information on Malaysia's healthcare system from health facilities, and the list of registered practitioners to registered medical products (Ministry of Health, 2013). Some other mobile applications such as Sime Darby Healthcare (Sime Darby Healthcare, 2013) provide free service to mobile users to book doctor appointments (at Sime Darby facilities). Malaysia telecommunication service providers such as Celcom (Celcom, 2013) and Maxis (Maxis, 2012) are also participating in innovative mobile healthcare solutions to dispense medical services more efficiently. Again, the question is: "Can environmental health surveillance systems be merged into mobile health technologies (in Malaysia)?"

RESEARCH PROBLEMS

There are some state-wide or regional health effect registries or surveillance systems that contain data of sufficient completeness, timeliness and quality to allow reporting of valid estimates of health effect prevalence, incidence, or mortality for a population, namely, CDC, HealthMap, Air pollutant index management system, Wisconsin Environmental Public Health Tracking, Air pollution monitoring system, California Environmental Health Tracking Program (Brownstein & Freifeld, 2007; California Environmental Health Investigation Branch, 2012; Center for Disease Control and

Prevention, 2010; European Environment Agency, 2011; Wisconsin Department of Health Services, 2011;). Although real-time environmental health surveillance system is a promising area in improving public health, little attention has been paid to the use of the social media networks as sources of data input and real time collaboration. Besides, social media network is rife with real-time data that can help public users quickly anticipate demand for environmental health data, health services and prevention. Therefore, an environmental health information system was developed by embedding an integrated ontological model to serve as dictionary of pattern to attract data sources from social media networks and vice versa.

The environmental health data often comes in different data formats for different reasons by different environmental health tracking and monitoring systems (California Environmental Health Investigation branch, 2012). For example, some environmental health agencies such as healthcare providers are not required to report asthma-related office visits to the state. Hospital data are collected for the purpose of tracking health care quality, rather than for public health surveillance (California Environmental Health Investigation branch, 2012). Traditional environmental health surveillance systems do not collect data input from social media networks (Schmidt, 2012).

More than ever, people use social media networks to learn about what is happening in the world, and the traditional news outlets become increasingly less relevant to the digital generation (Laird, 2012). Some environmental health surveillance systems were not made accessible to the public, and the surveillance data are also not explicitly interpretable by public users, which can make it difficult for the public audiences to use. Most of the environmental health surveillance systems included only selected location in their systems to keep track on event location and this may become cumbersome without an ideal

channel to keep track the location (World Health Organization, 2008). In this research, it is proposed that with social media, it would be much easier to determine the true location of outbreaks.

Some of the surveillance systems have low adaptability to different electronic devices such mobile-based device (Robertson, et al, 2010). This reduces the accessibility of the public users to the environmental health surveillance systems for quick update and response. Some of the environmental health surveillance systems are not operated in real-time to deliver outbreak reports (Lemon, et al., 2007). Non-real-time reporting of environmental health is referred as batch reporting.

The data inputs are given by their own selected healthcare agencies, collaborative programs and partnerships, and it sometimes take weeks to process, filter, summarize and store them in the database before they can be released to the public. Despite a common interest in monitoring the impact of environmental health, due to the wide variety of environmental health issues existing everywhere in the world, researchers could only track a fraction of the environmental health issues (California Environmental Health Investigation branch, 2012), usually covering only the most emergent environmental health issues in their own countries – this is also referred to as categorical surveillance (Nsubuga, et al, 2006). Some systems do only "passive surveillance" (Center for Disease Control and Prevention 2011), i.e. only receive reports submitted from hospitals, clinics, public health units, or other sources (Nsubuga, et al., 2006).

With the supporting evidence, the research problems have been identified and we aim to develop a comprehensive Android mobile-based and real-time environmental health information source to achieve the goals and are committed to taking personal responsibility to manage and mitigate the impacts of their corporate, professional and daily living activities on the environment.

System Architecture and Methods

As social media is exploding, the networking activities do not end when one leaves the computer. Thus people can update it and get themselves updated by their mobile phones now. Various social media applications are available for all varieties of smart phones These make it easy to stay connected and share information with friends within minutes. However, accessing large portions of user's timeline data without proper filter and classification can be tedious. Android mobile-based application of environmental health information source is proposed in this research. The proposed solution involves several study areas:

- Multi-tier architecture (also known as N-tier approach) (Jain, Dahlin & Tewari, 2005) as a classifier to identify location and Environmental Health Data from social media networks,
- Word-level N-gram approach (BodHuin & Totorella, 2003; Caynar & Trenkle, 1994) to be used as matching inputs against a known patterns dictionary (Environmental health ontological model),
- Android mobile application has to be designed, developed and installed in Android mobile (Android, 2012),
- Selected social media networks such as Facebook and Twitter are being used as target sources of inputs and sharing of outputs,
- Integrated environmental health ontological model in Malaysian context by various existing environmental health surveillance systems/ontological models.

The main purpose of this research is to provide an Android application that allows public users to access the desired environmental health data. The benefit of social media networks is they provide RSS feed just like the services widgets given by the online media news. This RSS feed eases data collection as it can track down the user post through Twitter/Facebook user account timeline. In return, the RSS feed can be shared across other social media networks.

The development of real-time environmental health source emphasizes collecting and disseminating reliable environmental health events to public population whenever there is internet connectivity, computers and smartphones in order to display the data. Since the early 1990s, the Geographical Information System (GIS) has grown substantially, and it was later adopted in the public health sector (Richards et al, 1999), especially epidemiologic studies (Zhang et al., 2009). Environmental Wellness/Environmental Health model plays an essential role as an indicator and to develop a holistic ontological model in aggregating the data from Social Media networks.

Proposed Ontological Model

A proposed ontological model is an integrated environmental health model from existing diseases surveillance systems, environmental health surveillance systems and environmental health ontological models presented by various vendors and researchers. The integration process of proposed ontological model development involves three stages:

In stage 1, develop priority environmental health issues in Malaysian context through literature review and observation of Malaysian-based environmental health-related systems such Air Pollutant Index Management System (APIMS). The literature review indicated various types of environmental health issues and potential health effects covered in different countries. The uncountable types of environmental health issues made it hard to identify them in detail. The most efficient way is to rely on the reliable publications to determine the priority environment health issues in Malaysia. Then the information was used to develop the most appropriate direction and flexible ontological model for environmental health issues in Malaysia without making tricky and tedious work on the model's structure. Stage 1 aims to determine the primary scope of environmental health topics in Malaysia and later the keywords will be extracted and compared with other existing environmental health surveillance system and ontological models in stage 2. For example, many studies (CIA World Factbook, 2012; Department of Environment, 2009; Ministry of Health Malaysia, 2007; Mokhtar & Murad, 2010; WHO, 2005) mentioned "infectious diseases", "air pollution", and "water pollution" as the most critical environmental health issues, therefore these keywords will be collected in a new proposed ontological model in Malaysian context. Table 1 shows a proposed environmental health ontological model that covers major topics in Malaysia. Precisely, it is a summary of environmental health topics from several publications such as Malaysia environmental health country profile (WHO, 2005), Malaysia environmental quality report (Department of Environment, 2009), Issue and framework of environmental health in Malaysia (Mokhtar & Murad, 2010), CIA World Factbook (CIA World Factbook, 2012), and Communicable disease control information system (Ministry of Health Malaysia, 2007).

In Table 1, the left column indicates the major environmental health topics or dimensions while the right column indicates their attributes or properties. The attributes or properties refer to dimension's sub-indicator. For example, sulphur dioxide (SO_2) is part of air pollution topic. All these keywords are gathered and taken from the above mentioned publications (CIA World Factbook, 2012; Department of Environment, 2009; ; Ministry of Health Malaysia, 2007; Mokhtar & Murad, 2010; WHO, 2005;). It is essential to know that the stage 1 only illustrates the environmental health issues covered in Malaysia; however, it is the core work of the ontological model.

In stage 2, integrate with other six environmental health surveillance systems and two environmental health ontological models such as National

Environmental Public Health Tracking Networks by CDC (Center for Disease Control and Prevention, 2012), Malaysia Air Pollutant Index Management System (Department of Environment, 2011), California Environmental Health Tracking Program (California Environmental Health Investigation Branch, 2012), Wisconsin Environmental Public Health Tracking (Wisconsin Department of Health Services, 2011), Environmental Health Monitoring System (European Environment Agency, 2011), HealthMap (2012), MedlinePlus Health (n.d), and CRISP Thesaurus (2006). This task aims to collect alternative keywords described in other existing surveillance systems and ontological models. The alternative keywords are also referred as indicators or information objects (Center for Disease Control and Prevention, 2012). The integration process removes duplicate keywords and adds new keywords from various existing environmental health surveillance systems and ontological models. For example, "air" can be also named as "air pollutant", "air quality" or "air pollution". Table 2 shows identified alternate keywords for two environmental health dimension (Air pollution and Water pollution) from various ontological models listed.

Table 2 shows the "air pollution" and "water pollution" are alternate main keywords in various ontological models/surveillance systems. The left column represents the alternate keywords used by other surveillance systems/ontological models while the right column indicates the vendors' names. In this research, it is assumed that the more alternative keywords collected from other surveillance systems and ontological models, the higher chances for the new proposed ontological model to meet the keyword expectation from social media. In this case, "air quality", "air" and "air pollutant" are discarded. The keyword "air quality" is likely to indicate measurement of air pollutant index, therefore it is more suitable to be used as supporting keywords. The keyword "air" is likely to be vague when the ontological needs narrow the definition. The keyword "air

Table 1. Proposed environmental health ontological model

Environmental Health Dimensions	Attributes or Properties
air pollution	Sulphur dioxide (SO2), Carbon Monoxide (CO), Nitrogen Dioxide (NO2), Lead (Pb), Particulate Matter (PM10 and PM2.5), Ozone (O3)/ Ozone depletion, Air Pollution Index (API)/ Air Quality Index (AQI), Open burning, Haze, General air pollution, Industrial waste, smog
Water pollution	Biochemical Oxygen Demand (BOD), sewerage, Daily waste, ammonia, River water pollution, Marine ecosystem issue, Chemical organic demand
Soil pollution	Pesticide
Environmental Radiation	Radioactive waste
Noise pollution	*None*
Climate Change	Carbon Monoxide Co2
Deforestation	Illegal logging
Infectious Diseases	Cancroids, Cholera, Dengue fever (DF) & Dengue Hemorrhagic Fever (DHF), Diphtheria, Dysenteries, Ebola, Food Poisoning, Gonoccocal Infection, Leprosy, Malaria, Measles, Myocarditis, Plague, Poliomyelitis, Rabies, Relapsing Fever, Syphilis, Tetanus, Tuberculosis, Typhus & Other Rickettsioses, Typhoid & Paratyphoid Fevers, Viral Encephalitis, Viral Hepatitis, Whooping Cough, Yellow Fever, Any other life Threatening Microbial Infection, HIV infection
Occupational Health	Coordination of occupation health agencies
Road Safety	*None*
Traffic crashes	*None*
Cross cutting issues	Health care waste
Solid waste	*None*
Toxic, Chemical and Hazardous wastes	*None*
Death and Effects of warmer temperatures	Airborne, food-borne, waterborne, Insect/mosquito-borne infections,
Biodiversity	Number of species, Diverse, Genetic, Organism, Community, Ecosystem level, Loss of Biodiversity
Afforestation	*None*
Bio-indicators	*None*
Biomass	*None*
Dichloro-diphenyl-trichloro-ethane (DDT)	*None*
Ecosystem	Complex communities of organism and their specific environments
Endangered Species	*None*
Inuit Circumpolar Conference (ICC)	Long-range transport of pollutants, Sustainable development, Climate change
Noxious substances	*None*
Overgrazing	*None*
Ozone Shield	*None*
Poaching	*None*
Ultraviolet radiation (UV)	*None*
Water-borne disease	*None*

Table 2. Identified alternate keywords for air and water from various ontological models

Alternate Keywords Used	Existing Ontological Models/Surveillance Systems
Air Quality	National Environmental Public Health Tracking Networks by CDC
	Malaysia Air Pollutant Index Management System
Air	California Environmental Health Tracking Program
Air Pollutant	Wisconsin Environmental Public Health Tracking
Air pollution	CRISP Thesaurus, 2006
	Environmental Health Monitoring System by European Environment Agency
Water Pollution	MedlinePlus Health
	CRISP Thesaurus, 2006
Community Water	National Environmental Public Health Tracking Networks by CDC
Well Water	National Environmental Public Health Tracking Networks by CDC
Drinking Water	California Environmental Health Tracking Program
	Wisconsin Environmental Public Health Tracking
Water	Environmental Health Monitoring System by European Environment Agency

pollution" and "air pollutant" show different vocabularies but the same context. However, social media networks are used to decide which keyword can attract more results by constructing a query in the search field. The keyword "air pollution" was chosen as an appropriate keyword in the proposed ontological model rather than the keyword "air pollutant" as it has a higher rank of results than others. Besides, the keywords "community water", "well water", "drinking water" and "water" would be discarded because these words lack strong context to represent the issue of water. However, they are rather suitable to be sorted in the category of supporting keywords. Fuzzy keywords may attract irrelevant news from social media networks. Lastly, the keyword "water pollution" was chosen as the appropriate keyword in the new proposed ontological model.

In stage 3, while integrating with other environmental health surveillance systems and two environmental health ontological models, the next task is define the level of indicators and continue to search for second level of alternative keywords and indicators. For example, under the main indicator – air pollution — there are

various sub-issues related to air pollution such "lead poisoning", "passive smoking" and "energy sector air pollution". Alternative keywords for "lead poisoning" are "heavy metal lead", "lead" or "lead emissions" in other surveillance systems and ontological models.

Table 3 shows the identification of attributes or properties of environmental health dimensions from various ontological models/surveillance systems were sorted in "Air pollution" and "Water pollution". In this case, the duplicated keywords would be appropriately removed while the new keywords would be added into the proposed ontological model. Apart from general water issues mentioned by MedlinePlus Health, CRIPS Thesaurus, and Environmental Health Monitoring system by European environment agency, other ontological models/surveillance systems included relevant keywords that may help to form an ontological model in Malaysian context.

After the development of the proposed ontological model in Malaysian context, this new environmental health ontological model will serve as a known pattern dictionary in matching the input from social media by using word-level

Table 3. Attributes identification of environmental health dimension

Environmental Health Dimensions	Environmental Hazards, Exposures and Health
Air Pollution	Ozone, Particulate Matter 2.5, Arsenic, Haloacetic Acid, Nitrates, Trihalomethane (*Source: Wisconsin Environmental Health Tracking Program*)
	Carbon Monoxide, Dust, Engine Exhaust, passive smoking (*Source: CRISP Thesaurus, 2006*)
	Annual PM 2.5 Level (Monitor + Modeled), Annual PM 2.5 Level (Monitor only), Ozone Days above regulatory standard (Monitor + Modeled), Ozone Days above regulatory standard (Monitor only), PM2.5 - Days above regulatory standard (Monitor + Modeled), PM2.5 - Days above regulatory standard (Monitor only) (*Source: National Environmental Public Health Tracking Networks*)
	Habuk Halus (PM10), Sulfur Dioksida (SO2), Nitrogen Dioksida (NO2), Ozon (O3), Karbon Monoksida (CO) (*Source: Malaysia Air Pollutant Index Management System (APIMS)*)
	exposure to PM2.5, exposure to PM10, exposure to ozone, exposure to traffic pollution (*Source: California Environmental Health Tracking Program*)
Water Pollution	Arsenic, Disinfection Byproducts, Public water use, Domestic well water use, Levels of Contaminants in Domestic (self-supplied) well water (*Source: National Environmental Public Health Tracking Networks by CDC* and *California Environmental Health Tracking Program*)
	Nitrate Levels in Drinking Water (*Source: California Environmental Health Tracking Program*)
	Arsenic, Haloacetic Acid, Nitrates, Trihalomethane (*Source: Wisconsin Environmental Public Health Tracking*)
	General Water issues
	(*Source: MedlinePlus Health, CRISP Thesaurus, 2006, Environmental Health Monitoring System by European Environment Agency*

N-gram approach (BodHuin & Totorella 2003; Caynar & Trenkle 1994). In this research, there are 24 main indicators and 412 secondary indicators. It is worth to take note that keywords discovery and integration from stage 1 to stage 3 aimed to develop a suitable ontological model in Malaysian context before accuracy testing in part 1 and part 2. And this will be discussed in a later section.

Software Architecture

Figure 3 briefly illustrates the overview of the (Malaysian) Environmental Health Monitoring and tracking System, also named MyEHMS, that allows public access to monitor the trends, impacts, links, and effects in a national baseline tracking network for environmental health. This system is embedded with customized Google Maps in order to visualize the location and deliver the early warnings of critical environmental health threats. Public users (Social media users) would be able

to join the responsive feedback discussion, search for particular environmental health events, share the events through social network, and submit any critical environmental health threat which is not located in the system.

In Process, this level is where it handles *user request from Web Frontend, data acquisition from news feed sources*, and *text classifications*. The request from user is received and converted into a database query. The database then returns the alarm reports that match these queries. The query results are displayed on Google Map with built-in markers.

Data acquisition allocates data from News Feed Source based on several criteria. In general, the system identifies and converts each source of news feed into a standard report format, containing five main fields: title, link, description, location, and date. The title is the report title, link is the URL, location is the specific position in physical place, date is the date of issue of the report, and descrip-

Figure 3. The architecture of proposed environmental health information system

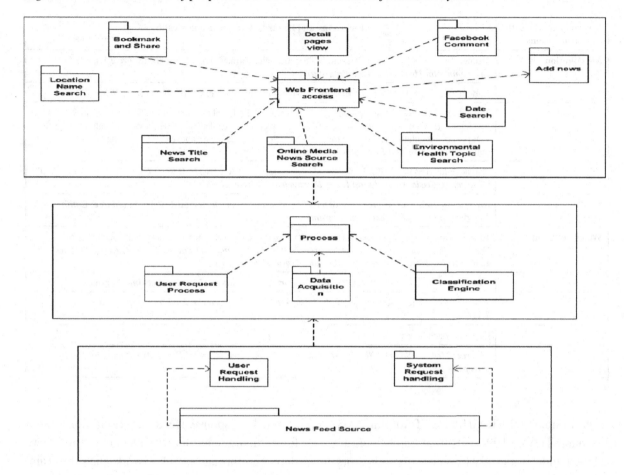

tion is a brief summary of the report. The parsing process involves extracting the elements from the documents that are useful. For instance, with Star Online News, the system extracts the parts according to the five main fields and removes the rest of the original publication. The Classification engine decides the primary locations and environmental data (exposure, hazard, and health) associated with each report acquired from web sources.

The classification engine has two modules that process the raw input and final output, which are the Reader module and Parser module. While the Reader module takes the raw input from the web source, segments it and prepares it for input to the parser, the Parser module takes segmented input and produces location and environmental data as output.

Reader module uses multi-tier architecture (also known as N-tier approach) (Jain, Dahlin & Tewari 2005) as a classifier to identify location and Environmental Health Data for each web source and Geocoding Web Services later generate coordinates for the identified location. In general, the Classifier examines every sentence and paragraph in the reports in order to match location name and Environmental Health categories against existing taxonomy of known patterns. This may cause multiple locations and multiple environmental health categories to be allocated to a single report.

Parser module uses a word-level N-gram approach (BodHuin & Totorella 2003; Caynar & Trenkle 1994) to match input against a dictionary of known patterns. After the initial data acquisition, the parser receives the input text, strips it of non-alphanumeric characters and splits it into word tokens. It then converts all capital letters to lowercase, except for those tokens that are only one or two characters in length. The parser then compares the input to its dictionary of place and environmental health category, mapping text patterns to the database IDs of all locations, environmental health categories, possible reactions and environmental dimensions known to the system. The dictionary patterns are stored in memory as a tree, where each node is a hash table that maps single tokens to either sub nodes or IDs (leaves), the system can look up each input token in constant time.

In News Feed Source, once the web sources are determined with location and environmental health data, the system stores them in a relational database (MySQL). User Request handling processes any request from public users whereas system request handling processes internal requests by the system.

System Implementation

The implementation uses Android integrated development environment software (IDE), which can be used to develop applications or plugs-ins. There are some major features in Android mobile-based environmental health information system: program startup, Google map view with three markers, web view output and list view output, and lastly search tab and setting tab.

Figure 4 shows the Android mobile-based environmental health information system program startup. The square highlighted icon represents the

Android mobile application. With the MyEHMS Android SDK file, the public users can install the file into Android platform.

Figure 5 shows the Google map view with three markers. These three markers are defined in three colors: blue, red and green. Each of these colours represents different contexts. The red marker is the default marker when the user initiates the program with GPS switched on in the smartphone. It detects the current location of the user and returns the results with exact location. The blue marker is the default preference marker when the user initiates the program. It provides the environmental health information with user's location preference set up in the preference settings. Lastly, the green marker refers to the search results performed by user.

Figure 6 shows the web view output and list view output. As shown in Figure 5, there are three markers that are pinned on the map containing environmental health information. When the user clicks on the marker, it shows a list of environmental health information in that particular location, also known as list view output. If the users would like to view original source of environmental health information, the users can click on "view full article" to have web view output.

Figure 7 shows the search tab and setting tab. The search tab refers to a search form that allows the public user to select the state and city and environmental health category. This allows the user to freely and randomly choose the location and environmental health information category. The settings tab refers to user's preference settings of preferred location and preferred environmental health information category. This allows the user to have easy access to the location and environmental health information for the next visit.

Figure 8 demonstrates how the public user can share, bookmark and comment the news. The public user is allowed to leave comments on the viewed alert page. Most importantly, the user is

Figure 4. Program startup

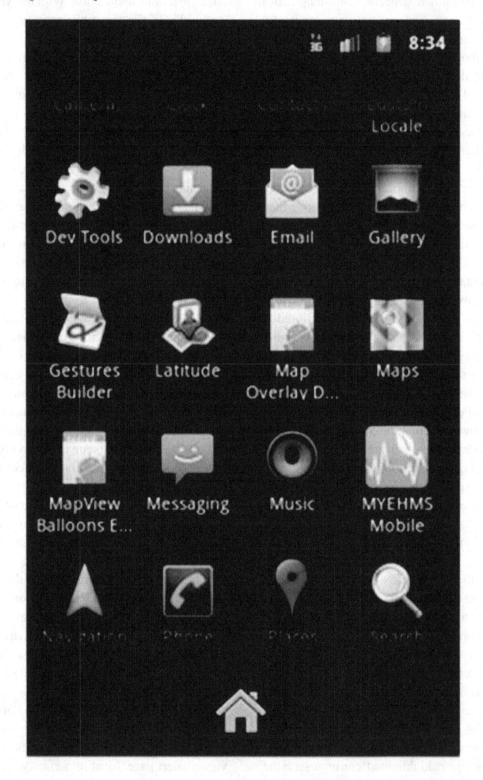

Figure 5. Google Map view with 3 markers

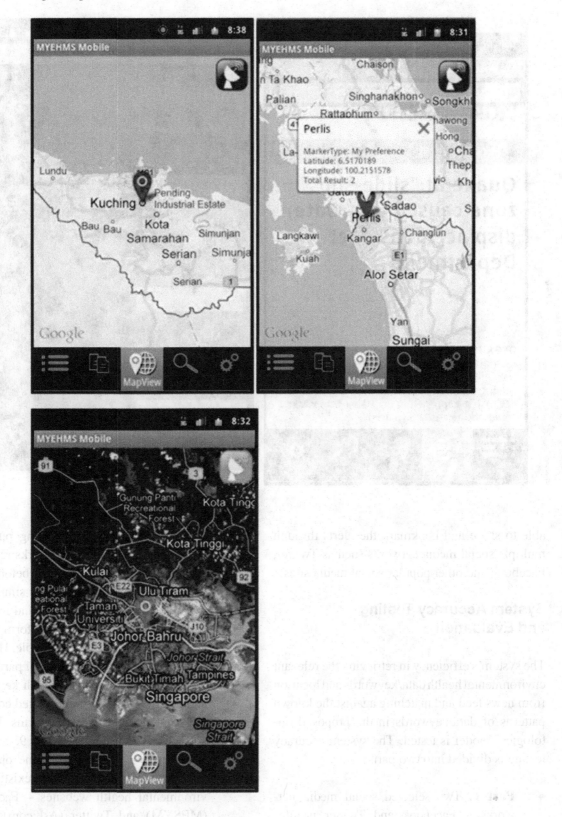

Figure 6. Web view output and list view ouput

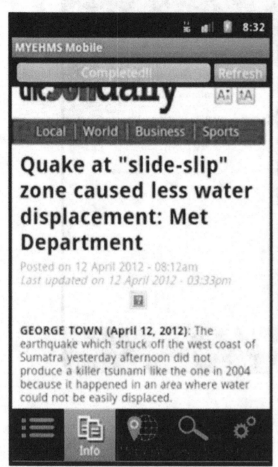 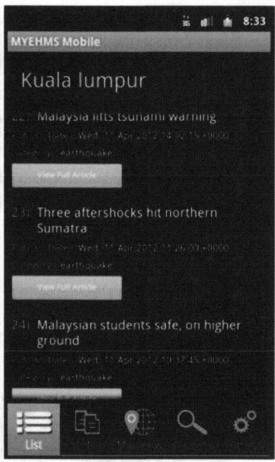

able to share and bookmark the alerts through multiple social media networks such as Twitter, Facebook and other popular social media sites.

System Accuracy Testing and Evaluation

The system's efficiency in retrieving the relevant environmental health data/keywords and location from news feed and matching against the known patterns of data/keywords in the proposed ontological model is tested. The system accuracy testing is divided into two parts:

- **Part 1:** Two selected social media networks – Facebook and Twitter profiles

– would be created for testing purpose. These two social media networks required user registration on their sites before conducting the experiment. Some simple environmental health keywords and location were filled in to provide a platform on social media networks. For example, H1N1 – Kuala Lumpur. The challenge of part 1 is to locate the environmental health keywords and location from the self-created contents on social media network platforms. The result will be described in Figure 9.

- **Part 2:** Two selected real time platform of social media networks with existing environmental health websites – Facebook (MESYM) and Twitter (Ask.com). They

Figure 7. Search and settings tab

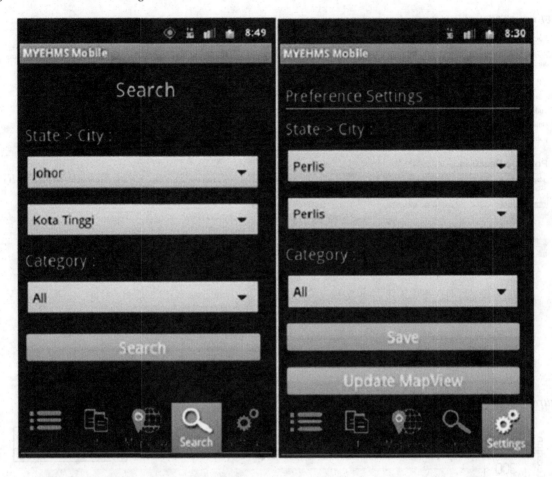

are also known as Malaysia Environment Sustainability Youth Movement (MESYM) and Ask.com. These two original sites have synchronized their daily information in their social media networks. The challenge of part 2 is to locate the environmental health keywords and location among the complex vocabularies posted by existing environmental health parties in their own social media networks. The results retrieved by the system will be compared to original websites searched results as shown in Table 4.

Figure 9 shows the number of returned results is 100% (436 keywords for both environmental health and location keywords) from social media networks (Facebook and Twitter) simulation test (part 1) with no intervention of irrelevant keywords. With this simulation test (part 1), the system has indicated the readiness of the proposed ontological model to go further in the accuracy testing to access complicated news feeds such as with real time platform that may contain highly irrelevant vocabularies and alternative vocabularies. This has also proved that the methods used such as multi-tier architecture (Jain, Dahlin & Tewari

Figure 8. Share, comment and bookmark news feed

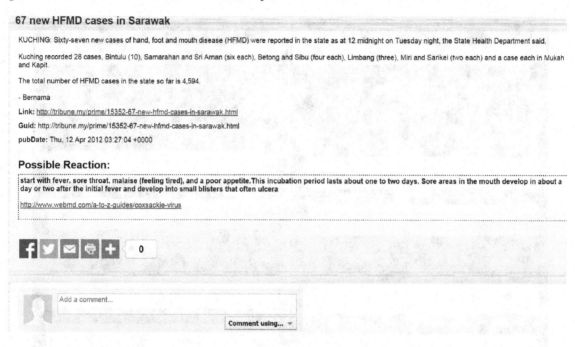

Figure 9. Social media networks simulation test

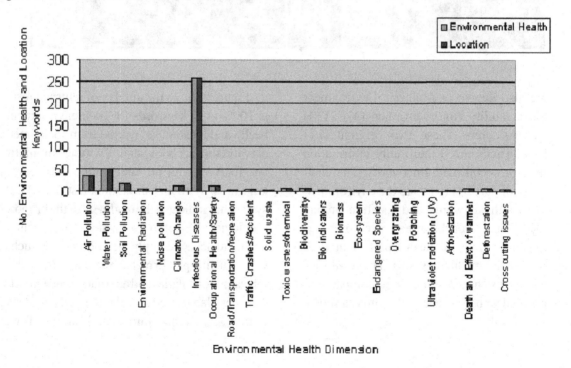

Table 4. Overview accuracy testing results of parsing social media networks

Environmental Health Dimensions	Environmental hazards, exposures and health	No. needed results	Before Keywords Refinement			After Keywords Refinement		List of Keywords refined and added to proposed ontological model
			No. news retrieved by MyEHMS	No. irrelevant news retrieved by MyEHMS	Accuracy in percentage (%)	No. news retrieved MyEHMS	Accuracy in percentage (%)	
Air pollution	Arsenic	14	12	0	86%	14	100%	rare earth, arsenic poisoning
	Dust	1	0	0	0%	1	100%	dusty
	Energy sector fly ash	1	0	0	0%	1	100%	fly ash
	Greenhouse gas	1	1	1	0%	1	100%	carbon footprint
	Lead	1	1	1	0%	1	100%	lead poisoning, lead emissions, heavy metal lead
	passive smoking	1	0	0	0%	1	100%	cigarettes, tobacco
	Slash-and-burn agriculture	1	0	0	0%	1	100%	slash and burn agriculture, slash and burn farming
	smoke/haze	1	0	0	0%	1	100%	smoky
	Trans-boundary air pollution	1	0	0	0%	1	100%	Trans-boundary haze pollution
Water Pollution	Arsenic	14	10	0	71%	14	100%	rare earth, arsenic poisoning
	deteriorating water quality	1	0	0	0%	1	100%	deteriorating water security
	Energy sector sludge disposal	1	0	0	0%	1	100%	sewage sludge
	rapid growth in water demand	1	0	0	0%	1	100%	Water Crisis
	Rural development sector drainage and flood control	18	0	0	0%	18	100%	Drainage, Floods
	Siltation caused by infrastructure development	1	0	0	0%	1	100%	siltation
	Siltation caused by logging	1	0	0	0%	1	100%	Siltation and logging
	Urban development sector drainage and flood control	18	0	0	0%	18	100%	Drainage, Floods

continued on following page

Table 4. Continued

Environmental Health Dimensions	Environmental hazards, exposures and health	No. needed results	Before Keywords Refinement			After Keywords Refinement		List of Keywords refined and added to proposed ontological model
			No. news retrieved by MyEHMS	No. irrelevant news retrieved by MyEHMS	Accuracy in percentage (%)	No. news retrieved MyEHMS	Accuracy in percentage (%)	
Soil Pollution	Energy sector sludge disposal	1	0	0	0%	1	100%	sewage sludge
	Slash-and-burn agriculture	1	0	0	0%	1	100%	slash and burn agriculture
	Soil degradation	5	2	0	40%	5	100%	environmental degradation
Climate Change	Droughts	7	0	0	0%	7	100%	drought
	Effects of Climate change	5	3	0	60%	5	100%	climate change
	flood	50	50	24	52%	50	100%	flash floods, flash flood, heavy flooding
Infectious Diseases	Avian Influenza	2	0	0	0%	2	100%	bird flu, avian flu, H5N1
	Hand, Foot and Mouth Disease	10	1	0	10%	10	100%	HFMD, Coxsackieviruses, Coxsackie A HFMD, Hand-foot-and-mouth, Coxsackie A, Coxsackie B, Pleurodynia, Bornholm disease
	Swine Flu H1N1	5	2	0	40%	5	100%	H1N1, Swine Flu, Swine Influenza A Virus
	Viral Hepatitis	1	0	0	0%	1	100%	Hepatitis A, Hepatitis B
Solid waste	Waste disposal	1	1	1	0%	1	100%	Industrial waste disposal
Biodiversity	number of species	1	0	0	0%	1	100%	Number of Orang Utan
Death and Effect of warmer temperature/ Global Warming	insect and mosquito-borne infections	1	0	0	0%	1	100%	mosquito borne, insect borne
Deforestation	Deforestation and destruction of biodiversity caused by logging	4	0	0	0%	4	100%	Forest clearing, Deforestation, Deforestation issues, deforestation rate

continued on following page

Table 4. Continued

Environmental Health Dimensions	Environmental hazards, exposures and health	No. needed results	Before Keywords Refinement			After Keywords Refinement		List of Keywords refined and added to proposed ontological model
			No. news retrieved by MyEHMS	No. irrelevant news retrieved by MyEHMS	Accuracy in percentage (%)	No. news retrieved MyEHMS	Accuracy in percentage (%)	
	Deforestation and destruction of biodiversity caused by conversion to other land use	4	0	0	0%	4	100%	Forest clearing, Deforestation, Deforestation issues, deforestation rate
Total	32 keywords being refined							61 new keywords

2005) and word-level N-gram approach (BodHuin & Totorella 2003; Caynar & Trenkle 1994) can efficiently read and parse the social media news feed without error. This has also indicated that the proposed ontological model processed in stage 1, 2 and 3 is considered mature for accuracy testing.

Part 2 result is described in Table 4 and keyword refinement is part of the testing. The sources used for keyword refinement relies on the relevant keywords suggested by original websites and search engines. For example, MESYM and Ask.com used Facebook and Twitter as their alternatives in news publishing and besides they synchronized the latest articles and news in social media.

Table 4 shows that fewer keywords and locations were detected and retrieved by the system (before keyword refinement) from social media networks when compared to the returned results of original sites (No. of needed results). The number of returned results from the system is not consistent with the returned results from the original sites. This has indicated that those keywords structured in the proposed environmental health ontological model are not holistic enough to cope with the large amount of social media web sources. In order for the system to achieve the same results made by different original sites

search, alternative keywords would be added into the proposed ontological model to gain same amount of news returned by the original sites. In this accuracy testing, the improvements were made when there were irrelevant alerts retrieved by the system. The improvements were conducted by refining and adding more alternative keywords to the ontological model. About 60 keywords were updated accordingly to the ontological model. These newly added 60 keywords were discovered when conducting the manual search on original site such as MESYM and Ask.com. Search on these original sites may benefit the researcher to discover relevant news and keywords suggested by the search features.

In Table 4, the environmental health keywords under the air pollution, water pollution, soil pollution, and climate change tend to have low accuracy due to the high number of irrelevant results retrieved by MyEHMS. This has indicated that those environmental health keywords are very common and vague in most of the news written by publishers. Besides, some environmental health keywords under noise pollution, road/transportation/recreation safety, traffic crashes/accident, toxic wastes/chemical wastes/hazardous wastes, bio-indicators, biomass, ecosystem, endangered species, overgrazing, poaching, and ultraviolet radiation (UV) were not able to extract any news from original sites. This has again indicated that choosing the relevant news feed may achieve reliable results, especially the real-time platform that specializes in reporting specific environmental health topics. To date, it does not fail to retrieve relevant news with exact keywords matching.

Discussion

Table 4 shows the accuracy testing results of My-EHMS by retrieving from social media networks like Facebook and Twitter. It also indicates the comparative results before and after keyword refinement. Last but not least, it also shows a list of refined keywords that have been added to the proposed ontological model as improvements. It also indicates some environmental health dimensions and some environmental health hazards, exposures and health keywords that were successfully being improved in terms of keyword refinement. At this stage, there were nine environmental health dimensions and 32 environmental health hazards, exposures and health keywords. Accuracy testing of matching the social media networks – Facebook and Twitter – against the existing ontological model was calculated based on (100%/ no. needed results x no. news retrieved by MyEHMS). Before keyword refinement, there were only four keywords which achieved above 50% accuracy: Arsenic under air pollution (86%); Arsenic under water pollution (71%); effects of climate change under climate change (60%); and flood under climate change (52%). Besides, there were three keywords which achieved 10% to 40% accuracy: soil degradation under soil pollution (40%); Hand, foot, and mouth disease under infectious diseases (10%); and lastly Swine flu H1N1 under infectious diseases (40%).

The other 25 environmental health keywords were not successfully matched with any relevant news from social media networks. There were two reasons behind this: the different authors in social media networks may be using different vocabularies for the same topic. The vocabulary is not standardized in such an open platform and it may be difficult to find the exact keywords by the system. Therefore, keyword refinement was conducted on these 25 environmental health keywords in order to increase the number of retrieved results by the system.

FUTURE RESEARCH DIRECTIONS

This research has several areas for future improvement: user testing on the system effectiveness, prediction of environmental health patterns, integration with more healthcare-related systems, sorting and classification in environmental health ontological model at a deeper level.

- User testing on the system effectiveness.

One of the objectives in this research is to develop a comprehensive mobile-based environmental health information system that can serve public mobile users. Apart from accuracy testing, it is necessary to test the effectiveness of the system in improving the public health. Public health concerns for environmental health information system can be addressed in the evidence gathered regarding the performance of the system. Evidence of the system's performance must be viewed as credible. For example, the gathered evidence must be reliable, valid, and informative for its intended use. Many potential sources of evidence regarding the system's performance exist, including survey data collected from public users. This user testing involves reusing the accuracy testing records mentioned above and also identifying eligible stakeholders. Stakeholders refer to participants selected from random people with little knowledge of public health.

- Prediction on environmental health patterns through social media.

In future, investigation can be conducted by integrating more reliable medical sources supported by local and state level healthcare agencies. In knowledge discovery and data mining field, this is an essential element to develop a comprehensive environmental health management system that helps to predict the environmental health patterns. Prediction on environmental health patterns can be illustrated with a chart event. According to the collected data in MyEHMS, most of the environmental health information is considered post-event. Post-event refer to the incident that had already happened or just happened. In order to achieve the prediction concept, a forecasting model can be developed through integrating various valuable sources. For example, social media networks play a critical role to predict the environmental health patterns. Regular users of social media networks may post illness-related news. For example, a regular user makes a post that "today he is sick". With this, MyEHMS can collect and sort them into relevant groups and location. When the location and the particular disease are determined, it is assumed that the future incidents can be predicted. Apart from social media networks, weather forecast report may help to predict environmental health patterns. For example, 10% chance of showers today, but 70% chance of getting flu next month.

- Integrate with existing healthcare systems.

MyEHMS is only a prototype of tracking and monitoring environmental health issues in Malaysia. It is believed that the number of new diseases and toxic chemicals are growing every day. The growing number far exceeds the ability to test them on possible toxic effects on people, plants and animals in every place. It is unlikely for MyEHMS to detect all possible environmental health issues on a short term basis without improving the existing environmental health ontological model. However, it will be possible with support from other local healthcare-related systems from both private and public sector such as Total Hospital Information System (THIS), Personal Health Record (PHR), Teleprimary care, Clinical Information System (CIS), Oral Health Clinical Information System (OHCIS), and PrimaCare in Malaysia (Ministry of Health, 2012).

- Improve the Mobile-apps development.

More than ever, mobile apps are now looked upon as a robust tool that can make a big difference to tracking and monitoring environmental health issues. MyEHMS has a mobile-app version that allows tablet-users and mobile-users to keep track on environmental health issues in any places they want. The improvement shall be made when there is an opportunity to conduct user testing on the effectiveness of MyEHMS mobile-app. There is a potential for MyEHMS to receive voice command and response with environmental health issues. Voice recognition in mobile may help those users to speak on phone while the phone can process the instruction and response with retrieved results from MyEHMS.

- Self-learning module.

The method of collecting the data, including numbers and types of reporting sources, and time spent on collecting data are critical for MyEHMS. Sometimes, mistakes cannot be made when reporting the environmental health information when it is critical. There is a potential for MyEHMS to get self-learning module such as keyword self-refinement or correction. Self-learning module refer to learning activities designed for MyEHMS to work independently when it meets suggested new keywords or alternative keywords in web sources. The research can be deployed state-of-art at self-learning algorithms that automatically figured out which keywords in the database of tweets were associated with elevated levels of diseases. The self-learning module is an essential element for MyEHMS to continually grow and serve not only public users but also patients and physicians. This may improve the availability and utility of existing data but also facilitate the creation of new data to ensure the accessibility of core and other environmental health related issues.

According to California Environmental Health Investigation Branch (2012), although the environment is known to play an important role in human health, no comprehensive, integrated, state or national system exists to track the countless hazards, exposures, and ensuing health effects that could be due to environmental factors. There are tens of thousands of chemicals, and researchers are still learning about the toxic effects of many of them (California Environmental Health Investigation branch, 2012). For example, when environment is broadly defined to include air pollution and infectious disease, we will be able to assess the status of local air as good, moderate, unhealthy, very unhealthy and hazardous (Malaysia Department of Environment, 2009), or we will be able to identify disease transmission through air, water, food or other communicable media. There is growing scientific evidence that environmental factors are strongly linked to many chronic diseases such as asthma, birth defects, and cancer (Center for Disease Control and Prevention, 2012). The current systems in Malaysia (Air Pollutant Index management and communicable disease control information system) are insufficient to track some hazards and chronic diseases.

In response to this challenge, many healthcare agencies and researchers have developed environment health surveillance systems that involve the on-going collection, integration, analysis, interpretation, and dissemination of data on environmental hazards; exposures to those hazards; and related health effects in their own countries. The goal of tracking is to provide information that can be used to plan, apply, and evaluate actions to prevent and control environmentally related hazards, exposures and health. Undeniably, the social media networks and mobile technologies now provide absolute alternatives for monitoring the environmental health effect. They have absolute means of instant information mobility, real time update, forecast visualization, and prevention role in environmental health disaster.

CONCLUSION

We have seen that the Android mobile-based environmental health information source is a research stepping-stone in utilizing the social media networks and mobile technologies as data inputs and sources to understanding the effect of environmental health issues. Based on the accuracy testing results, data shows that the system is able to match exact environmental health keywords after keyword refinement was conducted and improved. This has also indicated that part 2 testing is rather more complicated than part 1 when it comes to evaluating the accuracy of parsing news feed data. It is believed that in real time platform social media users tend to use different vocabularies on the same topic. The vocabulary is not standardized in such an open platform and it may be difficult for the system to find the exact keywords. Further research is needed to have better control of ambiguity environmental health information by integrating with existing surveillance systems and ontological models that are much more constructive.

REFERENCES

Android. (2013). *Android application*. Retrieved March 4, 2013, from http://www.Android.com/

Avnet, L. (2013). Twitter could be useful in tracking disease outbreaks, study suggest. *Mashable*. Retrieved February 5, 2013, from http://www.huffingtonpost.com/2013/01/24/twitter-disease-outbreaks_n_2543495.html

Bautista, C. (2013). Twitter can help health officials track outbreaks. *Mashable*. Retrieved March 5, 2013, from http://mashable.com/2013/01/24/twitter-can-track-disease-outbreaks/

BodHuin. T., & Totorella, M. (2003). Using grid technologies for web-enabling legacy systems. In *Proceedings of Eleventh Annual International Workshop on Software Technology and Engineering Practice (STEP'03)*, (pp. 186-195). STEP.

California Environmental Health Investigation Branch. (2012). California Environmental Health Tracking Program. *Environmental Health Investigation Branch*. Retrieved June 4, 2012, from http://www.ehib.org/project.jsp?project_key=EHSS01

Cayzer, S. (2004). Semantic blogging and decentralized knowledge management. *Communications of the ACM, 47*(12), 47–52. doi:10.1145/1035134.1035164

Celcom. (2012). Celcom focuses on innovative mobile healthcare solutions. *Celcom*. Retrieved July 8, 2012, from http://www.theborneopost.com/2012/06/08/celcom-focuses-on-innovative-mobile-healthcare-solutions/

Centres for Disease Control and Prevention. (2010). *National environmental public health tracking network*. Center for Disease Control and Prevention. Retrieved June 5, 2012, from http://ephtracking.cdc.gov/showLocationLanding.action

Chunara, R., Andrews, J. R., & Brownstein, J. S. (2012). Social and news media enable estimation of epidemiological patterns early in the 2010 Haitian cholera outbreak. *The American Journal of Tropical Medicine and Hygiene, 86*(1), 39–45. doi:10.4269/ajtmh.2012.11-0597 PMID:22232449

Department of Environment. (2011). Air Pollutant Index Management System (APIMS). *Department of Environment Ministry of Natural Resources and Environment*. Retrieved June 5, 2011, from http://www.doe.gov.my/apims/

Department of Health New York. (2009). Glossary. *Department of Health*. Retrieved June 15, 2011, from http://www.health.ny.gov/environmental/public_health_tracking/about/glossary.htm

European Environment Agency (EEA). (2011). *Air Pollution monitoring system*. Retrieved June 8, 2011, from http://www.eea.europa.eu/maps/ozone/map

Facebook. (2013). Retrieved May 7, 2013, from https://www.facebook.com/

Factbrowser.com. (2012a). Malaysia has 34MM mobile subscribers and 17.5MM internet users. *Factbrowser*. Retrieved May 6, 2013, from http://www.factbrowser.com/facts/6143/

Factbrowser.com. (2012b). 87.9% of Malaysians on the Internet access Facebook. *Factbrowser*. Retrieved May 6, 2013, from http://www.factbrowser.com/facts/3404/

Factbrowser.com. (2012c). Malaysia's mobile penetration is more than 100%, compared to 59% for internet and 41% for social media. *Factbrowser*. Retrieved May 6, 2013, from http://www.factbrowser.com/facts/4159/

Firefly. (2013). Social animals on the move in Asia: A social media & mobile perspective. *Firefly*. Retrieved May 5, 2013, from http://www.fireflymb.com/Libraries/Papers_and_Presentations/FireflyMillwardBrown_AMAP_Social_Animals.sflb.ashx

Freifeld, C., & Brownstein, J. (2007). *HealthMap*. Retrieved June 7, 2011, from http://www.health-map.org/about/

Garrett, J. J. (2005). Ajax: A New Approach to Web Applications. *Adaptive Path*. Retrieved July 12, 2011, from http://www.adaptivepath.com/ideas/ajax-new-approach-web-applications

Google. (2012). Google Flu Trends. *Google.org*. Retrieved August 25, 2011, from http://www.google.org/flutrends/about/how.html

Health Protection Agency. (2010). Introduction to environmental public health tracking. *Health Protection Agency*. Retrieved May 8, 2013, from http://www.hpa.org.uk/webc/HPAwebFile/HPAweb_C/1287143109858

Healthmap. (2012). Healthmap. *Boston Children Hospital*. Retrieved June 4, 2012, from http://healthmap.org/en/

Jain, N., Dahlin, M., & Tewari, R. (2005). TAPER: Tiered approach for eliminating redundancy in replica synchronization. In *Proceedings of the 4th conference FAST 2005 on USEUNIX Conference on File and Storage Technologies*. USEUNIX.

Laird, S. (2012). How social media is taking over the news industry. *Mashable*. Retrieved May 20, 2013, from http://mashable.com/2012/04/18/social-media-and-the-news/

Lemon, S. M., Hamburg, M. A., Sparling, P. F., Choffnes, E. R., & Mack, A. (2007). Global infectious disease surveillance and detection: Assessing the challenges – Finding solutions. *Forum on Microbial Threats*. Retrieved May 8, 2013, from http://www.ncbi.nlm.nih.gov/books/NBK52867/pdf/TOC.pdf

Lowensohn, J. (2008). Google now tracking flu trends via search. *CNET*. Retrieved August 18, 2011, from http://news.cnet.com/google-now-tracking-flu-trends-via-search/

Maxis. (2012). Maxis and IJN establish partnership to bring healthcare content and awareness to maxis customers. *Maxis*. Retrieved 15 May, 2013, from http://www.maxis.com.my/mmc/index.asp?fuseaction=home.article&aid=618&status=1

MedLinePlus Health. (n.d.). Environmental Health Ontology. *BioPortal*. Retrieved June 10, 2011, from http://bioportal.bioontology.org/search

Ministry of Health. (2007). Communicable Disease Control Information System. *Ministry of Health*. Retrieved July 15, 2011, http://www.unescap.org/idd/events/2007_REM-avian-influenza/Surveillance-of-infectious-diseases-in-Malaysia.pdf

Ministry of Health. (2013). MyHealth. *Ministry of Health*. Retrieved 8 May, 2013, from http://www.myhealth.gov.my/v2/

Mokhtar, M. B., & Murad, M. D. W. (2010). Issues and framework of environmental health in Malaysia. *The Free Library by Farlex*. Retrieved June 1, 2011, http://www.thefreelibrary.com/Issues+and+framework+of+environmental+health+in+Malaysia.-a0222252556

New York Department of Health. (2009). Glossary. *Environmental Health Tracking*. Retrieved May 20, 2013, from http://www.health.ny.gov/environmental/public_health_tracking/about/glossary.htm

Nsubuga, P., White, M. E., Thacker, S. B., Anderson, M. A., Blount, S. B., & Broome, C. V. ... Trostle, M. (2006). *Public Health Surveillance: A tool for targeting and monitoring interventions disease control priorities in developing countries* (2nd ed.). Retrieved May 20, 2013, from http://www.ncbi.nlm.nih.gov/books/NBK11770/

O'Reilly, T. (2005). What is Web 2.0: Design patterns and business models for the next generation of software. *O'Reilly*. Retrieved July 16, 2011, from http://oreilly.com/web2/archive/what-is-web-20.html

Richards, T. B., Croner, C. M., Rushton, G., Brown, C. K., & Fowler, L. (1999). Geographical Information Systems and Public Health. *The Long Island Breast Cancer Study Project*. Retrieved March 10, 2011, from http://healthcybermap.org/HGeo/res/phr.pdf

Robertson, C., Sawford, K., Daniel, S. L. A., Nelson, T. A., & Stephen, C. (2010). *Mobile phone-based infectious disease surveillance system, Sri Lanka*. Retrieved May 13, 2013, from http://wwwnc.cdc.gov/eid/article/16/10/pdfs/10-0249.pdf

Schmidt, C. W. (2012). *Trending now: Using social media to predict and track disease outbreaks*. Retrieved May 15, 2013, from http://www.ncbi.nlm.nih.gov/pmc/articles/PMC3261963/

Sime Darby Healthcare. (2013). *Sime Darby Healthcare*. Retrieved May 15, 2013, from http://www.simedarbyhealthcare.com/

Taylor, C. (2013). *250,000 social media users in U.S. said they got the flu*. Retrieved May 18, 2013, from http://mashable.com/2013/01/16/facebook-twitter-flu/

Thesaurus, C. R. I. S. P. (2006). Environmental Health Ontology. *BioPortal*. Retrieved June 11, 2011, from http://bioportal.bioontology.org/search

Twitter. (2013). *Twitter Inc*. Retrieved May 18, 2013, from https://twitter.com/

Vodafone. (2012). *Disease outbreak*. Retrieved May 22, 2013, from http://mhealth.vodafone.com/solutions/access_to_medicine/disease_outbreaks/

Wisconsin Department of Health Services. (2011). *Wisconsin Environmental Public Health Tracking*. Retrieved June 8, 2011, from http://www.dhs.wisconsin.gov/epht/DataInfo.htm

Woodfin, G. (2011). *How to find your twitter RSS Feed & Profile ID Number*. Retrieved August 25, 2011, from http://www.glenwoodfin.com/rss/how-to-find-your-twitter-rss-feed-in-2011/

World Fact Book, C. I. A. (2012). The World Factbook Environment: Current issues. *Central Intelligence Agency*. Retrieved June 7 2011, from https://www.cia.gov/library/publications/the-world-factbook/fields/2032.html

World Health Organization. (2005). Malaysia Environmental Health Country Profile. *World Health Organization*. Retrieved June 8, 2011, from http://www.environment-health.asia/fileupload/malaysia_ehcp_07Oct2004.pdf

World Health Organization. (2008). *Foodborne disease outbreaks: Guidelines for investigation and control*. Retrieved August 29, 2011, from http://www.who.int/foodsafety/publications/foodborne_disease/outbreak_guidelines.pdf

Zhang, J., Shi, H., & Zhang, Y. (2009). Self-organizing map methodology and Google maps services for geographical epidemiology mapping. In *Proceedings of Digital Image Computing: Technique and Application 2009* (DICTA '09) (pp. 229-235). DICTA. doi:10.1109/DICTA.2009.4610.1109/DICTA.2009.46

KEY TERMS AND DEFINITIONS

Android: A type of operating system developed by Google for Mobile phones.

Environmental Health Surveillance/Information System: A surveillance system involving the collection, analysis, and dissemination of data for use in public health practices.

Environmental Health Tracking: The ongoing collection, integration, analysis, and interpretation of data about environmental hazards, exposure to environmental hazards and human health effects potentially related to exposure to environmental hazards.

Geocoding: A process of finding associated geographic coordinates (often expressed as latitude and longitude) from other geographic data.

Google Map: A web mapping service application and technology provided by Google.

Mobile Health Technologies: A term used for practice medicine and public health, supported by mobile devices.

Ontological Model: A domain ontology (or domain-specific ontology) models a specific domain, which represents part of the world.

RSS News Feed: A family of web feed formats used to publish frequently updated works such as blog entries, news headlines, audio and video.

Social Media: A media for social interaction, using highly accessible and scalable publishing techniques.

Chapter 12
The Introduction and Evaluation of Mobile Devices to Improve Access to Patient Records:
A Catalyst for Innovation and Collaboration

Jonn Wu
BC Cancer Agency Vancouver, Canada

Shaina Reid
IMITS Provincial Health Services Authorities, Canada

John Waldron
IMITS Provincial Health Services Authorities, Canada

Jeff Barnett
BC Cancer Agency Vancouver, Canada & University of Victoria, Canada

ABSTRACT

Prompt and efficient access to patient records is vital in providing optimal patient care. The Cancer Agency Information System (CAIS) is the primary patient record repository for the British Columbia Cancer Agency (BCCA) but is only accessible on traditional computer workstations. The BCCA clinics have significant space limitations resulting in multiple healthcare professionals sharing each workstation. Furthermore, workstations are not available in examination rooms. A novel and cost-efficient solution is necessary to improve clinician access to CAIS. This prompted the BCCA and the Provincial Health Services Authority (PHSA) Information Management Information Technology Services (IMITS) team to embark on an innovative provincial collaboration to introduce and evaluate the impact of a mobile device to improve access to CAIS. The project consisted of 2 phases with over 90 participants from multiple clinical disciplines across BCCA sites and other PHSA facilities. Phase I evaluated the adoptability, effectiveness, and costs associated with providing access to CAIS using desktop virtualization via Citrix. Citrix is a server solution that provides remote access to clients via the Web or to dummy terminals in a network. Phase II incorporated the feedback and findings from Phase I to develop a customized mobile application. Phase II also addressed privacy and security requirements and included additional users and workflows. This is explored in this chapter.

DOI: 10.4018/978-1-4666-6150-9.ch012

INTRODUCTION

The BC Cancer Agency (BCCA) provides a population-based cancer control program for the residents of British Columbia (BC) and the Yukon, two large regions in Canada, serving a population of over 4.5 million. The BCCA operates six regional cancer centres, and 56 community chemotherapy clinics. Patient health information is currently stored in a paper chart as well as an electronic clinical data repository (CAIS, Cancer Agency Information System). Although the paper chart functioned as the traditional patient record, it often does not travel as quickly as patients do as they move between cancer centres and clinics; furthermore, charts are often not up to date, compared to CAIS. In recent years, BCCA clinicians have become more reliant on CAIS, although access to the electronic record is limited to desktop computers in crowded physician work spaces; additionally, computer workstations are not available in patient encounter rooms or at the point of care. The inability to access the right information at the right time impacted clinical workflows and patient care. This chapter will discuss a successful health information technology implementation on the basis of a collaborative effort between clinicians who were empowered to drive the solution, and willing IT partners who acted as technology enablers.

BACKGROUND: THE IMPETUS FOR CHANGE

The BC Cancer Agency (BCCA) provides a population-based cancer control program for the residents of British Columbia and the Yukon (Canada), serving a population of over 4.5 million. Its mandate includes prevention, screening, diagnosis, treatment, and survivorship. The BCCA operates six regional cancer centres which provide the full spectrum of cancer care, from assessment and diagnostic services, to chemotherapy, radiotherapy and supportive care delivered by provincially standardized protocols. To properly serve the population which is dispersed over a large geographic area (1.4 million square kilometers, or 550,000 square miles), the six full service centres are supported by 56 community chemotherapy clinics so patients can receive portions of their cancer treatments closer to home.

Similar to other health organizations, patient health information was historically stored in a traditional paper chart. However, due to the potential distributed nature of cancer treatment delivery in BC i.e. a patient from a smaller community may be seen in consultation in their home community cancer clinic, followed by radiotherapy at a larger cancer centre, and complete their chemotherapy at their home clinic, the paper chart may not always follow the patient's whereabouts in a timely fashion. Furthermore, updating the paper chart with reports and results is a time consuming and resource intensive manual procedure which results in charts that are out of date.

In 1992, the BCCA started to develop CAIS (Cancer Agency Information System) initially as a patient scheduling system; since then, it has become a robust and rich multi-disciplinary electronic clinical data repository (Henkleman 2003). In addition to a multi-disciplinary scheduling system, CAIS also consolidates patient demographics, clinical documentation and other reports, and laboratory data from over 40 clinical sources. Other functions include an imbedded eFilm viewer for diagnostic images, a centralized population based cancer registry and patient outcomes data for survivorship research. Thus, it is understandable that BCCA clinicians have become more reliant on CAIS, rather than the paper chart, to provide timely and current information for a patient.

Unfortunately, two major issues prevent adequate access to the electronic record. Firstly, access is limited to bulky desktop computers in over-crowded physician workspaces. These workspaces were configured over 20 years ago to accommodate two physicians. Care teams have since expanded to include medical trainees, clinical fellows, nurses and other allied health care professionals. These workspaces can only accommodate two or three workstations, which result in multiple team members having to share a desktop. Secondly, computer workstations are not available in patient encounter rooms or at other points of care. Since the paper chart is often not available for a patient encounter, the clinician must transcribe salient pieces of information to a piece of paper that they can bring into the examination room; often, this is incomplete as it is difficult to anticipate what information is required until one has interacted with the patient. The inability to access the right information at the right time has significant impact on clinical workflow and patient care.

To address some of these issues, an early pilot project was initiated and run by Medical Oncologist, Dr. Kevin Murphy in 2007. His pilot project deployed and evaluated a small number of early tablet computers (Toshiba 200M Portege, 12" screen) to clinicians at the Fraser Valley Cancer Center, one of the six full service BC cancer centres. He had no formal information technology (IT) support during the pilot and was limited to the mobile devices available at the time. Participants expressed reluctance to engage with the tablet computers after seeing some of the early testers struggle with network access, connectivity, initializing the tablets, plugging in battery chargers and using a digital pen that was required for use of the device (Murphy, 2007).

Since that time, mobile information and communication technologies (ICT) have experienced significant advancements, with improved usability and increased wireless network coverage; this has resulted in the proliferation of mobile phones (smart phones), handheld devices (personal digital assistants, tablets), and mobile applications in general use (Bosivert, 2012). However, the future of mobile computing technologies and the realization of their full benefits in health care depend on integrating the current mobile solutions with

clinical workflow and the electronic health record (EHR). Many reports in the literature describe well intentioned but unsuccessful initiatives, or discuss descriptive outcomes that do not provide objective evidence to support the impact of mobile devices on workflow (Pan-Canadian Change Management Network, 2012, Keshavjee *et al*, 2006). However, one successful example is the Ottawa Hospital; in 2010, they successfully deployed a native iPad application to support clinicians' information and communication needs (Marin, 2011). They recently became the first hospital in the world to enable computerized provider order entry on the iPad. These success stories help identify key factors in successfully implementing and adopting information technologies. A key element includes documenting the users' workflow and information requirements: "The extent to which mobile technology will be adopted….will depend on how well the technology can support their day-to-day work routines" (Chatterjee et al 2009).

In response to limitations in accessing up to date clinical information, and spurred by the growth of mobile devices in everyday use, clinicians have increasingly requested solutions to provide mobile access to health records. One such group was the radiation oncologists at the Vancouver Cancer Centre (VCC). The VCC is the oldest of the 6 campuses, with many of the clinic areas built over 30 years ago, before planners had an opportunity to realize the growth in health care team members and desk space requirements for computers. Thus, any improvement in workflow would have a major impact at VCC. In early 2012, the clinical leadership at VCC recognized these challenges and endorsed an initiative to examine the use of mobile devices to improve access to electronic health records at the point of care. The authors assembled a project team including a clinician champion, clinical informatician, partners from Information Management Information Technology Services (IMITS), and other clinical leaders. To maximize the adoption of mobile devices in this initiative, the project team recognized that the objectives and directions of the application must be clinician driven, with our IT partners acting as important technology enablers. This chapter will review our collaborative effort, which resulted in a high adoption rate, and significant improvement in clinical workflow.

MOBILE ACCESS: PROJECT OVERVIEW

The mobility project was designed in two phases. Both phases would consist of a pre-usage survey, followed by 3 months of usage, and a post-usage survey. One on one interviews were also conducted for further impressions.

Phase I was an introductory mobility pilot which leveraged existing software solutions and campus-wide Wi-Fi to provide 34 clinicians read-only access to CAIS via Citrix. This was meant to be a fiscally efficient pilot where the only costs were purchasing the tablet devices. As well, since no customization of the software solutions were necessary, Phase I was able to launch very quickly, on April 1st, 2012.

The goal in Phase II was to develop a customized software solution specifically for the mobile device. Clinical requirements and design elements of the software application consisted of feedback from Phase I, as well as input from 8 clinicians who participated in the development phase. On July 30st, 2012 Phase II was expanded first to 50 clinicians across multiple BCCA facilities, then to a further 40 clinicians at other hospital sites. Pre- and post-usage surveys and interviews were conducted to assess feedback and post-usage adoption.

The following sections will provide greater detail as well as discuss the pre- and post-usage evaluations for each phase.

PHASE I: INTRODUCTION TO MOBILITY

Proposed Solution

During the project planning phase, the clinical leadership recognized the value in assessing mobile solutions to improve access to electronic health records. However, during Phase I of the project, resources were only available to purchase mobile devices; resources were not available to purchase any software solutions, software customization, network hardware, data access, user training or technical support. This limited the scope of potential software/hardware solutions. This caveat was the main driver when determining the proposed solution for Phase I.

Given the resource limitations, the clinicians' requirements were limited but very clear i.e. the chosen mobile device would need to be small, portable and easy to use. As well, they did not want any additional login accounts i.e. User access must be linked to their existing enterprise Windows login account. Since the project lacked on site support during this first phase, the operating system would need to be intuitive, and one that most clinicians would already be familiar with. Thus, the project team selected the Apple iPad2 as the mobile device. At the time of the project planning phase in early 2012, the iPad tablets were the clear market leaders accounting for 80-90% of all internet traffic on tablet devices (Sterling, 2013). This was clearly evident in health care too, since most of the physicians who participated in Phase I already owned an iOS device (iPhone, iPad, or both). These trends continue to date, as a recent survey in the US revealed 68% of physicians own an iPhone, 59% own an iPad whilst 31% owned other smart phones or tablets (The Year of the Big EHR switch 2013). It was hypothesized that if participants were already familiar with using an iOS device, this would help facilitate adoption of its use in the clinic. Early reports in the non-academic literature have suggested that iPads have a high degree of user-friendliness and are easy to clean; a report from a large pediatric hospital suggested that these devices have a promising potential in healthcare and help provide for portability, convenience and quick access (Teves, 2013). Despite the lack of technical support, we employed a research assistant to write a series of How-To documents that were available on an intranet set; these documents were also given to participants prior to commencing the project. Topics included: how to create an iTunes account, how to connect to our wifi network, how to access Outlook/Exchange Server, and how to use the Citrix application. Remarkably, despite not having any previous experience with iOS, our research assistant was able to learn how to use the operating system, and create the documents, within a week.

The lack of resources proved to be more challenging when considering technical issues for Phase I. In terms of software solutions, the BCCA and IMITS have a site-wide license for Citrix. All BCCA clinicians have access to CAIS via Citrix on their clinic desktops, and were well versed with using Citrix when information was required remotely. Thus, we leveraged the existing Citrix infrastructure to install the iOS Citrix application on the tablets. Users may only log into Citrix if they have a valid Windows login account. No further user management was necessary for this initial phase.

Data access was provided through campus-wide wifi networks, which had been recently installed at all six regional cancer centres in late 2011. All parts of the hospitals, including traditional "dead zones" in radiation shielded areas had wifi hotspots in order to support the use of chemotherapy "smart infusion pumps" (Dose Error Reduction devices, DERs). This meant tablet devices could access our secure wifi network from any part of the hospital, thereby providing data access at the point of care without incurring any further expenses.

Security was a significant concern during the life of this project. Fortunately, by leveraging existing IT solutions and user permissions, this provided some security solutions too. For example, a user cannot access the wifi network unless they have been authenticated with a valid and current PHSA Windows login account. Furthermore, one can only access the Citrix servers if the user has been granted the appropriate permissions to do so. Lastly, because Citrix is a viewer that provides "read only access" to CAIS, no patient information resides on the tablet.

At the time of the pilot project, the provincial Health Shared Services of British Columbia (HSSBC) and IMITS teams were in the midst of procuring a robust mobile device management (MDM) system. A MDM system is software that secures, monitors and helps support mobile devices deployed across an enterprise. This was not available for our project. Thus, we leveraged the existing MDM features in Microsoft Exchange Server, by forcing users to connect their tablets to the Exchange Server in order to access their corporate (Outlook) emails and calendars. This provided the project team the ability to force the use of passwords, mandatory time outs, and remote wiping of the device in the event the device was lost or stolen.

Study Design

All physicians who were present during the study period (April to June, 2012) were automatically enrolled into the study, to avoid any selection or other unintentional bias which might be present in early adopters. In total, 34 physicians from the Department of Radiation Oncology at the Vancouver Cancer Centre participated in Phase I.

All users completed a mandatory 16 question online survey, followed by a 30 minute introduction to the tablet to ensure users were able to create an iTunes account, connect to the WIFI network, access the Exchange Server to access their emails/calendars (to ensure the appropriate MDM settings were pushed to the device), and lastly the user was able to use the Citrix application to connect to CAIS. This was followed by a three month usage period (April 1st to July 1st, 2012). No formal onsite technical support was available; all assistance was provided by our research assistant, colleagues, or by contacting Apple Support. Phase I was concluded by an online post-usage survey (36 questions) and one on one interviews. See Appendix 1 and 2 for the surveys.

Results

The pre-usage survey confirmed our impression that our cohort of participants were relatively tech savvy. For example, 86% already use a mobile device on a daily basis, and 78% use a mobile device in their current clinical workflow. Furthermore, the survey also revealed that the majority were optimistic that mobile devices will enhance their clinical workflow (67%), and 91% were looking forward to adding a mobile device to the clinic setting.

The post-usage survey was completed by 32 of 34 participants (94%). Additional insight was provided by one-on-one interviews. For the most part, clinicians were pleased with the form factor (70% agreed the tablet was portable and easy to carry around), and the majority used the device for other purposes, including emails (96%) and other medical applications (60%). More importantly, 63% indicated the mobile device had a positive impact on their clinical workflow, and 76% confirmed access to CAIS provided more current information than what was available in the paper chart. Lastly, 83% of users had a positive experience with the device, and 73% believed it was useful in a clinical setting.

Despite the high rate of adoption and the belief that the tablet improved access to health informa-

tion, only 50% were satisfied with the screen size, 55% thought the resolution was sufficient to review electronic records appropriately, 55% thought the text was too small, and in the end, only 50% thought the screen was of an appropriate size. These results should not be surprising since the iPad2 screen is only 9.7" (diagonally), whereas the average desktop monitor used to access CAIS in the clinic is 21". Using Citrix to view CAIS on a significantly smaller screen without the opportunity to optimize how data was being displayed resulted in an equivocal user experience.

Summary

By leveraging existing software solutions and campus-wide WIFI, the introduction of mobile devices to view health information demonstrated an overall positive impact on clinical workflow while addressing space and access concerns. Because the software and data presentation could not be customized to the tablet's ideal form factor, usability was an important impediment to maximizing adoption amongst clinicians. Feedback from Phase I was then used to drive the solution in Phase II.

PHASE II: ACTING ON KEY FINDINGS

Proposed Solution

The goal of Phase II was to determine if an alternative approach to application delivery and information presentation on a mobile device would positively impact the findings in Phase I. The results of Phase I found 55% of clinicians would be willing to use the solution for review of clinical information. Phase II focused on improving the delivery and format of the views of clinical information on a mobile device. The goals were improving access to clinical information, solution usability, security and privacy requirements, as well as evaluation of the solution in different clinical settings.

The solution in Phase II was developed through partnership with a vendor who was tested and proven in the marketplace. The selected vendor focused on collecting data from multiple clinical information systems and presenting in a single, integrated patient-centric view. The innovative platform was originally developed with input from clinicians, administrators and IT experts at a Canadian hospital. The solution, while designed inherently to generically address the need to display clinical information on a tablet format, also allowed for flexibility in configuration to meet the specific requirement at BCCA and other PHSA facilities. Design, development and testing of the solution for PHSA involved various clinical and technical inputs over a 3 month period leading to the deployment and activation.

Study Design

There were ninety (90) participants in the study. Twenty-five (25) radiation oncologists from multiple BCCA sites, some of whom participated in Phase I, were included in Phase II. Additionally, twenty—five (25) medical oncologists from Systemic Therapy groups across all BCCA centers were invited to participate. Additionally, forty (40) clinicians from BC Children's and Women's Hospitals (C&W) participated.

Communication of the activation was primarily handled through an intranet website and email; participants were emailed the link to the intranet site which included the four steps required to enroll in the project. Step 1 provided information about the purpose of the study; Step 2 incorporated privacy and security requirements by having participants sign a privacy agreement developed specifically for the project; Step 3 provided a baseline survey that aligned with Phase I; and Step 4 provided instructions on how to launch the patient record viewer application on the mobile device.

As previously discussed, the project team recognized the importance of clinician engagement to ensure the product will support their workflows and provide the required information at the point of care. The clinician-driven design process invited users to participate at various levels, including: 1) the clinical design team, 2) as a usability tester, or 3) as a pilot user. We believe integrating end users in the design process will maximize the probability of producing a useful tool and ultimately drive adoption of an information technology solution. These sessions resulted in versions of the application to support workflows in different environments. One version of the mobile application presented information from CAIS and WORx (pharmacy system) targeting the BCCA participants. A second version presented information from EVE, the legacy clinical information viewer used at C&W. Both versions provided a user interface designed as a native iOS application (the operating system used by iPads). The application provided users with read-only access to all of the patient information available in the clinical applications. Also, the application provided access to clinicians' clinic schedule and patient appointments. The application has a user-defined configuration for the visual layout of the patient record.

Many of the elements of the patient chart were combined into a single view that was referred to as a patient dashboard made up of dashlets for each area of the patient chart (see Figure 1).

The application also presented the end user with laboratory values in a grid format that was easy to read and viewable as a time line (see Figure 2). The time period could be set by the end user to change how far back they wanted to look for results, in order to allow clinicians to find their own balance between speed and information available.

Patient medications were displayed in a grid showing all current medications (see Figure 3).

At the end of Phase II, participants were asked to complete a post-implementation survey to measure the effect of the mobile device and patient

Figure 1. Application showing a Patient Dashboard

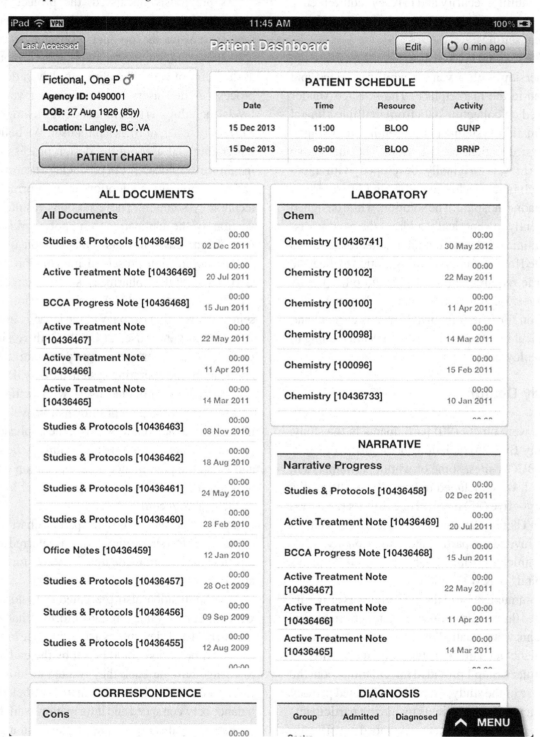

Figure 2. Laboratory results displayed in a grid format

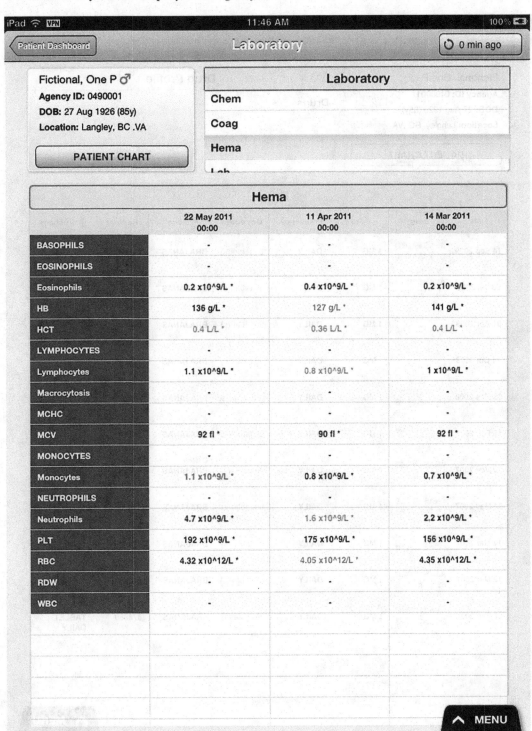

Figure 3. Medication display – all current medications

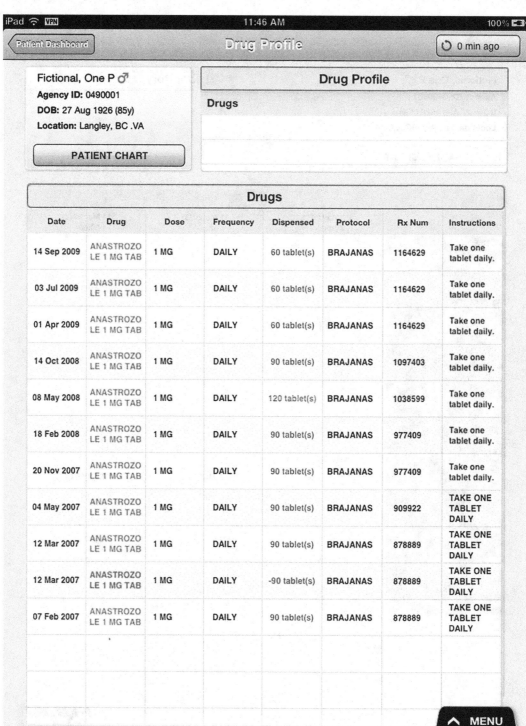

record application. A subset of participants was observed while using the current tools such as desktop computers and paper charts. This was compared to the post-pilot observations when the mobile device and patient record viewer application was available. The observations captured data about time required to access patient information, turnaround time between patients, and challenges with using the tools. Twelve semi-structured interviews were also conducted during the project period.

A multi-method research study was used for the evaluation that involved surveys, observational studies, and interviews. The responses to the post-implementation survey and interviews determined if and how mobile devices and the patient record viewer application are useful and effective in a clinical setting. The baseline survey results were compared to the post-implementation survey results. Similarly, the results of the baseline observations were compared to the post-implementation observation results. The interview results were analyzed using grounded theory methodology to identify the major themes.

Results

In general, the results show that clinicians are among the early adopters of mobile computing technology according to Rogers' Diffusion Theory (with more than 90% of the respondents are using mobile computing technology in their clinical practice). The majority of the respondents (> 80%) are either very comfortable or comfortable with using mobile computing technology.

Clinicians highly appreciate the in-time availability of information (98%), a privilege peculiar to mobile technologies that subsequently offer clinicians the ability to access information when and where it is needed. Other highly ranked and expected functionalities include: using the mobile device for patient education, communication purposes, and for clinical decision-making. Moreover, almost all respondents (98%) expect the iPad and

other mobile computing technology become a larger part of the patient care experience for both clinicians and patients.

The majority of the post-implementation survey respondents (92%) are either highly or moderately satisfied with the solution (see Figure 4). Clinicians rated their overall satisfaction with the solution between 4 and 5 with 5 being extremely positive. The iPad application user interface, multiple functionalities, and ease of use were the main drivers for clinicians' positive feedback.

Based on the results of the post-pilot survey, most of the post-implementation survey respondents (92%) found that the response time, security and reliability of the iPad and the mobile application to be either moderately or highly acceptable (see Figure 5).

In terms of the information quality (completeness, relevance, accuracy, format, comprehensiveness), most of respondents (92%) found the information within mobile application to be either highly or moderately acceptable (see Figure 6).

Similarly, most participants (90%) agree that there were sufficient technical support and training resources for the solution.

In general, most of the respondents (95%) rated the service quality (implementation process, technical support, and training) either moderately or high acceptable (see Figure 7).

In terms of productivity and efficiency, clinicians reported reduction in the number of interruptions during patient visits and a reduction in the need for printing (reports, conference documents). Most of the survey respondents (> 80%) believe that the mobile device improved their workflow as it facilitated the retrieval of information. This allowed the clinicians to involve the patients in care planning, increase collaboration with other healthcare providers and enhance support in decision.

The goal in Phase II was to improve usability and chose to evaluate an application solution built specifically for the mobile device, in this case using a native iOS application. Clinical requirements and design elements of the software

Figure 4. Post-pilot survey: Clinicians level of satisfaction

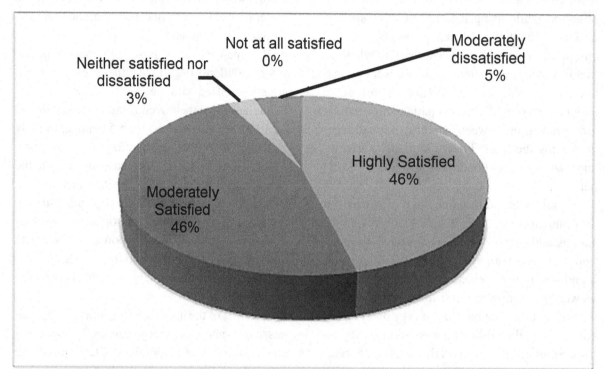

Figure 5. Post-pilot survey: System quality

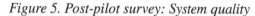

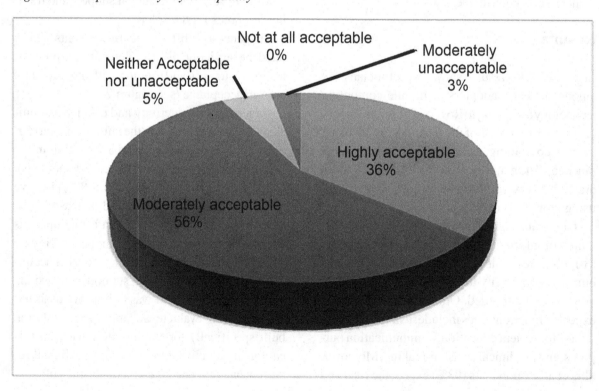

Figure 6. Post-pilot survey: Information quality

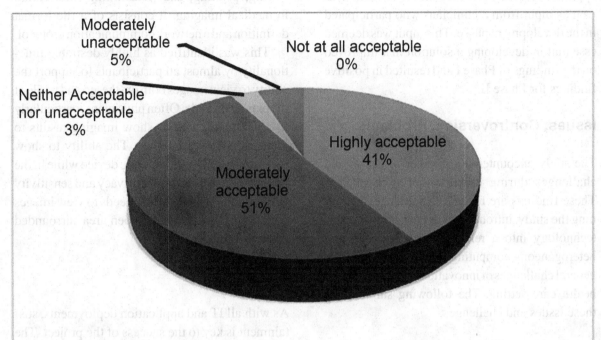

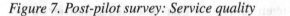

Figure 7. Post-pilot survey: Service quality

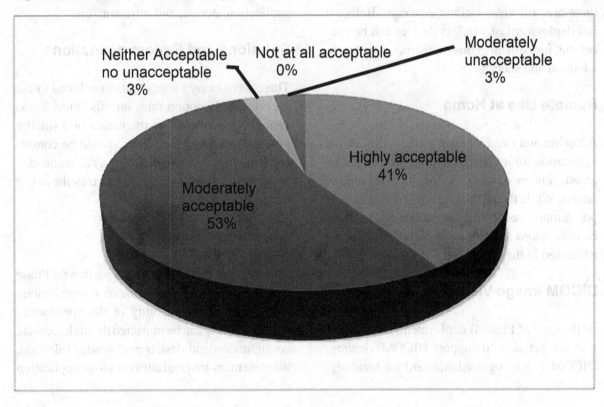

application consisted of feedback from Phase I, as well as input from 8 clinicians who participated in the development phase. This input was deemed essential in developing a solution that improved on the findings of Phase I and resulted in positive findings for Phase II.

Issues, Controversies, Problems

The study encountered a number of issues and challenges during execution of both phases. These findings are related to challenges in running the study, introduction of new, non-standard technology into a relatively conservative, and heterogeneous computing environment, and the general challenges of innovation in a public-sector health care setting. The following summarizes these issues and challenges.

Wi-Fi Access

While the issue of incomplete wireless network access had been addressed at BCCA, at C&W there are still areas lacking coverage. Before a full deployment of wireless devices can be successful, investment in this infrastructure is key to adoption and success.

Remote Use at Home

Adoption and satisfaction with the utility of the application for a variety of workflows would be greatly enhanced with the addition of remote access. While the technology available does support remote access, there are privacy and security considerations and risk assessments that must be addressed in the future.

DICOM Image Viewing

At the time of Phase II deployment, the solution was not yet able to support DICOM viewing. DICOM is a recognized standard for handling, storing, printing, and transmitting information in medical imaging. It consists of a file format definition and a network communication protocol.

This was identified as highly desirable functionality by almost all participants to support the ability to view images both on-the-go and while at the patient bedside. Often physicians, particularly in cancer care, wish to show imaging results to their patients and families. The ability to show these images through a mobile device while in the patient room would ensure privacy and sensitivity to the patient who currently needs to view images with their physician in an open area surrounded often by other staff.

Sustainment

As with all IT and application deployments, sustainment is key to the success of the project. The pilot nature of this initiative did not make accommodations for ongoing support of the application. Moving forward successfully will require a support team with training and knowledge transfer on the application, device, and infrastructure.

Solutions and Recommendations

There were many factors that contributed to the success and adoption rates on this study. Some factors were inherent in the nature of a smaller pilot project while the others should be considered for similar deployments as a recommended approach. The following summarizes these key success factors.

Application Usability

The process to select the vendor partner for Phase II of this project included market research along assessment of the usability of the application. While usability can be impacted through accurate configuration and design post vendor selection, there are many inherent attributes to an application that cannot be modified. It is crucial to select a partner vendor whose usability has been tested and proven. Various methods to usability evaluation are possible such as think aloud, surveys, interviews, focus groups, design or cognitive walk-throughs. The usability of the system, in this project, led to the elimination of formal training as part of the project, further increasing adoption and satisfaction for busy physician schedules.

Device Selection

The decision to focus on iPads was a deliberate decision that led to high adoption rates. The iPad is currently the most popular tablet computer on the market; many had previously used the device, were familiar with the functionality and did not require training. The iPad is also fast to log on to in comparison to desktop computers in the current environment. The selection of iPads as the device of choice also meant the ease of obtaining test devices was simplified as many clinical areas were willing to purchase these devices with their own funding in combination with trial devices offered by Apple. Future deployments in conjunction with a "Bring Your Own Device" (BYOD) approach, will also lend to high adoption since so many users already own iPads and iPhones.

Privacy Was Not an Obstacle

An important element to the design of the Phase II strategy was elimination of storage of patient data in any secondary location, including on the iPad or in a separate database. The use of mobile device management (MDM) functions also ensured privacy and security legislation was adhered to. Mobile device management software offer the ability to remote wipe the device to remove access to the clinical applications as well as can limit other features that pose a security risk. As this was a pilot project, very few iPad features were disabled, however in the future this risk assessment will need to be repeated to ensure a balance can be appropriately found between security risk and functionality restriction. Fewer restrictions on the iPad will lead to higher adoption.

Personal vs. Shared Devices

Mobile devices, particularly iPads are typically intended to be used as a one user personal device, as opposed to shared device. This deployment model, allows a user to stay logged into their device as the move between clinics, locations and patients. With desktop PCs, many people leave the PC "locked" thus requiring other users to reboot the PC to gain access. On the current state PC configuration, the length of time it takes to log on to the operating system to access the application is another inhibiting factor. Testing showed that log on to a newer desktop PC can take up to 1.5 minutes to access the clinical information system, versus less that 5 seconds for access to the iPad application.

Vendor Selection

In the mobile application arena the vendor must be flexible, agile and fast paced while remaining low cost. In Phase II, the selected vendor used a prototyping approach effectively and was very adaptable to changing requirements with strong ability to communicate with our clinical design team.

Clinical Engagement

The time given up by physicians and other clinical stakeholders was integral to the speed of the design phase and overall satisfaction and ownership of the end product. The project team outlined various levels of engagement available to clinical volunteers in the project. Depending on availability, clinicians participated on 1) the clinical design team, 2) as a usability tester, or 3) as a pilot user.

Research Component

This pilot initiative included academic diligence, through a partnership with the University of Victoria. This element to the project provided the ability to collect baseline and post implementation data to show the value provided to clinicians for decision makers at the executive level to determine the next steps.

FUTURE RESEARCH DIRECTIONS

The study findings suggest mobile access to clinical information in a usable format is beneficial for the care provider. While this study focused on a particular application running on a specific form-factor (iPad), future research should consider alternative form factors with the goals of identifying the best means to provide the right information, in the right format, at the right time and place for the clinician. Considering at this time technologies such as Google Glass, and "smart watches" or more generally referred to as "wearable computing", there is further research needed to understand the applicability of these form-factors in a clinical setting including usability as a primary concern.

Future research should focus on providing both read and data entry functionality in a mobile solution. The ability to take action, with as few impediments as possible, upon reading information is key to efficient processes. In theory, providing order entry and charting functions in the clinical application would increase adoption and derive workflow efficiencies.

Further to providing data entry functionality for the clinician, there are a growing number of opportunities to use a mobile device as a biomedical device. For example, peripherals can be attached to a tablet and with the appropriate application, collect data such as vital signs, blood pressure, and even generate ECG tracings. The integration of the biomedical data directly into the electronic health record and made available immediately to all providers may have benefits for patient care. There may be opportunities to leverage that biomedical data for decision support, alerts, and notifications.

Future research should consider the role of the mobile device as a primary communications tool for clinicians and their care teams. There is potential to provide means for clinicians to engage others through instant messaging, video chats, and simple online presence detection. Reducing the technical limitations to intra-provider communications may facilitate consultations and hand-offs in the care setting.

Many clinicians, and the general public, now own some form of mobile device. For many, they access their personal mobile device throughout the day both at work and home. There has been demand in organizations to allow use of personal devices for work purposes. This notion is referred to as "Bring Your Own Device" or BYOD. The concept is focused on people using any device of their choice at work. It is then the organization's responsibility to provide secure access to the applications and data. In general, this is achieved using web browser-based applications or remote-access software such as Citrix. The nature of BYOD and effectively managing such solutions in a health care setting is not well researched. There are a myriad of issues and solutions to address many of them; however, future research should be considered on how best to deliver an effective BYOD solution without jeopardizing privacy and delivering a sustainable solution.

CONCLUSION

In healthcare, timely access to patient information at the point of care is vital in the care process. At BCCA an electronic repository called CAIS is used to store patient information alongside the traditional paper chart. Due to limitations of the paper chart, clinicians prefer using CAIS to access information. Unfortunately, access is limited to computer workstations in overcrowded work spaces; furthermore, workstations are not available in patient encounter rooms.

The proliferation of mobile devices in recent years prompted clinicians and investigators at the BCCA to partner with the PHSA IMITS team to investigate the potential of these devices to improve clinical workflow. The project consisted of 2 phases with over 90 participants from multiple clinical disciplines across BCCA sites and other PHSA facilities. Phase I leveraged existing software and hardware infrastructure at the BCCA to provide mobile access to 34 clinicians, using a generic viewer (Citrix). Although feedback was largely positive, the end users' main complaints were related to usability. Phase II incorporated the feedback and findings from Phase I, and invited clinicians to participate on the design team to develop a customized mobile application. Phase II also addressed privacy and security requirements and included additional users and workflows. Despite adding significant complexity by expanding the user base to over 90 users across multiple and different health care environments, the post-usage surveys revealed over 90% of users successfully adopted the solution in their daily workflow.

We believe key success factors in this and other solution transformation projects include engaging the end users to ensure their workflow, information and usability requirements are included in the design of the tool. In our project, the key ingredient for success was the collaborative partnership between clinicians and the IMITS team within PHSA. The clinicians fully understood the clinical workflow and information requirements. However, they realized they could not implement a technology solution on their own, and embraced the concept of partnering with the IMITS team from the conceptual design phase to the execution of a solution. To that end our PHSA IMITS partners recognized the importance of empowering clinicians to drive the development of the product, which allowed the development

team to act as technology enablers. This was an example of how a partnership between the clinical and the technical realms could ensure the success of a potentially complicated health information technology project.

ACKNOWLEDGMENT

The authors wish to acknowledge the contributions from the following individuals: Dr. Mohamed Khan, John French, and Adam Kahnamelli from the BC Cancer Agency, and Dr. Omid Shabestari, Shadi Melhem, and Stacey Slager from the University of Victoria.

REFERENCES

Boisvert, S. (2012). An enterprise look at mHealth. *Journal of Healthcare Risk Management, 32*(2), 44–52. doi:10.1002/jhrm.21094 PMID:22996431

Henkleman, D. (2003). The Evolution of a Health Information Brokering Service in the Province of British Columbia. *Electronic Healthcare, 2*(2), 16–21.

Keshavjee K. Bosomworth J. Copen J. Lai J. Kucuky-azici B. Lilani R. Holbrook A. M. (2006). Best Practices in EMR Implementation: A Systematic Review. In Proceedings of AMIA Annual Symposium. AMIA.

Martin, R. (2011). *Onsite: The iPad Revolution at the Ottawa Hospital Deploying Mobile Technology in a Large Hospital*. Retrieved from http://www.mobilehealthcaretoday.com/onsites/2011/01/the-ottawa-hospitals-ipad-revolution.aspx

Murphy, K. (2007). *Evaluating the Use of Tablet PCs in an Ambulatory Clinic Setting*. Retrieved from http://www.medicalcomputing.org/mcr/openaccess.php

Pan-Canadian Change Management Network - Communications Working Group. (2012). *Why Change Matters - Investing in Change Management*. Retrieved from https://www. infoway-inforoute.ca/index.php/resources/tool-kits/change-management/national-framework/governance-and-leadership/resources-and-tools/doc_download/1330-why-change-matters-investing-in-change-management-healthcare-information-management-communications-hcim-c-2012-26-3-44-46

Sterling, G. (2013, May 29). *Tablet Market Share iPad Remains Dominant, Samsung Shows Growth*. Retrieved from http://marketingland.com/tablet-market-share-ipad-remains-dominant-samsung-shows-growth-45974

Sutirtha, C., Suranjan, C., Saonee, S., Suprateek, S., & Lau, F. (2009). Examining Success Factors For Mobile Work In Healthcare: A Deductive Study. *Decision Support Systems*, *46*(3), 620–633. doi:10.1016/j.dss.2008.11.003

Teves, J., Chaparro, B., Chan, R., Copic, N., Riss, R., & Simmons, J. (2013). *Exploring iPad Usage by Healthcare Professionals in a Pediatric Hospital*. Retrieved from http://usabilitynews.org/exploring-ipad-usage-by-healthcare-professionals-in-a-pediatric-hospital/

Year of the Big EHR Switch Confirms Physicians Favor iPad and Mobile Applications. (2013, May 30). Retrieved from http://www. prweb.com/releases/2013/5/prweb10553455. htm?PID=6150547

KEY TERMS AND DEFINITIONS

BYOD : Bring Your Own Device; concept whereby people use a personal device in a corporate or enterprise setting. Considerations need to be made for how a range of devices will access systems.

CAIS: Cancer Agency Information System; application used by BC Cancer to manage patients, schedules, reports, scanned documents, other EMR functions.

Citrix: Citrix Corp. manufacture a family of products that provide access to server-based hosting of desktop applications and environments. See http://www.citrix.com.

Computerized Provider Order Entry: A computer application that provides functionality to enter and track orders for a patient (e.g. lab order, imaging order) and review the status and results of an order. The order placer can be a nurse, a doctor, a clerk or anyone with appropriate permissions to create an order for the given patient.

Customized Mobile Application: A computer application that runs on portable device such as a laptop, tablet or smartphone. Customized implies the application was configured to the specific needs of its users.

Form Factor: Refers to the physical geometry of a computer device. Describes the shape and style of a computer device. E.g. laptop, tablet, phone.

MDM: Acronym; Mobile Device Management. Software solution used to manage mobile devices (e.g. tablets, smartphones); provides features to apply security settings, administer operating systems, track and apply changes to devices as required by IT policy.

Mobile Device: A computer that can travel with the user without need to be physically connected to a power source or network; no wires or other physical constraints. General term to describe computers such as tablets, smartphones and laptops.

Usability: The ease of use and learnability of a human-made object such as a computer application.

APPENDIX 1

Phase I iPad Pilot Project: Pre-Usage Survey

General Experience with Mobile Devices

1. I would describe my comfort with using mobile devices (iPad, PDA, Blackberry, tablet) as"
    a. Very comfortable.
    b. Comfortable.
    c. Somewhat comfortable.
    d. Not very comfortable.
2. In my personal life, I use a mobile device:
    a. Every day.
    b. A few times a week.
    c. A few times a month.
    d. Not at all.
3. I find mobile devices _____ in my personal life.
    a. Extremely useful.
    b. Useful.
    c. Somewhat useful.
    d. Not at all useful.
4. I would say that mobile devices are _____ in my professional practice.
    a. Extremely useful.
    b. Useful.
    c. Somewhat useful.
    d. Not at all useful.

Thoughts about the iPad in Clinical Practice

5. I think that having an iPad as a part of my clinical practice will greatly enhance my work flow.
    a. Strongly agree.
    b. Agree.
    c. Neutral.
    d. Disagree.
    e. Strongly disagree.
6. I already know what functions I will use the iPad for.
    a. Strongly agree.
    b. Agree.
    c. Neutral.
    d. Disagree.
    e. Strongly disagree.
7. It will take a bit of time to get familiar with how the iPad works.

    a.   Strongly agree.

    b.   Agree.

    c.   Neutral.

    d.   Disagree.

    e.   Strongly disagree.

8.   I am looking forward to using the iPad in my clinical practice.

    a.   Strongly agree.

    b.   Agree.

    c.   Neutral.

    d.   Disagree.

    e.   Strongly disagree.

9.   I have heard from colleagues that have used the iPad in their clinical practice.

    a.   Strongly agree.

    b.   Agree.

    c.   Neutral.

    d.   Disagree.

    e.   Strongly disagree.

10.   Overall, the feedback I hear about iPads in clinical practice is positive.

    a.   Strongly agree.

    b.   Agree.

    c.   Neutral.

    d.   Disagree.

    e.   Strongly disagree.

11.   I have independently looked into using the iPad or other mobile devices in my clinical practice.

    a.   Strongly agree.

    b.   Agree.

    c.   Neutral.

    d.   Disagree.

    e.   Strongly disagree.

12.   I think patients are starting to expect more mobile devices and a greater presence of information technology as a part of their health care experience .

    a.   Strongly agree.

    b.   Agree.

    c.   Neutral.

    d.   Disagree.

    e.   Strongly disagree.

13.   I plan to use the iPad to ONLY review charts before I visit the patient.

    a.   Strongly agre.e

    b.   Agree.

    c.   Neutral.

    d.   Disagree.

    e.   Strongly disagree.

14. I plan to use the iPad to ONLY discuss medical imaging and test results with the patient during the patient interview.
    a. Strongly agree.
    b. Agree.
    c. Neutral.
    d. Disagree.
    e. Strongly disagree.
15. I plan to use the iPad before and during the patient interview.
    a. Strongly agree.
    b. Agree.
    c. Neutral.
    d. Disagree.
    e. Strongly disagree.
16. I expect that iPads and other devices like it will becoming a larger part of cancer care experience for patients as well as health care professionals.
    a. Strongly agree.
    b. Agree.
    c. Neutral.
    d. Disagree.
    e. Strongly disagree.

APPENDIX 2

Phase II iPad Pilot Project: Post-Usage Survey

General Experience

1. Overall, I had a _____ experience in using the iPad.
    a. Very positive.
    b. Positive.
    c. Neutral.
    d. Negative.
    e. Very negative.
2. I found the iPad got in the way of my practice rather than enhanced it.
    a. Strongly agree.
    b. Agree.
    c. Neutral.
    d. Disagree.
    e. Strongly disagree.

Practical and Logistic Issues with the iPad

3. I found the iPad easy to carry around.
   a. Strongly agree.
   b. Agree.
   c. Neutral.
   d. Disagree.
   e. Strongly disagree.
4. I had concerns about how to keep the iPad clean and free from infection.
   a. Strongly agree.
   b. Agree.
   c. Neutral.
   d. Disagree.
   e. Strongly disagree.
5. I had concerns about the battery life of the iPad, that it might not make it through the day without being charged.
   a. Strongly agree.
   b. Agree.
   c. Neutral.
   d. Disagree.
   e. Strongly disagree.
6. I had no problem with connectivity to the network for Internet access.
   a. Strongly agree.
   b. Agree.
   c. Neutral.
   d. Disagree.
   e. Strongly disagree.
7. I had no problem logging in to the PHSA network.
   a. Strongly agree.
   b. Agree.
   c. Neutral.
   d. Disagree.
   e. Strongly disagree.

Usability Issues with the iPad

8. I found the resolution of the screen for viewing images to be satisfactory.
   a. Strongly agree.
   b. Agree.
   c. Neutral.
   d. Disagree.
   e. Strongly disagree.

9. I prefer to use an external keyboard when using the iPad.
    a. Strongly agree.
    b. Agree.
    c. Neutral.
    d. Disagree.
    e. Strongly disagree.
10. I found the screen size to be:
    a. Way too large.
    b. A bit large.
    c. Just the right size.
    d. A bit too small.
    e. Way too small.
11. I found the font size to be:
    a. Way too large.
    b. A bit large.
    c. Just the right size.
    d. A bit too small.
    e. Way too small.
12. I found it _____ to enter patient data into the iPad.
    a. Very easy.
    b. Easy.
    c. Neither easy nor difficult.
    d. Somewhat difficult.
    e. Very difficult.
13. I found it _____ to check and write email on the iPad.
    a. Very easy.
    b. Easy.
    c. Neither easy nor difficult.
    d. Somewhat difficult.
    e. Very difficult.
14. I found it _____ to review labs on the iPad.
    a. Very easy.
    b. Easy.
    c. Neither easy nor difficult.
    d. Somewhat difficult.
    e. Very difficult.
15. Was the iPad you were using lost or stolen?
    a. Lost.
    b. Stolen.
    c. Neither.
16. Did you at any time feel the need for a supplementary power adaptor?
    a. Yes.
    b. No.

17. How would you say using the iPad in your practice impacted your workflow process?
    a. Significantly impacted.
    b. Somewhat impacted.
    c. Neutral.
    d. Barely impacted.
    e. Not at all impacted.

Functionality of the iPad

18. I only used the iPad before seeing the patient but not during the consultation.
    a. Strongly agree.
    b. Agree.
    c. Neutral.
    d. Disagree.
    e. Strongly disagree.
19. I used the iPad before seeing the patient and during the consultation.
    a. Strongly agree.
    b. Agree.
    c. Neutral.
    d. Disagree.
    e. Strongly disagree.
20. I used the iPad only during the patient consultation.
    a. Strongly agree.
    b. Agree.
    c. Neutral.
    d. Disagree.
    e. Strongly disagree.
21. I used the iPad to take notes during the patient consultation.
    a. Strongly agree.
    b. Agree.
    c. Neutral.
    d. Disagree.
    e. Strongly disagree.
22. During the consultation with the patient, I placed the iPad:
    a. On my lap.
    b. On the counter in the examining room.
    c. Somewhere else (please specify).
23. The patient seemed not to be bothered by my use of an iPad during the consultation.
    a. Strongly agree.
    b. Agree.
    c. Neutral.
    d. Disagree.
    e. Strongly disagree.

24. I think the patient appreciated being able to see laboratory results and medical imaging on the iPad.
    a. Strongly agree.
    b. Agree.
    c. Neutral.
    d. Disagree.
    e. Strongly disagree.
25. I find that CAIS is more up-to-date than the paper chart, which is helpful when using the iPad in the patient consultation
    a. Strongly agree..
    b. Agree.
    c. Neutral.
    d. Disagree.
    e. Strongly disagree.
26. I used the paper chart in conjunction with the iPad.
    a. Strongly agree.
    b. Agree.
    c. Neutral.
    d. Disagree.
    e. Strongly disagree.

Overall Opinion on iPad Use

27. On the whole, I would say that the iPad is a valuable and useful tool for my clinical practice.
    a. Strongly agree.
    b. Agree.
    c. Neutral.
    d. Disagree.
    e. Strongly disagree.
28. There are some functions I still prefer a desktop or laptop computer for (please list).
29. Please check the items below for which you used the iPad:
    a. Scheduling.
    b. Email.
    c. Medical imaging.
    d. Reviewing imaging reports.
    e. Reviewing pathology reports.
    f. Reviewing previous clinical notes.
    g. Reviewing lab results.
    h. Accessing web-based knowledge.
    i. Accessing more up-to-date information through CAIS.
    j. Taking notes.
    k. Other (please state).

Other iPad Apps

30. I found that once I got the hang of it, I started searching out other medical apps to use on the iPad.
    a. Strongly agree
    b. Agree..
    c. Neutral.
    d. Disagree.
    e. Strongly disagree.
31. Did you use the iPad for your narrative? If so, which app did you use?
32. What other functions did you seek apps for?
33. Would you like to see a special iPad application specially made for CAIS?
    a. Yes.
    b. Maybe.
    c. No.
34. If we made a customized app for CAIS, what would you like to see? Eg. bigger buttons, bigger text, etc.

Expectations of the iPad

35. The iPad _____ my expectations in terms of its functionality in my practice.
    a. Greatly exceeded.
    b. Somewhat exceeded.
    c. Met.
    d. Failed to meet.
    e. Greatly disappointed.
36. Please feel free to leave any further comments about your experience using the iPad below.

Chapter 13

Analysis and Linkage of Data from Patient–Controlled Self–Monitoring Devices and Personal Health Records

Chris Paton
University of Oxford, UK

ABSTRACT

This chapter outlines the recent advances in self-tracking technology both for wellness and healthcare purposes. It addresses one of the key challenges in mobile health: how to link the data from self-tracking devices with data in clinical data systems, such as Personal Health Records and Electronic Health Records systems. This chapter also discusses advances in visualisation and analysis for personally controlled data from self-tracking and PHR systems.

INTRODUCTION

In recent years, a large number of personal self-tracking devices have emerged onto the consumer marketplace (Swan, 2009). Self-tracking devices cover a wide range but include devices that measure activity using accelerometers to disposable stick-on patches that measure ECG readings. The vast majority of these devices are used for the purposes of monitoring exercise for fitness and weight-loss, but a significant minority is used for monitoring a range of health conditions including diabetes (Gross, Levin, Mulvihill, Richardson,

& Davidson, 1984), COPD (Koff, Jones, Cashman, Voelkel, & Vandivier, 2009), heart failure (Klersy, De Silvestri, Gabutti, Regoli, & Auricchio, 2009) and Parkinson's disease (Little, McSharry, Hunter, Spielman, & Ramig, 2009), to choose a few examples.

In this chapter, we discuss the current landscape of self-tracking devices and examine how the data collected from such devices could be integrated into the clinical health record of the patient or consumer thereby making the data more useful for management of chronic conditions and maintaining good health.

DOI: 10.4018/978-1-4666-6150-9.ch013

Self-Tracking for Wellness

By far the most prevalent group of self-trackers are the fitness fanatics, dieters and "worried well". Arguably, this is also the group where self-tracking can have the largest impact on the health of the individuals and the state of the healthcare system. The personal health benefits of keeping fit and active have long been established (Franco et al., 2005). These include a lower risk of cardiovascular disease (Thompson et al., 2003), cancer (Thune & Furberg, 2001) and diabetes (Manson et al., 1991). From wider societal point of view, by remaining fitter for longer healthy individuals present a lower burden on healthcare services, take less sick-days (Proper, Van den Heuvel, De Vroome, Hildebrandt, & Van der Beek, 2006) and are able to take up caring and support roles longer into their retirement than individuals who take less exercise.

Evidence is emerging that self-tracking offers an increased incentive to keep fit and healthy over not self-tracking by increasing motivation through a process of feedback and a range of gaming effects (Swan, 2009). It will always be difficult to determine a clear link between increased take up of self-tracking technology for health and fitness and the general trend to increased exercise and health-consciousness among affluent consumers. However, recent behaviour change models may be able to demonstrate why this type of technology is enabling people to lead healthier lives. The Fogg behaviour model (Fogg, 2009) outlines a combination of three factors that influence whether or not an individual is likely to change behaviour: motivation, ability and triggers.

Self-tracking equipment has effects in all three of these domains:

Motivation

Many self-tracking tools have a "gamification" (McCallum, 2012) element built into them that can motivate users to compete both with themselves and other users through social networking platforms. For example, the Nike+ Fuelband® will display "points" on the LCD display mounted on the wristband that users can earn through increasing activity levels.

GPS tracker users can upload their GPS data from recent runs and share them with the community of users at Runkeeper.com. This could prove to be a powerful source of motivation as they become part of a community that congratulates and challenges each other to run further and faster.

Ability

Adopting a healthy lifestyle is a difficult challenge for most people. Certain types of self-tracking technology can make this transition easier by offering simple tools that replace the more difficult to maintain paper based systems of recording weights or activity levels. As discussed later in this chapter, the integration of data from self-tracking devices with clinical IT systems may be able to make the transition easier through advice from healthcare professionals on easier and more effective ways to maintain health and fitness that may not have been previously identified by patients.

Triggers

The Fogg model identifies triggers as a key to behaviour change (Fogg, 2009). Even if an individual has a high level of motivation and user-friendly tools that make the behaviour change easy to do, they still require a well-timed trigger to initiative the change. By using reminders and alerts, an ecosystem of technology that uses self-tracking devices, smartphone applications and web-based portals, individuals will be able to create triggers for exercise and activity that fit in with their daily regimens.

Self-Tracking for Long Term Conditions

Many of the positive behaviour changes established for currently healthy self-trackers also apply for patients with long-term conditions. There is increasing evidence that adoption of a healthy diet and exercise regime can help alleviate symptoms in a wide variety of long-term conditions from heart failure to diabetes (Stewart et al., 1994).

However, patients with long-term conditions may also gain additional benefits from self-tracking such as better management and adherence to medications (Smith et al., 2006) and informed decision making by their healthcare professionals who may have access to more accurate and more highly granular data. A short vignette outlines some of these benefits:

Mrs X is a patient with hypertension who is often nervous when her doctor takes her blood pressure. Over the past six months, she has been using a bluetooth home blood pressure monitor that connects wirelessly to her phone. She pulls out her phone and taps on the blood pressure app that shows the doctor her readings since her last visit. Even though her blood pressure was recorded as high by the doctor, the fact that most of her home recordings were within an acceptable range reassures the doctor that he doesn't need to prescribe any new medications or increase her dosage of medications.

Remote monitoring for patients with long-term conditions has a long and venerable history (Picot, 1998). Many patients with diabetes have long been adjusting their medication doses based on readings from home blood glucose monitors (Kovatchev, Cox, Gonder-Frederick, & Clarke, 2002), patients with COPD often alter their daily dose of steroids depending on readings from a home spirometer or peak flow meter (Khdour et al., 2011) and patients with heart failure often use daily weight readings to adjust the level of diuretics they require to keep their fluid levels in check (Klersy et al., 2009).

With more modern tools, these patients and more are now using a range of portable and connected electronic devices to make taking these measures less burdensome and allowing more rapid use of the data by health professionals. Instead of needing to bring in a long list of recordings on a piece of paper, the doctor can often view from her office the current readings of patients who are monitoring them through a web-based portal.

SELF-TRACKING TECHNOLOGY

Self-tracking technology is rapidly advancing and a variety of different types of sensor can be integrated in a number of configurations. In this section, we outline some of the commonly used sensors by health-trackers although there are many more highly specific sensors becoming available for certain diseases and conditions.

Self-Tracking Using Built in Smartphone Sensors

Probably the most accessible item of self-tracking hardware is the one a significant proportion of people already own: the smartphone.

Since the introduction of the iPhone in 2007, the smartphone sector has accelerated rapidly with fierce and growing competition between the Apple iOS operating system and the Google-backed Android Open Source platform. Data on smartphone uptake has shown that the majority of phones now being sold are Smartphones, with Android at more the 80% market share (but with Apple taking the lion's share of the profits).

GPS

Most smartphones now include the Global Positioning System (GPS) method of tracking location. Although primarily used for driving directions, GPS can also be harnessed for self-tracking for health and wellness purposes. For example, using the RunKeeper app, a wellness enthusiast can generate maps of runs completed with timings. These can also be shared with other users of RunKeeper on their website.

The GPS sensor can also be used in a number of long-term conditions. For patients suffering from dementia, the GPS sensor on their phone could be used to alert carers if they have wandered off and may need assistance (Bail, 2003). The GPS sensor could also be used to determine whether or not patients are becoming less active and more housebound - this could be an indication of a general deterioration in physical or mental health.

Accelerometer

As well as tracking location through GPS, smartphones are also equipped with an accelerometer that measures the acceleration of the devices across multiple axes of movement. By combining this data with computer algorithms, it is possible to detect the number of steps a person makes during a day, transforming the phone into a pedometer.

This can be used by runners, but also by people with long term conditions such as heart failure who want to maintain a reasonable level of activity but are not wanting to track a pre-determined route.

The accelerometer function can also be used to power sleep-tracking applications. If the smartphone is placed on the bed, the accelerometer can detect movement and hence calculate periods of deep sleep, light-sleep or wakefulness during the night.

Camera

The smartphone camera has a number of applications for self-tracking from the relatively basic snapping of photos of food to keep a food diary to the relatively advanced photoplethysmography applications that use a smartphone camera to determine a patient's pulse rate by the changes in colour caused by tiny blood vessels in their face.

One example is the Foodswitch application that uses the smartphone's camera to scan barcodes in supermarkets to help individual choose healthier meal options (Armstrong, 2012).

Microphone

The smartphone's microphone can also be used as a sensor, picking up ambient sounds to track activities such as mealtimes, exercise or bodily functions. Sonouroflow uses the smartphone's microphone to listen to micturition noises to diagnose prostatic hypertrophy (Zvarova et al., 2011), for example. With improving machine learning algorithms, it is anticipated that the microphone will be able to interpret more activities of daily living and begin to pick up other diagnostic indicators such as heart sounds and breath sounds (Comtois, Salisbury, & Sun, 2012).

Peripheral and Independent Self-Tracking Devices

A number of home monitoring devices and pieces of self-tracking equipment can now be linked via bluetooth to a smartphone (Bluetooth, 2007). This enables users of the devices to use the smartphone to store their readings and view their data. Data collected in this way also offers the opportunity to be linked to electronic health records (described later in this chapter).

Health and Fitness Devices

These types of devices are normally targeted at well individuals looking to increase their fitness and general level of health.

Some of the most commonly used pieces of self-tracking equipment are activity trackers that often take the form of a wristband, pendant or bracelet. These devices usually contain an accelerometer which can be used to track steps and other forms of activity such as time spent in various stages of sleep. By linking with a smartphone via bluetooth, data collected by these devices are immediately viewable and can be edited, annotated or stored by users.

The number of devices classified as 'wearable technology' is rapidly increasing and there are now a number of manufacturers of items of clothing that contain sensors that can be linked to a smartphone. These so called "smartclothes" can detect heart rate, breathing rate and activity when worn as a bra, vest or t-shirt. Socks have been developed that can track activity and numerous other smartclothes are under development with more advanced medical applications. Even diapers are now available as 'smartdiapers' that electronically record an infants bowel and urinary functions (Yambem, Yapici, & Zou, 2008).

Devices for Patients with Medical Conditions

Home monitoring equipment, such as a home blood pressure monitor or weighing scales, have been used by patients to track their health for many years. These devices used to require patients to record their readings in a journal that they could then take with them to their healthcare provider to get advice on managing their conditions.

More recently, however, it has become possible to link such devices with smartphones and tablet PCs to enable the automatic recording of readings and provide feedback to patients when they review their data.

Devices such as implantable cardioverter-defibrillators (ICDs) often contain transmitters that enable the collection of data from the devices. Home monitoring equipment is available that enables patients to transmit the data from their implanted devices on a continuous or intermittent basis.

DATA LINKAGE

Most self-tracking and self-monitoring equipment is designed to be used as a stand-alone device or in a relatively closed ecosystem. For self-tracking bands and pendants, this usually involves the device, and smartphone app and sometimes a website, where data from the smartphone is uploaded into the "cloud" for viewing on the site.

Personal Health Records and Patient Portals

There have been several attempts over recent years of better integrating home monitoring devices used by patients with long-term conditions to clinical IT systems. Some of these show significant promise and appear to be growing in popularity. These systems are often described as Personal Health Records. As well as uploading data, individuals have been encouraged to add descriptive information about their health status and updates on their symptoms or subjective assessment of the health state.

Some of the more high profile PHR endeavors include:

HealthVault

HealthVault (www.healthvault.com) made available a proprietary standard that allowed device manufacturers to allow their users to upload data from their devices to their computers and on, through a internet connection, to the HealthVault website.

Dossia

Dossia (www.dossia.com) is a PHR platform that uses Open Source software to integrate data from a wide variety of healthcare systems with the aim of providing patients with a view of their data, even if it is stored in different organisation's systems.

Google Health

Google Health was a web-based portal that aimed to give patients a place to manually enter details about their health status and to access to health records stored in providers systems that had partnered with Google.

In addition to specific PHR platforms such as those described above many electronic health record vendors and healthcare providers are offering a portal service to patients. These "patient portals" may prove easier to implement and adopt as they are often included as standard in many new EHR installations and, particularly in the UK, the government mandates seem more directed towards providing a view into the patients data rather than a method of contributing data to the system.

Standards for Data Linkage

A wide range of standards has been developed in the healthcare sector of a period of many years. Theses standards were initially developed as messaging protocols to allow medical information to be securely transferred from one system to another. For example, if a hospital laboratory wanted to send their results from their computer system to the system used to administer patients they could format the message in a standardised format that could be read by the other system. Over time, these standards have evolved to include storage as well as messaging and common language or terminology structures have been developed.

HL7 is the most dominant standards set in use in medical informatics today although there are many others with various degrees of overlapping and extended functionality including OpenEHR, IHE, DICOM and CEN. In its latest incarnation (Version 3), HL7 offers an XML based protocol linked to a reference information model (RIM) and common terminology descriptions (using SNOMED-CT) to ensure that medical information conveyed in HL7 messages adhere to a common structure. This means that, for example, a Blood Pressure reading (or any other measurement or term) is recognised as a well-defined concept in other systems that are connecting using HL7 messaging or storage. These allow "semantic interoperability" where the different systems share an understanding of the meaning of the data in the medical context.

Non-Standard Meta-Data

Although many medical systems are adherent to standards like HL7, many home-based monitoring devices and almost all self-tracking devices are not compliant. However, it is not necessary for systems to adhere to the standards as long as appropriate meta-data are attached to data. This is because data can easily be translated using an integration engine such as Mirth from one structure to another as long as the data structures are adherent to a meta-data format that means that mapping can take place.

It is often argued that a lack of health IT standards it the reason why patient-held information is not integrated into clinical systems, but as long as the data are described in meta-data, it should not be an impediment to integration.

DATA ANALYSIS

As these data are collected and integrated there is a danger that both patients and clinicians will become overloaded with the information generated.

Data Visualisation

Instead of presenting data as long lists or tables, it is often more useful for both patients and doctors to present data in the form of charts and diagrams. There has been good progress on data-visualisation by self-tracking equipment providers and PHR providers.

Algorithms

If the data is especially complicated and difficult to understand, it is often useful to reduce the data down using algorithms to a score or summary of the activity or health state. For fitness users, the Nike + Fuelband generates a score rather than the number of steps or GPS route a person has taken. This score is calculated by means of a proprietary algorithm that the manufacturers feel represents a "good" or "bad" level of activity. For patients with long term conditions, there are a number of well established risk scoring systems in the medical literature that can not only summarise complex data but that can be predictive for future events such as risk of heart attack, stroke or hospital admission.

Decision Support Systems

As algorithms become more advanced it may be possible to further reduce the need to present the data to patients and clinicians. What is really needed by users are appropriate alerts and messages that convey the information about the current health state of an individual and trends that may indicate a need for action or intervention. This means that instead of presenting data, either as a chart or table of numbers, it may be preferable to provide alerts and suggestions for altering current treatments, dosages or activities.

For example, if a patient with heart failure begins to become fluid overloaded due to a decrease in the heart function, it may be preferable to simply suggest an increase in dose of medication to the patient while the trend could be presented to the clinician as alert in case a more drastic change in management is required.

One interesting possibility for decision support is the generation of interventions based on "all the data" mapped to health outcomes. The deterioration of a patient is often the result of a multitude of factors some of which may be measured and some of which will not be. With appropriate machine learning technology, it may be possible to data-mine a population of patients to work out correlations between patterns across a range of data inputs (wearable sensors, clinical data form the EHR, demographic data, genomic data, etc.) that do not currently fit our medical model of diagnoses and treating disease. If certain patterns are highly correlated with certain outcomes, it may be possible to intervene with treatment at an earlier stage in a disease process to reduce negative outcomes for patients by spotting the development of these patterns in real time.

DISCUSSION

Two major developments have presented the potential for a merging of personally collected health and lifestyle data and clinical data collected by healthcare professionals:

Wearable Technology

Following Moore's Law, microprocessors are getting smaller and cheaper at an exponential rate. The technology that enables the collection and wireless transmission of data from biometric sensors is now of a small enough size and costs that devices can be manufactured that can fit comfortably into a wristband or wearable pendant. These tiny sensors can be linked to smartphones and tablet computers to enable transmission of the data to the cloud for further review and analysis.

Electronic Health Records

Countries around the world have now adopted Electronic Health Records in their national hospital systems and individual doctors and clinicians use Electronic Medical Records for managing their patients and record keeping. These systems are now becoming increasingly interconnected and many large-scale data aggregation projects are now in motion.

In the US, the HITECH Act (Blumenthal, 2010), part of the Obama stimulus package, has given doctors and hospitals access to over $20 billion to enable them to purchase and install electronic health records systems. As part of the conditions of these grants, these hospitals have to open up their systems for access by patients and be able to share their records with the government and other healthcare providers. This data sharing has promoted the adoption of terminology and interoperability standards such as Health Level 7 and SNOMED-CT.

In the UK, the NHS has been digitising hospital records systems for the last 10 years and is now in the process of creating new data extraction services to pull data from GP systems (Health and Social Care Information Centre, 2013). They have also created a mandate to allow patients access to their electronic health records and have a number of projects that utilise health IT standards to enabling better access to services and transparency of data.

As these two technology trends proceed, it will become inevitable that the demand for data integration will increase. The standards and tools discussed in the previous section will be important for allowing this to happen but a number of socio-political issues will also need to be addressed including data security and privacy and how to better provide personalised services to patients based on their longitudinal readings and lifestyle choices.

CONCLUSION

The rapid growth in wearable technology and the use of electronic clinical systems offers a significant opportunity to provide personalised care to more patients based on data they are collecting about themselves. Whether individuals are simply seeking to prevent the possible onset of future healthcare problems through lifestyle change or if they are trying to mitigate the symptoms of a long term condition such as heart failure or COPD, the linkage of personally generated data with data collected and stored by the healthcare system has the potential to improve clinical decision making and empower patients to make more informed decisions about their treatment or lifestyle options.

REFERENCES

Armstrong, R. M. (2012). App. review-Food-Switch. *The Medical Journal of Australia*, *196*(3), 207. doi:10.5694/mja12.10203

Bail, K. D. (2003). Electronic tagging of people with dementia: Devices may be preferable to locked doors. *BMJ*, *326*(7383), 281. doi:10.1136/bmj.326.7383.281 PMID:12560288

Bluetooth, S. I. G. (2007). *Specification of the Bluetooth system.* Core Version 1.1. 1 February 22, 2001.

Blumenthal, D. (2010). Launching HITECH. *The New England Journal of Medicine*, *362*(5), 382–385. doi:10.1056/NEJMp0912825 PMID:20042745

Comtois G. Salisbury J. I. Sun Y. (2012). A smartphone-based platform for analyzing physiological audio signals. In Proceedings of Bioengineering Conference (NEBEC), 2012 38th Annual Northeast (pp. 69–70). IEEE. 10.1109/NEBC.2012.6206966

Fogg B. J. (2009). A behavior model for persuasive design. In Proceedings of the 4th International Conference on Persuasive Technology. ACM.

Franco, O. H., de Laet, C., Peeters, A., Jonker, J., Mackenbach, J., & Nusselder, W. (2005). Effects of physical activity on life expectancy with cardiovascular disease. *Archives of Internal Medicine*, *165*(20), 2355–2360. doi:10.1001/archinte.165.20.2355 PMID:16287764

Gross, A. M., Levin, R. B., Mulvihill, M., Richardson, P., & Davidson, P. C. (1984). Blood glucose discrimination training with insulindependent diabetics: A clinical note. *Biofeedback and Self-Regulation*, *9*(1), 49–54. doi:10.1007/BF00998845 PMID:6487674

Health and Social Care Information Centre. 1 Trevelyan Square. (2013, September 26). *Care. data. standard*. Retrieved April 10, 2014, from http://www.hscic.gov.uk/article/3525/Caredata

Khdour, M. R., Agus, A. M., Kidney, J. C., Smyth, B. M., Elnay, J. C., & Crealey, G. E. (2011). Cost-utility analysis of a pharmacy-led self-management programme for patients with COPD. *International Journal of Clinical Pharmacology, Therapy and Toxicology*, *33*(4), 665–673. PMID:21643784

Klersy, C., De Silvestri, A., Gabutti, G., Regoli, F., & Auricchio, A. (2009). A meta-analysis of remote monitoring of heart failure patients. *Journal of the American College of Cardiology*, *54*(18), 1683–1694. doi:10.1016/j.jacc.2009.08.017 PMID:19850208

Koff, P. B., Jones, R. H., Cashman, J. M., Voelkel, N. F., & Vandivier, R. W. (2009). Proactive integrated care improves quality of life in patients with COPD. *The European Respiratory Journal*, *33*(5), 1031–1038. doi:10.1183/09031936.00063108 PMID:19129289

Kovatchev, B. P., Cox, D. J., Gonder-Frederick, L., & Clarke, W. L. (2002). Methods for quantifying self-monitoring blood glucose profiles exemplified by an examination of blood glucose patterns in patients with type 1 and type 2 diabetes. *Diabetes Technology & Therapeutics*, *4*(3), 295–303. doi:10.1089/152091502760098438 PMID:12165168

Little, M. A., McSharry, P. E., Hunter, E. J., Spielman, J., & Ramig, L. O. (2009). Suitability of dysphonia measurements for telemonitoring of Parkinson's disease. *IEEE Transactions on Bio-Medical Engineering*, *56*(4), 1015–1022. doi:10.1109/TBME.2008.2005954 PMID:21399744

Manson, J. E., Stampfer, M. J., Colditz, G. A., Willett, W. C., Rosner, B., & Hennekens, C. H. et al. (1991). Physical activity and incidence of noninsulin-dependent diabetes mellitus in women. *Lancet*, *338*(8770), 774–778. doi:10.1016/0140-6736(91)90664-B PMID:1681160

McCallum, S. (2012). Gamification and serious games for personalized health. *Studies in Health Technology and Informatics*, *177*, 85–96. PMID:22942036

Picot, J. (1998). Telemedicine and Telehealth in Canada: Forty Years of Change in the Use of Information and Communications Technologies in a Publicly Administered Health Care System. *Telemedicine Journal*, *4*(3), 199–205. doi:10.1089/tmj.1.1998.4.199 PMID:9831745

Proper, K. I., Van den Heuvel, S. G., De Vroome, E. M., Hildebrandt, V. H., & Van der Beek, A. J. (2006). Dose–response relation between physical activity and sick leave. *British Journal of Sports Medicine*, *40*(2), 173–178. doi:10.1136/bjsm.2005.022327 PMID:16432007

Smith, C. E., Dauz, E. R., Clements, F., Puno, F. N., Cook, D., Doolittle, G., & Leeds, W. (2006). Telehealth services to improve nonadherence: A placebo-controlled study. *Telemedicine Journal and e-Health*, *12*(3), 289–296. doi:10.1089/tmj.2006.12.289 PMID:16796496

Stewart, A. L., Hays, R. D., Wells, K. B., Rogers, W. H., Spritzer, K. L., & Greenfield, S. (1994). Long-term functioning and well-being outcomes associated with physical activity and exercise in patients with chronic conditions in the medical outcomes study. *Journal of Clinical Epidemiology*, *47*(7), 719–730. doi:10.1016/0895-4356(94)90169-4 PMID:7722585

Swan, M. (2009). Emerging patient-driven health care models: An examination of health social networks, consumer personalized medicine and quantified self-tracking. *International Journal of Environmental Research and Public Health*, *6*(2), 492–525. doi:10.3390/ijerph6020492 PMID:19440396

Thompson, P. D., Buchner, D., Piña, I. L., Balady, G. J., Williams, M. A., & Marcus, B. H. et al. (2003). Exercise and physical activity in the prevention and treatment of atherosclerotic cardiovascular disease a statement from the Council on Clinical Cardiology (Subcommittee on Exercise, Rehabilitation, and Prevention) and the Council on Nutrition, Physical Activity, and Metabolism (Subcommittee on Physical Activity). *Circulation*, *107*(24), 3109–3116. doi:10.1161/01.CIR.0000075572.40158.77 PMID:12821592

Thune, I., & Furberg, A.-S. (2001). Physical activity and cancer risk: dose-response and cancer, all sites and site-specific. *Medicine and Science in Sports and Exercise, 33*(6 Suppl), S530–50, discussion S609–10.

Yambem, L., Yapici, M. K., & Zou, J. (2008). A new wireless sensor system for smart diapers. *IEEE Sensors Journal*, *8*(3), 238–239. doi:10.1109/JSEN.2008.917122

Zvarova, K., Ursiny, M., Giebink, T., Liang, K., Blaivas, J. G., & Zvara, P. (2011). Recording urinary flow and lower urinary tract symptoms using sonouroflowmetry. *The Canadian Journal of Urology*, *18*(3), 5689–5694. PMID:21703041

KEY TERMS AND DEFINITIONS

Electronic Health Records (EHR): Used by clinicians to store data and information about patients.

Personal Health Records (PHR): Used by patients to record their health information online.

Self-Tracking: Measuring subjective and objective measurements about oneself to keep track of changes over time.

Chapter 14
Social Media for Health Communication:
Implementation Issues and Challenges for Italian Public Health Authorities

Elisabetta Cioni
Università Degli Studi di Sassari, Italy

Alessandro Lovari
Università Degli Studi di Sassari, Italy

ABSTRACT

The aim of this chapter is to highlight the current issues and the challenging process of the adoption of social media by Italian local health authorities (ASL). After a literature review of the role of social media for health organizations, the authors focus their attention on how social network sites are modifying health communication and relations with citizens in Italy. They conduct an exploratory study articulated in three stages: after mapping the presence of local health authorities on the most popular social media platforms (Facebook, Twitter, YouTube), they carry out a content analysis to describe the prevalent kinds of messages published in the official Facebook timelines; in the third phase, using several interviews with healthcare directors and communications managers, the authors investigate implementation issues, managerial implications, and constraints that influence proper use of these participative platforms by Italian public health organizations. Limitations and further steps of the research are discussed.

INTRODUCTION

Social media are becoming very popular and are widely used in Italy. New interactive media, and in particular social network sites such as Facebook, Twitter and YouTube, are rapidly gaining importance in people's media consumption patterns:

indeed much research, at both the national and international level, has emphasized the growing role that participatory media is assuming in the search for information and to connect and engage with peers and organizations (Censis-Ucsi, 2013; Istat, 2013a; Nielsen, 2011). For these reasons private organizations, such as companies and

DOI: 10.4018/978-1-4666-6150-9.ch014

brands, and public institutions such as municipalities, universities and governmental agencies have begun to inhabit the social web by opening official accounts, pages or channels to interact and dialogue with customers and citizens (Comunello, 2012; Lovari et al., 2011; Lovari & Parisi, 2012). The social media wave has also begun to impact Italian health organizations, such as Local Health Authorities (ASL), hospitals and University hospitals (ICCR). This process is happening in the private and public health sector, at different rates, and using a variety of approaches (Fattori & Pinelli, 2013; Santoro, 2011). It is interesting to observe the organizational decision to open an official social media presence on popular platforms, whereby the owner directly manages content and relationships with a digital audience, composed of citizens, patients, associations, and media. This process of social media colonization (Lovari, 2013) strictly depends on the specific characteristics of the Italian healthcare framework, and it is influenced by the particular approach to communication and technology innovation in general (Contini & Lanzara, 2009; Ingrosso, 2008; Rubinelli, Camerini, Schulz, 2010). For this reason it is important to focus on the identifiable characteristics of the Italian healthcare framework and its organization at the national and regional levels.

During the Nineties, the Italian National Healthcare System (SSN), founded in 1978 (Law n. 23, 833), was reformed twice (in 1992 and 1999) and henceforth acquired its current organizational structure. The Italian SSN is governed at both the national and regional levels. At the national level, matters regarding fundamental health principles and the determination of the essential levels of healthcare provision are set down by the central Government and the Ministry of Health, through laws and guidelines established in 2001. The SSN provides health services, and it is expected to deliver them to all citizens, free of charge at the point of access or upon payment of a co-pay fee (ticket) and for which the Ministry of Health is guarantor at national level. At the local level,

services are provided through nineteen Regions and two autonomous Provinces, as the general legislative and administrative authorities for the establishment and organization of health structures and services. The Regions are directly responsible for local healthcare provision, which should relate to specific territorial requirements. The provision of health services at the local level is ensured primarily through the Local Health Authorities (ASL), 143 legal public bodies that have organizational, administrative, fiscal, financial, managerial and technical independence. They organize and provide healthcare services within their territorial areas through public facilities or accredited private structures, including preventive activities, primary care, pharmaceutical services, specialized diagnostic services, home-delivered health care for elderly and chronic patients, mental health, and housing for the elderly, disabled, and drug users. An important role in the Italian National Healthcare System is also played by University Hospitals (IRCCS), hospitals of excellence that have a commitment to research in the field of biomedicine and managing healthcare services, in addition to medical care for patients. The Ministry of Health exercises supervision over the University Hospitals in order to guarantee that research carried out is in the public interest and that it has a direct effect on patient care. They also give technical and operational support to other National Health Service bodies that provide health care in order to achieve the objectives set down in the National Health Plan regarding health research and staff training.

The National Health Plan, prepared by the Ministry of Health, the Regions, syndicates and other stakeholders, identifies the guidelines for the Italian health policy, which must be approved by the Conference State-Regions. In turn, the Regions also stipulate Regional Health Plans that must be in accordance with the National Plan. Finally, Local Health Authorities must prepare business plans and regulations to be approved by the regional authorities.

The Italian Healthcare System is clearly inspired by the methods of New Public Governance (McLaughlin, Osborne & Ferlie, 2002; Osborne, 2010). However, after more than ten years of implementation, there are still great differences between Regions in terms of both cost and quality of performance in healthcare services.

How does this highly elaborate healthcare system (that includes multiple actors with high managerial autonomy) face the challenges posed by the rapid spread of social media and social network sites?

The aim of this chapter is to highlight the current issues and the challenging process of the adoption of social media by Local Health Authorities (ASL) in Italy. To reach these objectives, we carried out a three-stage study, specifically addressed to different issues within our study. The first one was a quantitative study, mapping out the number of Italian local health units with an official presence on the three main social media platforms: Facebook, YouTube and Twitter. Secondly, a Facebook timeline content analysis was carried out to investigate the main communication strategies implemented by Italian health units on this social network site. Furthermore, qualitative interviews were conducted with top management and practitioners in charge of managing social media for Italian local health authorities in order to deepen the organizational implications, highlighting opportunities and constraints related to the use of these platforms for public communication and within the healthcare sphere.

BACKGROUND

To focus on this topic we have used a mix of scholarly and grey literature, such as white papers, surveys and technical reports. Many scholars worldwide have studied the use of the Internet as a tool to search for health information, since the end of the last century (Cline & Haynes, 2001; Houston & Ehrenberger, 2001). The first wave of research on the Internet emphasized uptake and the opportunities afforded by its implementation: indeed the Internet has the potential to supply a continuous health related information flow to satisfy consumer demand and increase personal knowledge on health issues. Moreover, there are also possible downsides of the Internet for health issues, such as the spread of misleading, inaccurate or inappropriate information that could constitute a public risk for citizens, or blurring the lines between health information and advertising, thus confusing patients (Eysenbach, 2008a; Houston & Ehrenberger, 2001).

The Internet is growing in importance as a medium to gather information about health. Research has focused on different aspects and traits of the Internet's potential for health information, with different methodologies and geographical samples (Fox, 2011; Fox & Jones, 2009; Fox & Duggan, 2013a; AlGhamdi & Moussa, 2012; Siliquini et al., 2011). The best source to evaluate the use of the Internet by European citizens is provided by Digital Agenda for Europe (DAE), that encapsulates the digital transformations that the European Union wants to achieve by the year 2020. Progress against these targets is measured in the annual Digital Agenda Scoreboard, according to which, in the first quarter of 2011, more than half of Internet users in the European Union looked for health related information (54%), with a significant increase compared to 2010, but with different values among countries (Eurostat, 2011). The Internet is not only used to search for health related information but also for making appointments with practitioners in health care centers and hospitals: in particular the proportion of European Internet users was 10%, with a higher percentage of use by the 25-54 and 55-74 age groups (Eurostat, 2012).

In addition to this data, the most comprehensive statistical framework on the use of the Internet for health in Europe is provided by the study conducted in 2011 by a group of researchers at the Joint Research Centre-Institute for Prospective

Technological Studies (Lupiañez-Villanueva et al., 2012). During this survey, a random sample of citizens aged from 16 to 74 years old who had used the Internet in the last three months in 14 EU countries, including Italy, were interviewed online (1,000 interviews per country, stratified by gender and age group). The surveyed citizens continued to consider direct interaction with doctors (75%) and nurses (40%) to be most relevant as sources of information about health, but the relevance of the Internet (35%) has become greater than that of pharmacies (32%). The perceived importance of the Internet as a main channel for health interaction is linked to women, to people aged between 25 and 54 years old, in the worst states of health, and suffering from a long-standing illness. Italy reported one of the highest percentages of people that consider the Internet as an important source of health information, equal to that of Sweden and surpassed only by Estonia, Slovakia, Slovenia and the United Kingdom. Very interesting for the purpose of our work is the data about perceived trust with respect to health information sources available to European citizens. According to this survey, Europeans, and Italians in particular, consider medical and health institutions the most trustworthy with respect to health information. Italy, however, also shows the highest percentage of trust in Internet-based health (48% of all participants), while Denmark reported 43%, Holland 41% and the United Kingdom 40%.

According to a survey in Italy, a questionnaire administered by physicians in six Italian hospital laboratories, 57% of respondents affirmed using the Internet to search for health-related information (Siliquini et al., 2011). The main motives cited were fast access and the possibility to gather a broad quantity of health information. Age, gender and education were associated with searching on the web: the most active users are young (30-41 years of age), female and well-educated.

In some cases, the Internet is also substituting the direct relations with doctors and health professionals: in fact, a PriceWaterhouseCoopers e-health study, carried out in ten countries, reports that 59% of patients use the Internet and smartphone applications to substitute medical examinations, and 43% of them prefer to contact doctors and public health organizations via the web and mobile devices (PriceWaterhouseCoopers, 2012).

The emerging use of technological innovations, such as self-quantified monitoring tools or health indicators (Fox & Duggan, 2013b), the development of web 2.0 and social media platforms are having a profound effect upon the relationship between health organizations and citizens, also attracting the attention of many scholars and practitioners interested in studying these new dynamics.

Social Media Use in Organizations

Social media (Kaplan & Haenlein, 2010) and specifically social network sites (boyd & Ellison, 2007) are widely used in our society. Several pieces of research highlight the pervasive growth of these media across the globe (Nielsen, 2011; Kout, 2012). Social network sites are no more the exclusive domains of teenage Internet activity -- they have become firmly established across socio-demographic groups and are increasingly used by adults and senior citizens (Nielsen, 2011; Zickuhr & Madden, 2012). The success of these platforms is rapidly increasing due to the connection with mobile phones. Social media access is becoming ubiquitous, since it increasingly happens on mobile networks, smartphones and wifi connected tablets, especially for teenagers and young adults.

Although these devices were initially adopted as personal communication tools, in the last five years we have seen a growing interest in using social media, such as blogs and social network sites, to enrich the organizational communication mix. Social media was initially used by companies to propagate information about products and services on the social web, to manage relations with customers, to listen to their needs, providing feedback, and stimulating e-commerce (Qualman, 2009; Shih, 2009; Solis & Breakenridge, 2009). At the same time, several studies have underlined the impact of social media in the public sector, investigating the adoption process and uses of these participative platforms by public administrations, federal government and municipalities (Mergel & Bretschneider, 2013). Some scholars have focused their attention on potential benefits, such as increasing transparency, openness, and access, and avoiding corruption (Bertot, Jaeger & Grimes, 2010; Bertot, Jaeger & Hansen, 2012; Bonsón et al., 2012; Mergel, 2013). Other scholars have focused on the impact of social media on communication strategies, allowing administrations to inform citizens about public services and opportunities in a new bidirectional way (Bryer, 2010; Lovari & Parisi, 2012); to promote and diffuse specific communication campaigns virally on the social web (Mergel, 2010); to enhance participation, to amass people's views about civic issues, disservices, and to find potential solutions to the inefficacy of administrations (Lovari, 2013; Nabatchi & Mergel, 2010; Noveck, 2009; Sirianni, 2009).

Social Media Use for Health

Digital technologies, and in particular social media, are becoming hot issues and research trends in health communication (Dutta, 2009; Kim et al., 2010). These platforms are also acquiring greater importance in health and medicine in general (Mayo Clinic Center, 2012; Meskò, 2013). This is the reason why some scholars started using the terms Medicine 2.0 (Eysenbach, 2008b) and Health 2.0 (Van De Belt et al., 2010). These definitions emphasize a new phase of health related organization, in which a strategic and relevant role is played by web 2.0 and social network sites in terms of both transparency of information and internal management. According to Eysenbach (2008b), Medicine 2.0 represents a new health system characterized by some major aspects such

as collaboration, participation, apomediation and openness, as opposed to the traditional and hierarchical structures within health care organizations. Social media are in fact profoundly changing the relationship between health organizations, health professionals and citizens (Andersen, Medaglia & Henriksen, 2012; Househ, 2013; Korda & Itani, 2011). These participative platforms are challenging traditional health promotion models prompting the advancement of innovative health communication patterns (Chou et al., 2009). Firstly, social media can be considered a strategic tool in order to empower citizens, giving them the possibility to explore many different data and sources of information, sharing thoughts and experiences with other people, exploring options, interacting with doctors and health structures in locations far away from where they live (Byron, Albury & Evers, 2013; Thielst, 2011; Eysenbach, 2008b; Lober & Flowers, 2011).

The relation between patients and medical personnel is also changing. Additionally, just as the Internet is becoming a familiar place, fully embedded in the everyday experiences of a great majority of the population, the very doctor-patient relationship is changing. In medical care practices, the traditional model described by Parsons (1951), which gives the doctor almost complete authority to make decisions in the patient's best interest, has been replaced in an increasing number of cases by greater patient control and relationships based on mutuality, more consistent with prevailing social values that emphasize individual autonomy and responsibility and somehow favor even consumerist attitudes (Morgan, 2003). Communication plays a decisive role for the achievement of the model of mutuality (Roher & Hall, 2006). Doctors and other health professionals have to interact with patients who have greater access to medical information through the media, internet and other sources, and who can become active seekers and producers of health related information. Patients are turning into e-patients, individuals who are enabled, empowered and engaged by technologies, and use social media to educate themselves and others to enhance health, especially accessing information from mobile platforms (Lober & Flowers, 2011; Perficient, 2013). Furthermore, patients can gather together on the social web, calling for other patients' participation and engagement, developing a community intelligence that can support a better use of knowledge and public data to improve health outcomes (Hesse et al., 2011). A negative consequence of this increasing use of social media for health by patients is that it could provoke an excess of alarm, eventually leading to an increase in pressure on the health care system with new service demands, or leading to a type of cyberchondria (Andersen, Medaglia & Henriksen, 2012; White & Horvitz, 2009).

Secondly, social media can represent a strategic tool for doctors, general practitioners, nurses and medical personnel. Besides personal use, social media can be used by doctors to search for updated information about health issues, to train medical fellows or to build up and maintain professional connections and a community of learning and practice. Doctors can also support patients and raise the visibility of their research or treatments (Levine et al., 2011; Popoiu, Grosseck & Holotescu, 2012; Yamout et al., 2011). Moreover, blogs and social networking sites could become pedagogical platforms to support medical education and to provide tailored messages to patients with specific illnesses (Shaw & Johnson, 2011). At the same time a relevant part of professionals remain skeptical in using these interactive media. For example, surgeons are hesitant to incorporate social media into their practices because of time constraints, but mostly for the security concerns and medical-legal risks associated with the use of these platforms with patients (Yamout et al., 2011).

From the health organization point of view, social media was originally used as a way to expand communication strategies, offering a new platform to spread health messages and give them visibility for specific targets (Harris, Snider & Mueller, 2013; Househ, 2013; Lobers & Flowers,

2011). Indeed social media use can help health authorities to build up an open communication infrastructure for exchanging information with traditionally hard-to-reach users, such as adolescents or immigrants (Bardus, 2011; Chou et al., 2009). These platforms can also be used by healthcare organizations to collect individual feedback, monitor patient conversations, and to proactively intercept and resolve complaints and possible disservice (CDC, 2012; Thielst, 2011). Furthermore, these platforms can be adopted to enhance a marked change in the organization's perspective, passing from a top-down, broadcast approach to a horizontal, side by side communication with citizens, giving them the voice to speak up on social media health organization profiles.

Besides the positive effects of social media, there are possible threats and dark sides in the use of these media by public health organizations: for instance, the possible augmentation of the digital divide and health disparities (Dutta, 2009; Shaw & Johnson, 2011); the underestimation of privacy and legal implications (Andersen, Medaglia & Henriksen, 2012; Househ, 2013); the risk of using a language suited for professional audiences rather than for a consumer audience (CDC, 2012; Hesse et al., 2011); the difficulties to balance user-generated health content and official institutional communication in the same social media platforms (Chou et al., 2009). Furthermore, there is little empirical evidence of the real effects of social media for changing behaviors: several scholars affirm that many journal articles are prescriptive, emphasizing the potential of these media for health campaigns, but there is still the need for specific analyses in order to isolate and determine social media effects on patient behavior (Bardus, 2011; Korda & Itani, 2011; Schein, Wilson & Keelan, 2011).

A YouGOv 2010 empirical study highlights how 25% of American citizens expected to connect with hospitals via social media at some point; 57% stated that hospitals' use of social media would be likely to have a strong impact on the decision to use their health services; and 81% reported that a strong social media presence indicates that the hospital's clinical functions operate better and are cutting edge (Thielst, 2011). Recently, PWC research (2013) revealed that more than half of American internet users read reviews of healthcare providers online, and 38% use blogs or social network sites, with doctors and hospitals being visited the most. Furthermore, according to a 1,350-consumer study carried out by the marketing agency Epsilon, social networking sites are increasing relevance in order to seek healthcare information (O'Mally, 2010). The study highlights how 40% of cyber surfers use social media for health information: 80% can be considered highly engaged users since they actively interact with other users of the platforms, while 20% are mostly passive, only reading contents. The study also found that participating in these platforms provides reassurance and intimacy for many users who can share health issues and concerns. Conversely, lack of participation is caused by difficulties of managing time in using these forums or by lack of trust in the digital information compared to a heavy reliance on direct medical advice from a doctor. Lastly, it is significant to highlight that most of the consumers feel that a direct endorsement by government could add credibility to social content (O'Mally, 2010).

We should consider that even if a health organization decides not to colonize social media, their services, doctors and general activities are, in any case, topics of discussion on the social web, in particular within blogs or social network sites. Indeed, health services have become the subject of public conversations on Facebook timelines or Twitter accounts whether or not hospitals or public health units are present on social media. This process also leads to the creation of several counterfeit social media pages in which external individuals use the logo of the institutions, acting and posting messages as if they were the health organizations. This could create possible risks and damage to the reputation of health authorities.

That is the reason why some scholars affirm that rather than remaining passive onlookers outside of the network, organizations should reside in the social web, contributing to discussions as peers rather than outsiders, adding their official voice to the conversation (Bonsón et al., 2012; Solis & Breakenridge, 2009).

Social Media for Health: The Italian Scenario

Italy is in a transition period toward digitalization, and there are many interesting features testifying the vitality of this digital revolution in the country. For example, the growing interest and use of social network sites and Facebook in particular.

According to a Censis-Ucsi study on Italian media consumption, Facebook is the most popular social network site (65.3%), followed by YouTube (53.1%), and Twitter at 21.3% of the sample, with a relevant increase (17%) in comparison with the previous research release (Censis-Ucsi, 2011). Social media is becoming transversal among the Italian population with the highest rates of new accounts and usage by adults and senior citizens (Censis-Ucsi, 2011; Istat, 2013a). A more recent study (Censis-Ucsi, 2013) reported how Italian citizens intensively rely on social media to search for information: 37.6% of the sample affirms gathering information via Facebook, with a peak of 71% in the age range of 14-29 years old; while 25.9% use YouTube to be informed (52.7% in the age range of 14-29 years old).

Facebook is also the most used social network site, with more than 23 million monthly active users (Cosenza, 2013). According to the observatory "Facebook and Social Media in Italy", 15 million active users connect daily to Facebook, 10 million surf it through smartphones or tablets, with an average monthly visit duration of more than 8 hours. Mobile Internet connectivity represents an increasing trend for the Italian market: 22.1% of the mobile audience accesses social media or blogs in a month (Digital Scoreboard Agenda,

2012), while 41% of the users navigate Internet from a smart phone connection and 10.1% from a tablet (Audiweb, 2013).

Within this scenario, few studies have been conducted in order to investigate the use of social media in health communication. As we have mentioned the Italian SNN is mostly a public health system: from this point of view, public health organizations follow a mandatory national law (n.150/2000), requiring public administrations to manage information and communication through specific structures such as the office for public relations (URP) and press offices. Public communication flows use different media, adopting a multichannel strategy to reach different public audiences with a variety of tools. It is evident how the Internet has profoundly changed Italian public health communication, attributable to specific laws stressing and enhancing organizational transparency and digital innovation for the quality of services. For these reasons the health communication mix has been enriched by thematic web sites and digital platforms. In the last report on the health status of the country, the Ministry of Health describes the main results of the online turn. For services provided online (e.g. the withdrawal of lab reports, the single booking centre, choice and change of doctor), 91.4% of users were satisfied, 4.2% indicated sufficiency and 4.4% dissatisfied. The reasons for dissatisfaction were: difficulty of access (48%), lack of clarity of instructions (43%), and failure to update information (9%). With regard to the content of the online pages, in February 2011, the Ministry of Health adopted a detection system for user satisfaction (with a scale from one to five stars) with the information available in the ministerial portal www.salute.gov.it in a web 2.0 format suggested by the Guidelines. In 2011, the number of votes cast were about 3,600. 36.5% of the voted pages scored an average of five stars, 18.2% received four stars, 22.1% three stars, 7.9% two stars and 15.3% one star. The pages that received the most votes were those containing information on health

care abroad, exemptions from the fees, lifestyles, communication campaigns, health professions, women's health, anti-doping, pharmacies, narcotic drugs and psychotropic substances. The pages that received five stars dealt with exemptions from the fees, the campaign for organ donors, tissues and cells, flu, health food and physical exercise, the campaign against AIDS, heat waves and infectious diseases. The Ministry's official YouTube channel had over 65,000 views in 2011, while the pages that received the most "I Like it" votes were those relating to videos on the life of nurses, the fight against the mistreatment of animals and the anti-smoking campaign. (Ministero della Salute, 2012).

The adoption of social media was recently acknowledged by the Italian Ministry of Health, which included some recommendations related to the use of these media and web 2.0 tools for health public bodies, for the first time. These recommendations, incorporated in a broader report on Internet website guidelines, highlighted the dialogical and interactive potential of these platforms but at the same time underlined the necessity to invest specific resources to manage these media in a strategic and participatory way (Ministero della Salute, 2012).

Social media and participative communities are frequently used by Italian citizens to search for health related information: indeed 34,7% of Internet users visit social network sites to find health information, with a value that is higher than that related to the use of institutional health websites (29,8%) (Censis-Forum per la Ricerca Biomedica, 2012). However, few Italian public health organizations have opened official accounts on social media. They do not seem attracted by these platforms like other Italian public administration areas such as municipalities, universities and Regions (Arata, 2011; Lovari & Giglietto, 2012). For instance Fattori and Pinelli (2013) investigated the use of Twitter in the Italian health system, mapping the presence of official accounts in the Italian SNN. In June 2013, there were a total of 33 health structures present in the Twittersphere:

the majority are located in the North East and Center of Italy, while the number of followers differ greatly from one structure to another, and from the public to the private sector. Regarding public health authorities: 16 have an official Twitter account, with an average number of tweets of 527, while the average number of followers is about 303. There are many differences between these accounts: some of those are publicized on the ASL web sites with a social bar or with some graphic icons. Twitter accounts are mostly used to propagate and give visibility to press releases and health promotion campaigns; only in a few cases, accounts are used strategically to engage followers or to create professional health networks (Fattori & Pinelli 2013).

Besides this specific study, we noticed a general lack of research in the area, in contrast with the growing attention and interest by citizens and mass media. It is paramount to advance research in this field to investigate strategies and uses of social media platforms by Italian SNN. The research should not only use quantitative data, useful in detecting usage patterns, but since this only outlines a general picture, it is vital to move forward with specific qualitative studies to better understand the meaning of certain choices, the social uses and the opportunities and threats of using social media for public health organizations.

MAIN FOCUS OF THE CHAPTER

Under this scenario we decided to study the main characteristics of the presence of Local Health Authorities, a specific branch of Italian SNN units, on social media. We chose to focus our attention on three platforms, Facebook, Twitter and YouTube, to map and detect the official presence of ASL in the social web (profiles, like pages, accounts, channels); to explore the communication strategies implemented within the social media message boards; and to investigate objectives, organizational implications, and the opportunities and threats related to the decision to colonize social media platforms by Italian Local Health Authorities.

Methodology

Our methodology adopted both quantitative and qualitative research tools, and it was articulated in three different phases aimed at diverse objectives.

In a first phase we visited all the 143 Italian Local Health Authorities web sites, using a list published on the Italian Ministry of Health website, to detect the presence of official social media channels. The search process followed three steps to ensure that the presence was officially managed by Local Health Authorities: firstly, we visited the homepage looking for a social bar, icon or widget promoting the presence of social media channels; secondly, we surfed the internal website pages, specifically searching the communication and administration sections, to detect the existence of news or links referring to social media; thirdly, we conducted a search on the main social media platforms using the internal search bar to find pages with the names of the Local Health Authorities. Once we found evidence of ASL accounts, groups or like pages, we directly contacted local health units to confirm whether the social media presence was official or not.

We mapped and detected all the various kinds of social media presence (official and unofficial like pages, groups created by employers or private citizens, thematic like pages, fake accounts) focusing our study on the official social media presence managed by Local Health Authorities. Information on the date of creation, the office in charge of managing the platforms, the number of messages published, profile biographies and information sections, the number of fans, followers and video comments was entered in a database and it was set in relation with other data such as local area population and the number of Local Health Authorities within the different Italian Regions.

In a second phase we manually counted the number of messages published by Local Health Authorities in the official Facebook presences over the course of about seven months of online activity, from January 1 to July 15, 2013. We decided to count only those posts explicitly written by health organizations and not all the messages that were simply shared without words and images to the links' address. We excluded Twitter accounts and YouTube channels from this type of content analysis. After collecting posts from Facebook timelines, we carried out a qualitative analysis categorizing the contents of each message. We slightly modified a typology tested in a previous study about Facebook communication strategies for Italian municipalities (Lovari & Parisi, 2012), modifying it to suit the health sector.

Finally in a third stage, we conducted telephone interviews with ASL general directors or communication managers for social media in order to better understand the reasons and motivations behind the launch and implementation of these platforms; the management of digital communication flows with citizens; and the opportunities and threats related to opening official presences on Facebook, Twitter and YouTube for health communication. All the Local Health Authorities with an official presence on social media were contacted via email, Facebook and Twitter message, or telephone call to find the right office in order to request the availability to collaborate in this qualitative part of the study. We carried out fourteen interviews with communications directors, press officers, and local health authority general directors. Interviews were conducted from July 10 to July 25, using a questionnaire with fifteen open questions: the average length of the interviews was 45 minutes. All the interviews were transcribed and thematically analyzed in order to better understand the complex process that guided Italian local health authorities to officially enter social media and the organizational implications related to the management of the official presences.

Mapping Italian Public Health Local Units in the Social Web

Among the 143 Italian Local Health Authorities (ASL), two out of three do not have, so far, (June 2013) any official presence on the most widespread social media platforms in Italy (Facebook, Twitter and YouTube). It is also noted that only a fraction (about half) of the healthcare institutions, which decided to be present on social media, located an icon or a social bar on the home page of their Internet portal, giving full visibility of their use of social media. In several cases, the presence is somehow hidden in the inside pages of the institutional portals, and it has to be searched for in the pages managed by the ASL communications and external relations offices, in the pages dedicated to specific targets (i.e. young people; pregnant women, etc.) or in the specific pages of particular communication campaigns (i.e. anti-smoking or other addictions, breastfeeding, etc.). In some cases, even if the Local Health Authority confirms the official presence, it is not shown within the portals, and only detectable through social media search functions.

A large group of Local Health Authorities, including those who have decided to use social media, use only one or two platforms, excluding other participative websites. The preferred choice is YouTube: in Italy one out of three ASLs has a YouTube video-channel. Moreover, only one in seven ASLs is on Facebook and even fewer on Twitter (one in nine).

There are considerable differences between the various Regions of Italy in terms of the use of the social web by the Local Health Authorities. These differences, however, are only slightly related to the traditional distinction between the Northern and Central Regions of Italy, where the majority of the population resides, where there are better living conditions and the Internet use by citizens is more frequent than in the South of Italy (Istat 2013a, 2013b).

Table 1. Percentage of internet users and percentage of local health authorities presence on social media by geographical area

Geographical Areas	Resident population (2013) (N=60 million)	% Internet use in the last 12 months (2013)	Number of ASL(N=143)	% Facebook presence on total n. ASL	% Twitter presence on total n. ASL	% YouTube presence on total n. ASL
North	45.8	59.1	51.7	13.5	14.9	33.8
Center	22.5	57.6	22.4	6.3	12.5	28.1
South	20.6	46.7	14.0	15.0	5.0	30.0
Islands	11.1	49.9	11.9	5.9	0.0	17.6
Italy	**100.0**	**54.8**	**100.0**	**11.2**	**11.2**	**30.1**

It seems to depend more on the choices made by the healthcare authority at the regional and even local level. While in one in three ASLs in Emilia Romagna uses Facebook, Twitter and YouTube (36%, the highest percentage in Italy), no official use is detected by the ASLs in Trentino, Tuscany, Marche and Molise, and in an intermediate position, Abruzzo (25%), Liguria (20%), Veneto and Puglia (17%). Consider the ASLs officially using at least one social platform, they are spread out in different Italian regions, with a higher concentration of experiences in Emilia Romagna (73%), followed by Campania (57%) Umbria (50%), and Basilicata (50%) and Lombardy (47%).

From this data no single clear regional direction appears, but rather a picture of scattered pilot

Table 2. Italian local health authorities' social media choice by geographical area

Geographical Areas	ASL on Facebook, Twitter & YouTube (%)	ASL at least on one social platform (%)	No ASL social media presence (%)	Total	N ASL
North	12.2	23.0	64.9	**100.0**	74
Center	6.3	25.0	68.8	**100.0**	32
South	5.0	35.0	60.0	**100.0**	20
Islands	5.9	17.6	76.5	**100.0**	17
Italy	9.1	24.5	66.4	**100.0**	143

experiences in different Italian Regions, revealing a substantial heterogeneity in choices, probably related to the different sensibilities and experiences of local actors.

How Health Authorities are Using Facebook Timelines: A Content Analysis

In the second phase of the research, we conducted a content analysis of the messages posted by Local Health Authorities in the Facebook official timelines. As showed in Figure 1, Italian Local Health Authorities officially present on Facebook posted 1367 messages from January to mid-July 2013. This number rapidly increases, passing to 2000 messages, if we count posts written by

other institutions, public administrations or local associations that have been simply shared by local health authorities in their timelines without adding any other information for the users.

The most active Local Health Authorities are N2 (249 posts), N5 (228 posts), N7 (199 posts), while S4, although having officially opened in April 2013, is more active in the timeline with 136 posts in less than four months of activity. The less dynamic Local Health Authorities appear to be located in the center of Italy: they tend to only share content from the corporate website without calibrating content for Facebook-'like' pages.

In the second stage, we manually classified all 1367 messages, using a content typology previously tested for another empirical study (Lovari & Parisi, 2012) and modifying it for use in public

Figure 1. Number of Facebook posts by 16 local health authorities (Jan-Jul 2013)

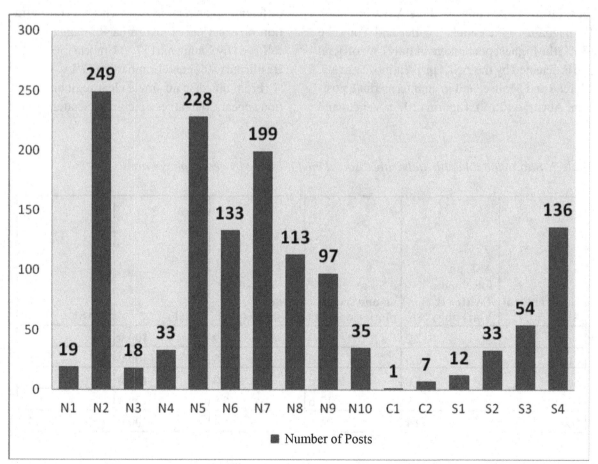

health communication. We used 7 categories to classify messages posted by ASLs in the their timelines:

- Information about public services and opportunities for citizens;
- Events promotion; health communication campaigns;
- Health authority life storytelling;
- Alerts about emergencies and disservices;
- Empowering citizens about health;
- Other.

As reported in Figure 2, the most recurrent category is "information about public services and opportunities for citizens" (n. 369; 26.99%) publicizing various services for the local population such as: working hours of some administrative offices; opening of new laboratories; launch of new medical services and examinations; pharmacies open during the weekends, or courses for painless childbirth or good parenting. The category "events promotion" (n. 202; 14.77%) contains posts launching or promoting conferences, meetings, and seminars addressed to the general public or to medical staff. These events are publicized in the Facebook timelines so as to increase their visibility, in addition to the web sites and press releases.

A relevant number of messages were collected in the category "health authority life storytelling" (n. 305; 22.31%) reporting information regarding ASLs, such as changes in the medical staff, new administrative roles assigned, and awards or ap-

Figure 2. Posts published in local health authorities' Facebook Like pages, by category

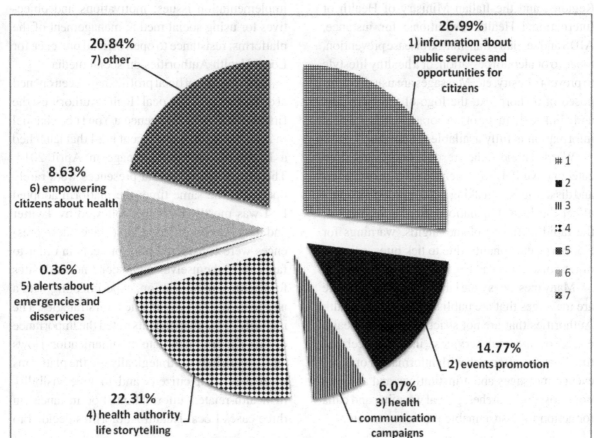

proved projects; it also publishes many pictures to describe specific events or everyday life inside the laboratories, territorial hospitals or administrative offices.

The category "empowering citizens about health" collects messages posted by Local Health Authorities to create awareness and engage citizens on issues that affect wellbeing in order to provide a sense of responsibility for their own health care. Through the publication of messages as well as videos and interviews, ASLs seek to raise awareness of special and delicate issues concerning health, disease prevention and wellbeing. These types of messages, although not frequently used by Local Health Authorities, are very important because they may allow citizens to make safer and healthier decisions.

Posts under the label "health communication campaign" (n. 83; 6.07%) illustrate specific health communication campaigns created by ASLs, the Regions, and the Italian Ministry of Health or International Health institutions: for instance, AIDS and sexually transmitted disease prevention, tobacco or alcohol cessation, or a healthy lifestyle to prevent obesity, etc. Messages are usually composed of a short text, the logo of the campaign and a link to thematic or corporate websites where information is fully available for citizens.

We also noticed the presence of an interesting category we defined "alerts about emergencies and disservices", breaking news reports that could affect the local population, such as measles or the rapid diffusion of meningitis, warnings for tick-borne encephalitis due to tick bites, or cases of rat poison in salad bags.

Many messages were labeled as "other". There are messages that are published by Local Health Authorities that are not strictly related to health issues or medical services: indeed Facebook timelines are often rich with information on local events, messages about institutions and associations, lost dog searches, global warming and calls for action for a sustainable environment, etc.

A Qualitative Focus: Listening to the Social Media Managers' Voices

In the third part of our research, we conducted telephone interviews with the people in charge of, or officially responsible for, the management of local health authorities' social network site presence. We focused our attention on those health units present on at least two social media platforms: in particular, we chose Facebook as a required platform, and then Twitter and/or You-Tube. Our decision was guided by the empirical evidence of timeline content analysis, with the aim of understanding how health organizations interact with the public on Facebook; the two other social network sites are indeed used more as broadcast media than participative ones. We decided to summarize the main evidence from the interviews in four sections thanks to a thematic analysis of the conversations with ASL personnel: implementation issues; motivations and objectives for using social media; management of the platforms; resistance to open official presence for Local Health Authorities on social media.

Social media official profiles have been opened at different times by Local Health Authorities: the first one was N8 who opened a YouTube channel in 2007, while the most recent is S4 that launched a Facebook official like page in April 2013. The official social media presences were rarely opened at the same time: the platform adopted first was mostly YouTube, followed by Twitter and then Facebook. In the first stage, these presences were considered pilot projects in order to familiarize themselves with social network sites for health communication, experimenting with a new language and communication strategies. The majority of our respondents noted the importance of this phase to calibrate communication flows and to learn how to strategically use the platforms to engage with citizens and to give visibility to health-related information. For instance, in three cases Local Health Authorities decided to open Facebook profiles and then modified them into 'like' pages (previously called fan pages), according to Facebook policies for non-profit organizations.

The idea to colonize social media was mostly developed by communications professionals, such as online communication managers, press office chiefs, public relations office directors, etc. Typically, these practitioners autonomously prepared a social media plan or a strategic report in order to present this opportunity to the top ASL management to obtain official approval or endorsement. There were also a few cases in which the idea was directly launched by the ASL general directors, who then involved communications staff to implement the task. These directors were familiar with digital technologies, personally using social media such as Facebook or Twitter to connect with their networks. Few of them are still so involved in the social media management that they have logins and passwords of the official pages to post or tweet together with the local health unit's communication staff.

In general, our informants reported that the decision to use social media for promoting services and health communication was accepted by the majority of the organizations. In particular, where the process was directly run and managed by top management, the implementation was simple and commonly agreed upon within the Local Health Authorities. This situation differs from that in which the idea to launch social media profiles was proposed and carried out by communications offices; in this case, our respondents highlighted the presence of some obstacles and sometimes a diffidence toward these participative platforms. Usually these negative attitudes came from the administration, specifically from the administrative personnel who are not allowed to access social network sites during working hours, due to Italian norms and regulations in terms of internet access for public administrations. For this reason, administrative employees are diffident about the use of

participative media and the activities carried out by their colleagues. On the contrary, doctors and medical staff showed an interest in collaborating with communication offices to record videos or deliver specific interviews about disease prevention and health campaigns to enrich Facebook, Twitter, and YouTube contents.

The decision to colonize social media platforms was driven by some specific motivations and objectives. First of all, the possibility to propagate health related information beyond traditional mass media such as press and television and outside of citizens' front offices and URP offices. Several respondents underlined how social network sites could give visibility to ASL's services, increasing awareness among the local population, or for citizens who prefer other healthcare units, such as private or university hospitals, to be fully informed about services.

Since we are a territorial authority we need to promote our health services via Facebook, Twitter and YouTube to foster their use by local inhabitants; most of them don't know about this opportunity and they just call the hospital (N5).

Analyzing the conversations with our informants, we noticed that a major reason to be on social media is the possibility to reach new targets, such as teenagers, high school students, or young adults who are frequent users of these platforms.

Facebook is populated by many adolescents and young people who are outside of traditional media patterns. We are using Facebook to propagate our health communication campaign since we can meet them in that place (N6).

Local Health Authorities try to intercept these groups by posting on specific topics such as health communication campaigns (i.e. drugs, HIV, sexually transmitted diseases, blood donation, obesity, etc.) or by promoting specific services addressed to them (i.e. counseling). This is the reason why some local health units decided to open thematic Facebook groups or other 'like' pages to support the official institutional one.

Moreover, a few respondents highlighted how opening a social media presence could also improve brand image and raise the reputation of ASL in the minds of citizens and the mass media. Furthermore, in only one case, the official social media presence was explicitly considered as a strategic tool to inform and engage internal staff such as administrative employers.

Beyond Facebook, YouTube channels were mostly opened as repositories for institutional videos already present in the ASLs' audiovisual archives; while Twitter accounts were launched to support press office activities and corporate communication in general, rather than to interact with citizens and patients.

The interviews allowed us to understand which structures are in charge of managing social media. Indeed, this information was not regularly present and published in the Facebook "information" or "bio" sections. There is a general heterogeneity in the management of social media by local health units: generally, it is managed by press offices, followed by URP offices and online communication offices. Posting for social media is only one of the numerous daily activities carried out by communication practitioners, in addition to writing press releases, organizing events or updating official ASL website. It is not an exclusive competence or skill: indeed dedicated structures - such as social media offices - have to be created in Italian public health organizations.

People in charge of managing and updating content on social media platforms vary in authority from one structure to another. On average, there are at least two individuals in charge of this activity. The majority of page administrators are journalists who work for the Local Health Authorities as employers or consultants. In some cases, social media staff are enriched by university students or graduates who are doing their internships in the

ASL communication structures. Content updates are made during working hours and via laptop or mobile connection outside of the office: we noticed how several local health structures have purchased smartphones and tablets to extensively manage social media presence overtime.

All of our informants recognized the importance of having a social media policy to inform citizens of the correct uses of the platforms, specifying conversation rules and types of inappropriate messages. However, only a few Local Health Authorities have already approved and publicized a social media policy: one local health unit mentioned the presence of the policy in the Facebook information section, linking it to the corporate web site for a complete reading; while another ASL has published a policy for Twitter, but not for Facebook.

Monitoring social media is an activity rarely carried out by health organizations. The evaluation of the social media activities is episodic and mostly quantitative, utilizing only statistics offered by the different platforms: i.e. 'Facebook Insights' dashboard, and number of followers and mentions displayed in Twitter. None of our respondents mentioned the use of qualitative tools, such as in-depth user interviews or web surveys to monitor the quality of the presence on Facebook.

In the last part of the interview, we asked our informants to identify the main constraints related to the adoption of social media for health communication. Three main obstacles for the use of social media for Local Health Authorities in Italy emerged from the thematic analysis of the conversations. The first and main reason, according to our respondents, is the lack of trained and specialized employees to manage these platforms: in particular, both communications directors and health authority general directors affirm confirm the difficulties of having qualified and skilled personnel dedicated to manage social media. Indeed, to be strategically active on Facebook or Twitter requires nurturing conversations and responding to public feedback all day: this means having specific communicators with the ability and the competence to quickly answer citizens' and patients' needs. For this reason, many health authorities prefer to select and colonize only one or two platforms, or to stay outside of the social web, since they do not have sufficient human resources at their disposal.

Why should we open the Facebook timeline if we don't have the resources to do it? It will be a bad service for citizens. It is better to be out of social media until we are ready to face this challenge (C1).

The second reason for resistance is related to the fear of receiving bad comments and critiques from citizens.

Being on social media means being in an open book where everybody can say whatever they want without any control (S4).

This factor can lead to fostering citizens' badmouthing, provoking a potential increase in claims against the authorities, and damaging reputations. This is the reason why many ASLs have decided to stay away from social media since they do not want:

to complicate the relations with citizens and patients, that are already complicated to manage (N10).

It is not only the scarcity of resources, but belief and a state of mind that impedes public health organizations to open themselves to the social web. This is the third factor mainly related to cultural aspects. In particular, some respondents highlighted how a large number of Local Health Authorities are run by general directors or top management who are not familiar with social media, and they are not able to fully understand the digital technological revolution in organizations. This is the reason why Internet websites are not built up with a user-centered approach

and why the majority of ASLs across the country have not yet officially opened official social media presences. The adoption of new technologies by organizations requires openness and commitment to face changes even if they complicate ordinary activities and the delivery of services. The decision to be on Facebook or Twitter relies on the complete understanding of these participative platforms that can reduce the distance between public health public organizations and citizens.

Solutions and Recommendations

Mergel and Bretschneider (2013) suggested analyzing the process of social media adoption in the public sector by applying a three-stage model: in the first stage, called intrapreneurship and experimentation, public agencies test informal social media presence, outside the organizational technology use policies, following the decision of creative employers who were attracted by these platforms through personal experience; the second stage, called order from chaos, underlines how organizations recognize the importance of these innovations and the need to draft norms and regulations for social media presence; in the third phase, named by the two scholars as institutionalization, public administrations have removed all of the variations in the use of social media, and they have approved a set of standards, rules, and processes in order to manage the process, indicating the resources associated with the enforcement of these protocols, with the advantage of reducing failure and misuse of these platforms.

On the basis of our research findings, the process of social media adoption by Italian health care local units is now facing the first stage indicated by Mergel and Bretschneider (2013). To hasten this stage and proceed, it is necessary to pay close attention to cultural and organizational differences. Inside the ASLs, there are still barriers to the use and development of communication between the three most relevant actors -doctors, administrative staff and communicators: each of them tends especially to respond to specific values belonging to their professional cultures. Doctors are interested mostly in the ways social media may change their clinical experiences and the relationship with patients and tend to consider the development of social media policies far from their main mission. Even among the director/managers of the communications offices we interviewed, we identified several differences between professional journalists and those who have received specific university training in public communication: the former are mostly inclined to use social media to increase overall institutional visibility, and the latter are inclined to dedicate more attention to interaction, listening and conversation with citizens and strategic publics.

Our research, as many others on Italian public administrations, detected at times a sort of distrust in citizen participation: bureaucrats tend to think it is unlikely that public interest can arise from direct interaction with citizens. In many cases, healthcare authorities believe that available resources should be used in more important sectors than for communication or that they are never sufficient to cover all communication activities (Househ, 2013). Somehow, the idea that the voice of the people corresponds to public complaints is still deeply rooted. From this point of view, it is understandable why healthcare authorities are inclined to use all communication tools, even the social media channels, in a broadcasted, unidirectional form. They do not seem very familiar with the proper use of social media platforms as valuable institutional tools to develop citizen empowerment about health. A very good example of this proper use can be retrieved in CDC's experiences (CDC, 2012). The underlying culture of social media use emphasizes one-to-one interaction and public discussion about decisions at both the individual and community levels. In cyberspace, there are many online support groups, digital communities concerned with specific diseases, or platforms created to share and to rank perceptions of health service quality. In the social web, citizens turn

into networked patients, patients who become active in the digital avenues not only to scout health-related information, but also to raise their voices toward healthcare organizations, doctors and other patients who share the same difficulties or diseases. Healthcare organizations cannot underestimate their roles and growing relevance inside and outside of the web.

A winning strategy to support the process of social media adoption will consider the specific point of view of each actor involved in this process, fostering them to explicate their positive and negative expectations, that may arise from different experiences and pertain to different facets of the process.

During the last decade of the twentieth century and the early years of the present century, there was a marked change in the organizational structure and the main mission of the Italian public administration. Then, much attention was devoted to the training and the exchanging of experiences between public personnel, to establishing and to sharing a strong sense of values related to the centrality of citizens. Somehow, in the following decade things changed, and a different perspective prevailed within public organizations, the mission of enhancing efficiency and accountability in order to reduce the government financial deficit.

In this framework, even the digitization of public administration was initially interpreted essentially as a way of reducing costs. Only recently has e-government been perceived in the light of an open government perspective, enabling citizen intervention and engagement (Contini & Lanzara, 2009; Lovari, 2013; Noveck, 2009; Sirianni, 2009). The challenge that social media pose to the Italian health care system as a whole, requires focusing once again on the empowerment of citizens. It seems unlikely that, in a period characterized by economic and fiscal crisis, public administrations and public healthcare authorities could find resources and invest efforts in training and exchange of experiences between all the actors involved to speed up this diffusion.

FUTURE RESEARCH DIRECTIONS

We are aware that this study has some limitations especially due to the choice to investigate only Local Health Authorities in the Italian National Healthcare System. This is a very specific case study. Quantitative data, however, are only useful to outline the traits of the phenomenon, which is subject to rapid change, therefore this can be used as basic knowledge to move on toward further qualitative research activities.

Further studies should be undertaken to investigate all the Italian SNN actors such as university hospitals (ICCR) and private healthcare organizations. Indeed, those belonging to the private health sector could be more disposed to strategically use social media in order to raise visibility, find new customers and generate money through fund-raising activities.

Other possible future stages of this research could include a comparison between Italy and other European countries, in order to capture the most interesting trends and organizational uses, aiming at defining social media guidelines for public health organizations in an international scenario. Much detailed research in this field and in health communication in general has also been carried out in the United States or by American university scholars (Hannawa et al., 2014; Kim et al., 2010). For this reason, there is a need to investigate these dynamics in different approaches and settings, with diverse national health systems, and other rates of social media use.

Furthermore, there is a need for empirical research to verify whether social network sites, and Facebook in particular, are activating innovative and participative communication practices between health organizations and citizens. Within this perspective, it would be interesting to deepen an understanding of the role that mobile technologies - such as the use of tablets and smartphones - play in accessing health communication and in connecting patients with health authorities.

CONCLUSION

Our study investigated the colonization and strategic use of social media by Italian Local Health Authorities, adopting a mix of quantitative and qualitative techniques such as adoption rate, post content analysis and telephone interviews with ASL communication managers.

From the empirical evidence, we can affirm that social media use for institutional health communication is still at an intrapreneurship and experimentation stage (Mergel & Bretschneider, 2013) for the quantity of official presences, and for the quality of social media presence related to platforms management.

First of all, we detected a limited number of ASLs' official profiles and pages in the main social networking sites such as Facebook, Twitter and YouTube. From the total 143 Italian Local Health Authorities, only one-third have an official presence on these platforms. The visibility of these presences is not well promoted in the ASL websites or in other official communication channels; in several cases, these pages are not clearly institutionalized, creating confusion and possible misinterpretation for citizens searching for ASL official presences in the social web.

ASLs can be divided into two categories: a) pro-active health authorities, those who have fully embraced web 2.0 philosophy, experimenting with social media as learning playgrounds for health communication; and, b) followers, those who are present on social media but not giving enough attention to the possibility to activate a dialogue with citizens. The majority of Italian Local Health Authorities fall into the second category: they use social media as a window to promote services and health campaigns but they do not seek to activate citizens' voices and engagement. During the interviews, communication managers clearly highlighted the difficulties in handling citizens' feedback, critics and flaming by online users; for these reasons they decided to implement broadcasting strategies instead of two-way communication strategies. This choice is clearly evident in the Facebook posting settings enabled by health authorities: only seven organizations allow users to post messages on their timelines.

In general, we noticed a broad constellation of uses of social media for Local Health Authorities: it seems that every ASL is following a proper specific strategy in order to inform and engage patients and citizens in general. Apart from a few cases (those coming from pro-active health authorities), these strategies create a traditional top-down flow of communication that does not favor user engagement. Indeed, Twitter and YouTube are used mostly as broadcasting media to propagate health information rather than stimulating users' participation. YouTube official channels diffuse videos previously recorded for other institutional activities or purposes; citizens' comments on videos are rarely activated in the platform, thus excluding the possibility to collect opinions and grassroots voices. Furthermore, ASL Twitter accounts are mostly used as online press tools, launching press releases and spreading health communication campaigns but with a rare use of interactive techniques such as hashtags, replies and mentions. Moreover, although Facebook affordances would allow the activation of a bidirectional communication with the public, the majority of the Italian ASLs present on this platform do not seem ready to take on this challenging opportunity. From the interviews, it is evident how worried ASL communication managers are about the possible consequences to open these conversational digital spaces to citizens' voices; while other practitioners attributed this unidirectional use to the lack of trained human resources able to strategically manage social media for health issues.

In conclusion, social media, and in particular social networking sites, seem to offer relevant opportunities for healthcare organizations to enrich communication within a multi-channel strategy, to rapidly inform and empower citizens about services and health issues, and to engage with hard-to-reach publics such as adolescents and marginalized people. In order to be effective and strategic, it is important to avoid a top-down, unidirectional use of these platforms, adopting a bi-directional communication strategy, planned and carried out by trained and skilled personnel. This is a strategic issue and an important challenge in the Italian health communication scenario.

ACKNOWLEDGMENT

The concept of the chapter is the result of a process of dialogue and sharing ideas between the authors. The attribution of each paragraph is the following: Elisabetta Cioni wrote "Introduction", "Solutions and Recommendations" and "Future Research Direction"; Alessandro Lovari wrote paragraphs from "Background" to "A Qualitative Focus: Listening to the Social Media Managers' Voices" (included). Abstract and conclusion of the chapter are written together. We would like to thank Ph.D candidate Claudia Pecorari for her help in collecting data.

This chapter has been produced as a part of the research project entitled "Communicating Health Through the Use of New Technologies", carried out at the University of Sassari, through the assistant professor's contract financed by P.O.R. SARDEGNA F.S.E. 2007-2013 – Objective regional competiveness and employability, Priority IV Human Capital, Measure 1.3.1.

REFERENCES

AlGhamdi, K. M., & Moussa, N. A. (2012). Internet use by the public to search for health-related information. *International Journal of Medical Informatics*, *81*(6), 363–373. doi:10.1016/j.ijmedinf.2011.12.004 PMID:22217800

Andersen, K. M., Medaglia, R., & Henriksen, H. Z. (2012). Social media in public health care: Impact domain propositions. *Government Information Quarterly, 29*(4), 462–469. doi:10.1016/j.giq.2012.07.004

Arata, G. (2011). *#TwitterPA T3/2011: Mapping the Presence and Activities of the Italian Public Bodies on Twitter.* Retrieved December 29, 2013, from http://t.co/lC5lEKMFK0

Audiweb. (2013). Online l'81% della popolazione italiana tra 11 e 74 anni. *Prima Comunicazione Online.* Retrieved July 28, 2013, from http://www.primaonline.it/2013/07/23/169869/online-l81-della-popolazione-italiana-tra-11-e-74-anni/

Bardus, M. (2011). The Web 2.0 and Social Media Technologies for Pervasive Health Communication: Are They Effective? *Studies in Communication Sciences, 11*(1), 119–136.

Bertot, J. C., Jaeger, P. T., & Grimes, J. M. (2010). Using ICTs to create a culture of trasparency: E-government and social media as openness and anti-corruption tools for societies. *Government Information Quarterly, 27*(3), 264–271. doi:10.1016/j.giq.2010.03.001

Bertot, J. C., Jaeger, P. T., & Hansen, D. (2012). The impact of policies on government on social media usage: Issues, challenges, and recommendations. *Government Information Quarterly, 29*(1), 30–40. doi:10.1016/j.giq.2011.04.004

Bonsón, E., Torres, L., Royo, S., & Flores, F. (2012). Local e-goverment 2.0: Social media and corporate transparency in municipalities. *Government Information Quarterly, 29*(2), 123–132. doi:10.1016/j.giq.2011.10.001

boyd, D. M., & Ellison, N. B. (2007). Social network sites: Definition, history and scholarship. *Journal of Computer-Mediated Communication, 13*(1), 210-230.

Bryer, T. (2010). Across the great divide: Social media and networking for citizens engagement. In J. H. Svara, & J. Denhardt (Eds.), *Connected communities, local government as partners in citizens engagement and community building* (pp. 73-79). Retrieved March 10, 2011, from http://www.tlgconference.org/communityconnectionswhitepaper.pdf

Byron, P., Albury, K., & Evers, C. (2013). It would be weird to have that on Facebook: Young people's use of social media and the risk of sharing sexual health information. *Reproductive Health Matters, 21*(41), 35–44. doi:10.1016/S0968-8080(13)41686-5 PMID:23684185

Censis –Forum per la Ricerca Biomedica. (2012). *Quale futuro per il rapporto medico paziente nella nuova sanità?* Retrieved June 28, 2013, from http://www.sanita.ilsole24ore.com/art/dibattiti-e-idee/2012-10-02/informazione-temi-sanitari-internet-130026.php

Censis-Ucsi. (2011). *I media tra crisi e personali nell'era digitale.* Retrieved July 10, 2013, from http://www.censis.it/17?shadow_pubblicazione=112567

Censis-Ucsi. (2013). *L'evoluzione digitale della specie.* Retrieved December 20, 2013, from http://www.censis.it/17?shadow_pubblicazione=120563

Center for Disease Control and Prevention (CDC). (2012). *CDC'S Guide to Writing for Social Media.* Retrieved July 10, 2013, from http://www.cdc.gov/socialmedia/tools/guidelines/pdf/guidetowritingforsocialmedia.pdf

Chou, W. S., Hunt, Y. M., Beckjord, E. B., Moser, R., & Hesse, B. W. (2009). Social media use in the United States: Implications for health education. *Journal of Medical Internet Research, 11*(4), 9–18. doi:10.2196/jmir.1249 PMID:19945947

Cline, R. J. W., & Haynes, K. M. (2001). Consumer health information seeking on the internet: The state of the art. *Health Education Research, 16*(6), 671–692. doi:10.1093/her/16.6.671 PMID:11780707

Comunello, F. (Ed.). (2012). *Networked Sociability and Individualism: Technology for Personal and Professional Relationships*. Hershey, PA: IGI Global.

Contini, F., & Lanzara, G. F. (2009). *ICT and innovation in the public sector: European studies in the making of e-government*. New York, NY: Palgrave.

Cosenza, V. (2013). *Osservatorio Social Media in Italia e Facebook*. Retrieved July 10, 2013, from www.vincos.it

Digital Scoreboard Agenda. (2012). *Life Online*. European Commission. Retrieved July 15, 2013, from https://ec.europa.eu/digital-agenda/sites/digital-agenda/files/scoreboard_life_online.pdf

Dutta, M. J. (2009). Health communication: trends and future directions. In J. C. Parker, & E. Thorson (Eds.), *Health communication in the new media landscape* (pp. 59–93). New York, NY: Springer Publishing Company.

Eurostat. (2011). Internet use in households and by individuals in 2011. *Statistics in Focus, 66*. Retrieved July 10, 2013, from http://epp.eurostat.ec.europa.eu/cache/ITY_OFFPUB/KS-SF-11-066/EN/KS-SF-11-066-EN.PDF

Eurostat. (2012). Internet use in households and by individuals in 2012. *Statistics in Focus, 50*. Retrieved July 10, 2013, from http://epp.eurostat.ec.europa.eu/cache/ITY_OFFPUB/KS-SF-12-050/EN/KS-SF-12-050-EN.PDF

Eysenbach, G. (2008a). Credibility of Health Information and Digital Media: New Perspectives and Implications for Youth. In M. J. Metzger, & A. J. Flanagin (Eds.), *Digital Media, Youth, and Credibility* (pp. 123–154). Cambridge, MA: The MIT Press.

Eysenbach, G. (2008b). Medicine 2.0: Social networking, collaboration, participation, apomediation, and openness. *Journal of Medical Internet Research, 10*(3), 1–9. doi:10.2196/jmir.1030 PMID:18725354

Fattori, G., & Pianelli, N. (2013). ASL e ospedali ai tempi di Twitter. *Il Sole24Ore Sanità, 16*(28), 8-9.

Fox, S. (2011). *Health Topics: 80% of users look for health information online*. Washington, DC: Pew Internet & American Life Project. Retrieved from http://www.pewinternet.org/Reports/2011/HealthTopics.aspx

Fox, S., & Duggan, M. (2013a). *Health Online 2013*. Washington, DC: Pew Internet & American Life Project. Retrieved July 20, 2013, from http://www.pewinternet.org/~/media//Files/Reports/PIP_HealthOnline.pdf

Fox, S., & Duggan, M. (2013b). *Tracking for Health*. Retrieved July 20, 2013, from http:pewinternet.org/Reports/2013/Tracking-for-Health.aspx

Fox, S., & Jones, S. (2009). *The social life of health information*. Washington, DC: Pew Internet & American Life Project. Retrieved from http://www.pewinternet.org/~/media//Files/Reports/009/PIP_Health_2009.pdf

Hannawa, A. F., Kreps, G. L., Paek, H.-J., Schulz, P. J., Smith, S., & Street, R. L. (2014). Emerging Issues and Future Directions of the Field of Health Communication. *Health Communication*. doi: doi:10.1080/10410236.2013.814959 PMID:24345246

Harris, J.K., Snider, D., & Mueller, N. (2013). Social Media Adoption in Health Departments Nationwide: The State of the States. *Frontiers in Public Services and System Research, 2*(1), art.5.

Hesse, B. W., O'Connell, M., Auguston, E. M., Chou, W. S., Shaikh, A. R., & Finney Rutten, L. J. (2011). Realizing the Promise of Web 2.0: Engaging Community Intelligence. *Journal of Health Communication: International Perspectives, 16*(1), 10–31. PMID:21843093

Househ, M. (2013). The Use of Social Media in Healthcare: Organizational, Clinical, and Patient Perspectives. In K. L. Courtney et al. (Eds.), *Enabling Health and Healthcare through ICT* (pp. 244–248). IOS Press.

Houston, T., & Ehrenberger, H. (2001). The Potential of Consumer Health Informatics. *Seminars in Oncology Nursing, 17*(1), 41–47. doi:10.1053/sonu.2001.20418 PMID:11236364

Ingrosso, M. (Ed.). (2008). *La salute comunicata: Ricerche e valutazioni nei media e nei servizi sanitari*. Milano: Franco Angeli.

Istat. (2013a). *Cittadini e nuove tecnologie*. Retrieved December 20, 2013, from http://www.istat.it/it/archivio/108009

Istat. (2013b). *Popolazione residente al 1° gennaio 2013*. Retrieved December 20, 2013, from http://demo.istat.it/pop2013/index.html

Kaplan, A. M., & Haenlein, M. (2010). Users of the world, unite! The challenges and opportunities of social media. *Business Horizons, 53*(1), 59–68. doi:10.1016/j.bushor.2009.09.003

Kim, J. N., Park, S. C., Yoo, S. W., & Shen, H. (2010). Mapping Health Communication Scholarship: Breadth, depth, and agenda of published research in Health Communication. *Health Communication, 25*(6-7), 487–503. doi:10.1080/1041 0236.2010.507160 PMID:20845126

Korda, H., & Itani, Z. (2011). Harnessing Social Media for Health Promotion and Behavior Change. *Health Promotion Practice, 14*(1), 15–23. doi:10.1177/1524839911405850 PMID:21558472

Kout, A. (2012). *Social Networking Popular Across Globe*. Washington, DC: Pew Internet & American Life Project. Retrieved July 15, 2013, from http://www.pewglobal.org/files/2012/12/Pew-Global-Attitudes-Project-Technology-Report-FINAL-December-12-2012.pdf

Levine, D., Madsen, A., Wright, E., Barar, R. E., Santelli, J., & Bull, S. (2011). Formative research on MySpace: online methods to engage hard-to-reach populations. *Journal of Health Communication, 16*(4), 448–454. doi:10.1080/10810730.201 0.546486 PMID:21391040

Lober, W. B., & Flowers, J. L. (2011). Consumer Empowerment in Health Amid the Internet and Social Media. *Seminars in Oncology Nursing, 27*(3), 169–182. doi:10.1016/j.soncn.2011.04.002 PMID:21783008

Lovari, A. (2013). *Networked citizens: Comunicazione pubblica e amministrazioni digitali*. Milano: Franco Angeli.

Lovari, A., & Giglietto, F. (2012). *Social Media and Italian Universities: An Empirical Study on the Adoption and Use of Facebook, Twitter and YouTube*. Retrieved July 20, 2013, from http://papers.ssrn.com/sol3/papers.cfm?abstract_id=1978393

Lovari, A., Kim, S., Vibber, K., & Kim, J.-N. (2011). Digitisation's impacts on publics: Public knowledge and civic conversation. *PRism, 8* (2).

Lovari, A., & Parisi, L. (2012). Public Administrations and Citizens 2.0: Exploring Digital Public Communication Strategies and Civic Interaction within Italian Municipality Pages on Facebook. In F. Comunello (Ed.), *Networked Sociability and Individualism: Technology for Personal and Professional Rellationships* (pp. 239–264). Hershey, PA: IGI Global.

Lupiañez-Villanueva, F., Maghiros, I., & Abadie, F. (2012). *Citizens and ICT for Health in 14 EU Countries: Results from an Online Panel.* Luxembourg: Publications Office of the European Union. Retrieved March 20, 2013, from http://is.jrc.ec.europa.eu/pages/TFS/documents/SIMPHS2_D3.2CitizenPanelfinal.pdf

Mayo Clinic Center. (2012). *Bringing the Social Media #Revolution to Health Care.* Mayo Foundation for Medical Education and Research.

McLaughlin, K., Osborne, S. P., & Ferlie, E. (Eds.). (2002). *New public management: Current trends and future prospects.* London: Routledge.

Mergel, I. (2010). Gov 2.0 revisited: Social media strategies in the public sector. *PA Times, 33*(3).

Mergel, I. (2013). *Social media in the public sector: A guide to participation, collaboration and transparency in the networked world.* San Francisco, CA: Jossey-Bass.

Mergel, I., & Bretschneider, I. (2013). A Three-Stage Adoption Process for Social Media Use in Government. *Public Administration Review, 73*(3), 390–400. doi:10.1111/puar.12021

Meskó, B. (2013). *Social Media in Clinical Practice.* London: Springer-Verlag. doi:10.1007/978-1-4471-4306-2

Ministero della Salute. Direzione Generale del Sistema Informativo e Statistico Sanitario. (2012). *Relazione sullo Stato Sanitario del Paese 2011.* Centro stampa del Ministero della salute. Retrieved March 20, 2013 from hhtp://rssp.salute.gov.it

Morgan, M. (2003). The Doctor-Patient Relationship. In *Sociology as Applied to Medicine* (5th ed., pp. 49–65). London: Saunders.

Nabatchi, T., & Mergel, I. (2010). Participation 2.0: Using Internet and social media: Technologies to promote distributed democracy and create digital neighborhoods. In J. H. Svara & J. Denhardt (Eds.), *Connected communities, local government as partners in citizens engagement and community building* (pp. 80-87). Retrieved March 10, 2011, from http://www.tlgconference.org/communityconnectionswhitepaper.pdf

Nielsen. (2011). *State of the media: The social media report.* Retrieved June 30, 2013, from http://blog.nielsen.com/nielsenwire/social/

Noveck, B. S. (2009). *Wiki government: How technology can make government better, democracy stronger, and citizens more powerful.* Washington, DC: Brookings Institution Press.

O'Mally, G. (2010, April 8). Study: Social Media Vital To Consumers Seeking Healthcare Information. *OnlineMediaDaily.* Retrieved July 25th 2013 from www.mediapost.com/publications/article/125801/?print

Osborne, S. P. (Ed.). (2010). *The New Public Governance? Emerging Perspectives on the Theory and Practice of Public Governance.* London: Routledge.

Parsons, T. (1951). *The social system.* Glencoe, IL: Free Press.

Perficient. (2013). *The Driving Force of Social Media in Healthcare*. Retrieved July 25th 2013 from http://www.perficient.com/Thought-Leadership/Perficient-Perspectives/2013/Social-Media-in-Healthcare

Popoiu, M. C., Grosseck, G., & Holetescu, C. (2012). What do we know about the use of social media in medical education? *Procedia: Social and Behavioral Sciences, 46*, 2262–2266. doi:10.1016/j.sbspro.2012.05.466

Price WaterHouse Coopers. (2012). *Emerging mHealth: Paths for growth*. Retrieved July 15, 2013, from http://www.pwc.com/en_GX/gx/healthcare/mhealth/assets/pwc-emerging-mhealth-full.pdf

PwC Health Research Institute. (2013). *Top health industry issues of 2013: Picking up the pace on health reform*. Retrieved July 15, 2013, from http://pwchealth.com/cgi-local/hregister.cgi/reg/pwc-hri-top-health-industry-issues-2013.pdf

Qualman, E. (2009). *Socialnomics: How social media transforms the way we live and do business*. Hoboken, NJ: John Wiley & Sons.

Roher, D., & Hall, J. A. (2006). *Doctors talking with patients/patients talking with doctors: Improving communication in medical visits* (2nd ed.). Westport, CT: Praeger.

Rubinelli, S., Camerini, L., & Schulz, P. J. (2010). *Comunicazione e salute*. Milano: Apogeo.

Santoro, E. (2011). *Web 2.0 e Social Media in medicina*. Milano: Il Pensiero Scientifico Editore.

Schein, R., Wilson, K., & Keelan, J. (2011). *Literature review on effectiveness of the use of social media: A report for Peel Public Health*. Retrieved June 25, 2013, from http://www.innonet.org/resources/files/socialmediaLitReview.pdf

Shaw, R. J., & Johnson, C. M. (2011). Health Information Seeking and Social Media Use on the Internet among People with Diabetes. *Online Journal of Public Health Informatics, 3*(1), 1–9. doi:10.5210/ojphi.v3i1.3561 PMID:23569602

Shih, C. (2009). *The Facebook Era: Tapping Online Social Networks to Build Better Products and Sell More Stuff*. Hoboken, NJ: Prentice Hall.

Siliquini, R., Ceruti, M., Lovato, E., Bert, F., Bruno, S., & De Vito, E. et al. (2011). Surfing the internet for health information: An Italian survey on use and population choice. *BMC Medical Informatics and Decision Making, 11*(1), 1–9. doi:10.1186/1472-6947-11-21 PMID:21211015

Sirianni, C. (2009). *Investing in democracy: Engaging citizens in collaborative governance*. Washington, DC: Brookings Press.

Solis, B., & Breakenridge, D. (2009). *Putting the public back in public relations*. Upper Saddle River, NJ: Pearson Education.

Thielst, C. B. (2011). Social Media: Ubiquitous Community and Patient Engagement. *Frontiers of Health Services Management, 28*(2), 3–14. PMID:22256506

Van De Belt, T. H., Engelen, L. J., Berben, S. A., & Schoonhoven, L. (2010). Definition of health 2.0 and medicine 2.0: A systematic review. *Journal of Medical Internet Research, 12*(2), e18. doi:10.2196/jmir.1350 PMID:20542857

White, R. W., & Horvitz, E. (2009). Cybercondria: Studies of the escalation of the medical concerns in web search. *ACM Transactions on Information Systems, 27*(4), 1–37. doi:10.1145/1629096.1629101

Yamout, S. Z., Glick, Z. A., Lind, D. S., Monson, R. A. Z., & Glick, P. L. (2011). Using Social Media to enhance surgeon and patient education and communication. *Bulletin of the American College of Surgeons*, *96*(7), 7–15. PMID:22315896

Zickuhr, K., & Madden, M. (2012). *Older adults and Internet use*. Pew Internet & American Life Project. Retrieved from http://pewinternet.org/Reports/2012/ Older-Adults-and-Internet-Use.aspx

ADDITIONAL READING

Bernstam, E. V., Shelton, D. M., Walji, M., & Meric-Bernstam, F. (2005). Instruments to Assess the Quality of Health Information on the World Wide Web: What Can Our Patients Actually Use? *International Journal of Medical Informatics*, *74*(1), 13–19. doi:10.1016/j.ijmedinf.2004.10.001 PMID:15626632

Dutta-Bergman, M. J. (2004). The Impact of Completeness and Web Use Motivation on the Credibility of e-Health Information. *The Journal of Communication*, *54*(2), 253–269. doi:10.1111/j.1460-2466.2004.tb02627.x

European Commission. (2004). e-Health - making healthcare better for European citizens: An action plan for a European e-Health Area. 2004, European Commission: COM 356 final, Brussels.

Eysenbach, G. (2002). Infodemiology: The Epidemiology of (Mis)information. *The American Journal of Medicine*, *113*(9), 763–765. doi:10.1016/S0002-9343(02)01473-0 PMID:12517369

Hesse, B. W., Moser, R. P., & Rutten, L. J. (2010). Survey of physicians and electronic health information. *The New England Journal of Medicine*, *362*(9), 859–860. doi:10.1056/NEJMc0909595 PMID:20200398

Lapointe, L., Mignerat, M., & Vedel, I. (2011). The IT productivity paradox in health: a stakeholder's perspective. *International Journal of Medical Informatics*, *80*(2), 102–115. doi:10.1016/j.ijmedinf.2010.11.004 PMID:21147023

Nettleton, S., Burrows, R., & O'Malley, L. (2005). The mundane realities of the everyday lay use of the internet for health, and their consequences for media convergence. *Sociology of Health & Illness*, *27*(7), 972–992. doi:10.1111/j.1467-9566.2005.00466.x PMID:16313525

Ratzan, S. C. (2001). Health literacy: communication for the public good. *Health Promotion International*, *16*(2), 207–214. doi:10.1093/heapro/16.2.207 PMID:11356759

Saleh, J., Robinson, B. S., Kugler, N. W., Illingworth, K. D., Patel, P., & Saleh, J. K. (2012). Effect of social media in health care and orthopedic surgery. *Orthopedics*, *35*(4), 294–297. doi:10.3928/01477447-20120327-05 PMID:22495836

Sneddon, E. (2012). Legally speaking: Social media and on-line conduct policies for medical practices. *The Journal of the Arkansas Medical Society*, *108*(9), 182–184. PMID:22435314

Taubenheim, A. M., Long, T., Smith, E. C., Jeffers, D., Wayman, J., & Temple, S. (2008). Using Social Media and Internet Marketing to reach Women with Heart Truth. *Social Marketing Quarterly*, *14*(3), 58–67. doi:10.1080/15245000802279433

KEY TERMS AND DEFINITIONS

ASL: Local Health Authority. It is a branch of the Italian Health National System, together with university hospitals (ICCR). ASLs are public bodies that have organizational, administrative, fiscal, financial, managerial and technical independence, offering health services for the local territory.

Civic Engagement: A variety of forms of citizens' activism and participation in the social and civic life of a territory. Civic engagement could be showed in the active presence in public debates and events, but also trough actions carried out in mass media (i.e. writing a letter to a newspaper, etc.), in the cyberspace (i.e. signing a on line petitions, etc.), and via social media, such as liking a Facebook page, writing a tweet or post messages for blogs and social network sites.

Facebook: Created in 2004, it is the most famous social network site supporting Internet mediated social interactions and communication. Nowadays over one million of people worldwide have Facebook accounts. This social media is the most heavily used social network site by companies, brands, universities and public administrations in general for communicating with their strategic publics and mass media.

Networked Patients: Patients who interact and become active in digital environments, such as blog o social network sites, to search for health related information and to raise their voices toward healthcare organizations, doctors and other patients who share the same difficulties and health issues.

Public Communication: The communication activities planned and managed by public administrations (i.e. municipalities, public hospitals, universities, etc.) aiming at informing citizens, media and other social and economic actors about public services and policies. Public communication is also important for enhancing participation in civic life via both offline and online tools and media.

Social Media: Web based platforms that allow to manage and foster relations, to develop sociability and increasing social capital. Thanks to social media citizens can not only read online contents but they are able to produce messages and upload imagines or videos. Social media started to be rapidly used by brands, companies and institutions as relational and communication tools to engage with clients and citizens. Social media embraces blogs, social network sites, content communities, wiki, and other web 2.0 platforms.

Social Network Site: Web 2.0 website used to stay in contact with peers and organizations. They are generally articulated in a profile with the possibility to visualize and traverse list of friends. Users can utilize social network sites for different aims such as social and professional relations, social commerce or entertainment.

Twitter: Launched in 2006, Twitter is a micro-blogging platform characterized by the possibility to publish short messages composed by 140 characters. Since fall 2012, Twitter has modified some features making it more similar to a social network site. It is mostly used to launch press releases and broadcasting messages.

Chapter 15
Social Media in Promoting HIV/AIDS Prevention Behaviour among Young People in Botswana

Tshepo Batane
University of Botswana, Botswana

ABSTRACT

This chapter explores the effects of social media in influencing the behavior of young people in relation to HIV/AIDS. The platform used for the project is an online discussion forum. The study is a One Group Pretest and Posttest inquiry. Formative evaluation is performed at the beginning of the study to establish participants behaviour, the intervention is introduced, then a summative evaluation is done to find out whether the intervention had any effect on the behaviour of the participants. The findings of the study indicate that there is a significant change in the behaviour of participants in relation to HIV/AIDS due to the use of the online forum. The study recommends that more efforts need to be directed to the use of various technologies that young people have at their disposal in the fight against HIV/AIDS as this can be very economical and effective.

INTRODUCTION

The idea of using technology to relate various forms of messages to promote prosocial ideas has been greatly adopted with success worldwide (Coleman & Meyer, 1990). Technology is an increasingly powerful tool for participating in global markets, enhancing the quality of education and improving basic services. Therefore it has become important for countries affected with

HIV/AIDS to harness the potential of these tools to assist in the fight against the disease. Studies show that educating young people on the risks of HIV and prevention strategies assist in modifying their behaviour to become less vulnerable. According to UNFPA (nd), targeted HIV education in young people has resulted in the delay in sexual debut, increased condom use and a decrease in HIV infection.

DOI: 10.4018/978-1-4666-6150-9.ch015

This study engaged the use of a social media platform in the form of an online discussion forum as an intervention strategy to promote HIV/AIDS prevention behaviour among young people. An online discussion forum allows users to post topics for discussion and other members can post their comments or their own topics. Discussions can either be public for all members of the forum to participate in or they can be private between a pair or selected number of people within a group. As Christopher (2004) says, interactive tools in the forums assist to develop a connection between the users, thus recreating the dynamics of a real conversation. In this study, the discussion forum was used as a place where participants interacted, shared information, experiences, asked questions and discussed various behavioural issues concerning HIV/AIDS. The postings in the forum were anonymous. This study was based on the premise that there is still a lot of stigma surrounding this disease which often makes it difficult for people to openly talk about their concerns. The anonymous feature of an online discussion forum gives people freedom to open up and discuss issues that they would otherwise not be able to share in face to face interactions. Thus, the objectives of the study were to: 1) investigate participants' behaviour in relation to HIV/AIDS, 2) assess the impact of an online discussion forum on this behaviour.

BACKGROUND

The development of technology in African countries has taken centre stage with countries working to broaden access to the internet and improving technical performance. Recent studies and reports indicate that there are plenty of technology resources in most African countries, however, most of these are not fully utilized to improve the lives of the people (Gerster Consulting, 2008; Kwankam & Ningo, nd; Ogungbure, 2011). In 2004, Adeyemi conducted a study on the use of Information Systems to prevent HIV/AIDS in La-

gos, Nigeria. The study surveyed health facilities in the state to find out how computer technology is used in the provision of health services. The study found out that 86% of the surveyed institutions possessed computers and other ICT tools, however, none of them used them in their work. The study concluded that even though there was reasonable ICT infrastructure in the area, there was gross underutilization of these resources. Therefore, there is need to train people to harness the potential of ICT to transform health care delivery and fight HIV/AIDS.

In the past, various mass media platforms such as television and radio have been used to deliver interventions and spread messages about HIV/AIDS. In recent years, social media has gained a lot of popularity among young people with leading social networking services reporting record breaking numbers of people using their services. Many authors agree that social networking sites are appealing because they satisfy a powerful human need to interact and communicate with other people, because after all, we are social beings (Altamirano 2011; Wavecrest Computing, 2009). Social networking also provides a form of entertainment to the users (Nations, 2011). This use of social media has also increased among the African youths (Affrinovator, 2011; Samie, 2011). Nowadays, most young people in the continent have sufficient access to the internet mainly through mobile phones and at their respective schools. Therefore, this paper contends that it is important to extend the use of these services to help in the fight against HIV/AIDS among young people. As Bouman (1998) says that entertainment media can play a great role in educating people on different social issues such as HIV prevention and other social ills, the only problem is that, this potential has not been sufficiently tapped.

The Intervention

The Discussion Forum used in this study was embedded in Blackboard 8.0 which was the Learning

Management System (LMS) used by the university where this research was based. Since the forum was already available in the LMS, there was not much done in contribution to its design, except to configure it to meet the purposes of the research such as; making the postings anonymous, enabling the Usage Statistical feature to assist determine the level of usage of the forum and making the forum accessible only to people participating in the project. When the users logged into the forum, they would find various discussion threads organized around particular topics and figures indicating the number of postings made on a particular thread. Participants would then click on a thread they wanted to follow or create new ones. They could either have a public discussion with everyone in the forum or engage in a private conversation with a particular member of the group. This forum was similar to many others available in that it provided the basic communication features that most discussion forums have. The only difference was that it was not a stand-alone forum but was part of a Learning Management System used by a university.

Theoretical Framework

This study was guided by Bandura's social learning theory which postulates that people model and role play their behaviour after others. The theory concentrates on the power of example. Social learning theory is generally a theory of human behaviour however; Bandura and people concerned with mass media communications have used it to specifically explain media effects. Bandura (1973,77,) say that Social Learning Theory is important in educating through entertainment because the intention is to modify behaviour and perception through role models that are socially acceptable or unacceptable. The hope is to prompt discussions among members concerning socially desirable behaviour that needs to be promoted. Such conversations are believed to have the capability to create a social learning environment

where people consider changing their behaviour to more desirable ones. Singal & Rogers (1999) say: "Collective efficacy emerges when people share ideas about social problems facing their system and discuss ways of confronting resistance to their plans for social change." (pp176).

Singhal et al. (1993), say that entertainment education seeks to capitalize in the appeal of proper media to show individuals how they can live safe, healthier and happy lives. The purpose is to instigate social change-defined as the process by which an alteration occurs in the structure of function of a social system. According to Singhal et al. (1993), embedding educational messages with entertainment assist to increase knowledge about the issues, create favorable attitudes and change overt behavior concerning the educational issue or topic. Social learning theory posits that behaviour change requires an informational component to increase awareness knowledge of risks to convince people that they can change their behaviour. The theory also asserts that social support is crucial for individuals as they engage in the new behaviour (Bandura, 1973). The Discussion forum in this study was used as a platform to promote positive behavior towards HIV/AIDS for young people to model and live responsibly.

Research Design and Data Collection Strategies

This study was a One Group Pretest and Posttest inquiry. The study triangulated both qualitative and quantitative techniques in obtaining data. Two sets of questionnaires containing both qualitative and quantitative questions were administered, one at the beginning of the study and the other one towards the end of the project. The questionnaires contained similar questions since the intention was to measure the before and after-effects of the same variables. At the beginning, a formative evaluation was performed through a questionnaire. Formative evaluation assists in identifying issues of interest, humor topics and topics that are too personal or sensitive to discuss, so that such issues can be handled with outmost caution, for example, as Singhal and Rogers (1999) point out an important advantage of before and after measurements is that they give the researcher opportunity to identify changes on variables caused by the intervention. Thus a formative evaluation is done on the participants before exposure on the intervention. Singhal and Rogers (1999) say that it is important to conduct formative evaluation while the activity, process or system is being developed or ongoing so as to improve its effectiveness. This exercise helped to establish the participants' behaviour patterns in relation to HIV/AIDS issues before the intervention. The results from the evaluation helped to guide in the design of the discussion forum and assisted to identify the main issues that needed to be addressed. However, participants were still free to discuss any topic of their interest.

After eight months, another survey was administered to test the effects of the online interactions on the participants' behaviour. During the follow up survey differences in the variables were identified to determine whether there were any changes as a result of exposure to the intervention. Summative evaluation was performed to determine the effectiveness of the intervention. Focus group discussions were conducted after administering the second round of questionnaires to obtain in-depth information; this assisted to understand the nuances of the various situations in the study.

Periodic checks were also performed to determine how much people used the forum in each month; a feature called Usage Statistics embedded in the discussion forum was used to do this. Quantitative data from the questionnaires was analyzed using Statistical Package for Research Software Program (SPSS). Cross tabulated results from the selected variables reported. Descriptive statistics and correlations were also used.

Content analysis was used to analyze data from the discussion forum, qualitative data from the questionnaires and focus group discussions. Since the intention of this study was to determine whether the intervention had any impact on the behaviour of the participants regarding HIV/AIDS, content analysis became a useful tool in assessing this change as (Corlazzoli, 2013) says that content analysis is an effective measurement of change. The unit of analysis in the study were the specific words, phrases and themes that described participants' attitudes, beliefs, knowledge and behaviour regarding HIV/AIDS, whether positive or negative. The words or themes that had similar meanings were grouped together to form categories. The material from the Discussion forum, qualitative data from the questionnaires and group discussions, was coded, highlighting the keywords and phrases and placing them in the identified categories. A tally sheet was kept to record the frequency at which the words were used in relation to the issue being discussed. Since the intention was to observe whether there was a change in the overall behaviour and attitudes of the participants, the frequency at which these keywords occurred was carefully monitored to see how their usage evolved over the period of the study to be able to determine whether there was change or not.

Site and Sample Population

Participants in this study were students from four different tertiary institutions in Botswana. The use of ICT presupposes access and basic understanding of ICT among the participants hence the chosen population; these were students with computer access at their institutions. Purposive sampling was used to select participants to ensure that the study targeted people who would be easy to locate for follow up investigations. Contact people from the institutions were used to identify participants. A total of 117 students participated in the project.

FINDINGS

Demographic Data

The following section presents the demographic data of the study. Tables 1 and 2 show the gender of the participants and the age of the participants respectively.

HIV Status and Testing

At the beginning of the study, 77% of the participants reported that they knew their HIV status, while 23% said they did not know. The percentage of females who knew their HIV status was higher than that of males within their gender brackets. From the total number of participants who had not tested for HIV, 50% of them cited lack of courage as the main reason for not testing with many indicating that they feared they may be HIV positive and were not ready to face that possibility. Others mentioned the stigma surrounding the disease as the problem. A topic was posted in the discussion forum for people to share their experiences with HIV testing and participants started relating their own experiences of how they went about testing and the benefit that came out of it. A majority of the participants reported that they

had tested for HIV more than once and admitted that going for the first test was the most difficult part, as one student stated: "nowadays, you find yourself having seconds thoughts about getting tested for the virus, however, you should know if something is wrong so everyone should take responsibility for their wellbeing and get tested no matter how hard". Another participant said "I also know that the first time I went for testing was not really easy but if you have gone once it becomes easy for you to go back there".

Students reported that the reason they were scared was because they were not ready to accept the results in case they were positive, however counselling and support from their partners helped them to go through with the testing. Getting the results was the most difficult part as one student stated "when the results came, I felt like running away and regretted why I did that".

Number of Sexual Partners

The study revealed that the majority of students had their first sexual encounter at the ages of 18 and 19 while 6% indicated that they were still virgins, and 5% said they had their first sexual encounter over the age of 21, see Figure 1.

On the issue of the number of sexual partners, 61% reported that they currently had one sexual partner, while 33% said they had more than one sexual partner and 12% saying they were not in a

Table 1. Gender of participants

Gender	Number	Percentage %
Male	54	46
Female	62	53
No response	1	1
Total	117	100

Table 2. Age brackets of participants

Age of participants	Number	Percentage %
18-21	42	36
22-25	34	29
26-29	25	21
30-33	11	9
No response	5	4
Total	117	100

Figure 1. Age of first sexual encounter for participants

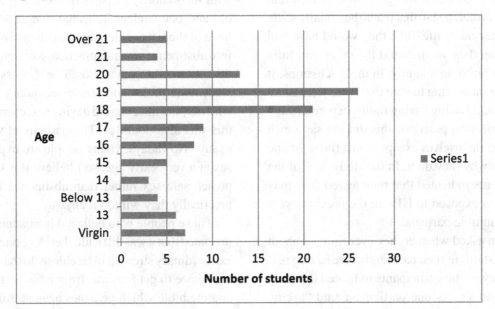

sexual relationship. Figure 2 shows a breakdown of the number of sexual partners that participants had.

The most popular reason stated for having more than one sexual partner was the other partner staying far away. Other reasons advanced for having multiple sexual partners were: economic

hardships, the need to satisfy sexual desire and unreliable partners, as one participant said "Sometimes it is just difficult to stick with one partner, especially if you suspect that your boyfriend has others on the side, you are tempted to also find more affection somewhere else". Some partici-

Figure 2. Number of sexual partners

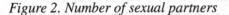

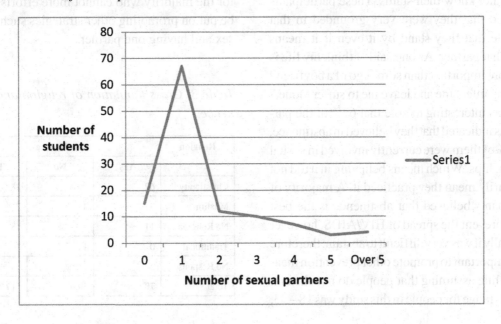

pants believed that it was good to have different partners at their age so that when they finally settle down later on in life, then they would have had all the fun they wanted, and then they can fully focus on building a family. In the discussions, it was very interesting to note that there were more voices condemning having multiple partners and the people who practiced this did not say much to defend themselves except to just throw in one sentence why they do it. In the study 15% of the participants indicated that they feared they may have been exposed to HIV in the previous year due to multiple partners.

When asked whether they ever find out about the HIV status of their partners before having sex, a majority of the participants indicated that they did not do so. As one participant said "asking someone of their HIV status is not an easy thing to do, that is why I prefer to just use a condom to protect myself in case there is a problem." A couple of participants indicated that they did try to go and find out their HIV status together with their partners before having sex, but that did not go down well, with one partner completely refusing and the other ending the relationship. There were only three participants in the study who reported that they refused to have sex with someone if they do not know their status. These participants indicated that they were very grounded in that principle that they stand by it even if it means losing that partner. As one said "I think my life is way more important than some ego of a boyfriend who may infect me and leave me to suffer alone."

It was interesting to note that 67% of the participants indicated that they believed in abstinence, but 78% of them were currently involved in sexual relationships. Which means believing in it did not necessarily mean they practiced it. A majority of participants believed that abstinence is the best way to prevent the spread of HIV/AIDS, however practically it was very difficult to abstain; therefore it was important to promote other prevention measures while assuming that people do not abstain. The age-range for people in this study was 18 – 33,

with the majority of participants being 20 years old and one student indicated that at this stage most of them were already sexually active, therefore abstinence was not practical for them, rather this is something that should be discussed with students at junior and senior secondary schools who may not have started having sex, even though this was also doubtful. The participant went on to say "Nowadays, young people are exposed to sex at a very early age, so I believe it is better to preach safe sex rather than abstinence because practically they will do it anyway".

Those people who believed in abstinence appreciated that it was difficult; therefore one needed extraordinary strength to be able to do that and the best place to get that was from believing in God and the bible which preaches against things like fornication. This is shown by the fact that a majority of people who believed in abstinence indicated that they practiced Christianity, see Table 3. They said if one deeply believes this then they would be able to withstand the pressures of having sex before marriage. Others stated the belief in the sanctity of marriage as the reason for abstaining and refraining from extra marital sexual activities. All in all students believed that it was good to preach abstinence for the few who could, but for the majority who cannot more efforts should be put on promoting other strategies such as safe sex and having one partner.

Table 3. Cross tabulation of religion and abstinence

Religion	Abstinence		
	Yes	**No**	**Total**
Christianity	62	26	88
Muslim	3	4	7
No Religion	11	7	18
Traditional	0	1	1
No Response	2	1	3
Total	78	39	117

Condom Use

At the beginning of the study, 78% of the participants reported that they were in a sexual relationship and 70% of them reported that they were using condoms. However, most participants indicated that it was easier to enforce condom use during the first few sexual encounters with a new partner, but from there they stopped using it. As one participant said "when you keep on demanding to use a condom, it's almost like you are saying I don't trust you." It was interesting to note that all the participants who indicated non-condom use were not married. 10 of them were females and two were males. In the discussions in the online forum, a majority of these participants expressed that they wanted to use the condom themselves but were often afraid to ask their partners. This fear of partners came across in a number of postings as one of the main reasons why people were not taking appropriate actions to protect themselves against HIV infections.

Alcohol

35% of the participants reported that they drank alcohol which was a troubling factor considering that HIV transmission has been closely connected to excessive alcohol consumption among young people. 20% of these participants regarded themselves as heavy drinkers, 2% as moderate drinkers, while 13% said they just drank occasionally. The 20% who were heavy drinkers indicated they were in sexual relationships and admitted that there had been times when alcohol impaired their judgement in responsible sexual behavior. However, it is worth pointing out that a high use of condoms was reported within this group of people who drank alcohol. Table 4 below shows a cross tabulations of alcohol, sexual relationships and condom use.

Effects of the Use of the Discussion Forum

At the end of the project, participants reported some behaviour changes which could be attributed

Table 4. Cross tabulations of alcohol, sexual relationships and condom use

Use Condoms			Sexual Relationship			
			Yes	No	No Response	Total
Yes	Drink alcohol	Yes	28	3	0	31
		No	48	2	1	51
		Total	76	5	1	82
No	Drink alcohol	Yes	5	1		6
		No	9	2		11
		Total	14	3		17
No response	Drink alcohol	Yes	0	2		2
		No	1	5		6
		Total	1	7		8
Not applicable	Drink alcohol	Yes		2		2
		No		8		8
		Total		10		10

to the use of the discussion forum. When the project started, 23% of the participants indicated that they did not know their HIV status, out of this number, 15% reported that they had since tested for HIV, making the total percentage of people who knew their status to be 92%. This 15% reported that the encouragement that they got from the forum was what helped them to gain courage to go and test, as shown by this quote "I am happy to announce that I did go for my HIV testing yesterday. I have never been so scared in my life, but I did it. It's not that I didn't know I had to do it, but all along I had decided to push it at the back of my mind but after talking about it so much in this forum, I decided it was time to take the bull by the horns, thanks guys for the encouragement". However, the remaining 8% indicated that they were still not ready to go through with the testing.

At the beginning of the study, 33% of the participants indicated that they had more than one sexual partner, and by the end of the project, this number had significantly declined to 11%. There were no significant changes in terms of abstinence as about the same number of participants practicing abstinence, with only 2% joining people in sexual relationships. There was a reported increase in condom use from 70% to 85%, however, there was also an increase in the number of people who drank alcohol from 35% to 37%. A majority of the postings in the forum indicated that people wanted to take more control of their lives in terms of sexual activities instead of letting their partners dictate to them what should happen.

Content analysis of the discussions in the forum was carried out to determine whether there were any changes in the attitude and behaviour of students to corroborate what they reported in the questionnaires. Through this analysis, negative, positive and changing attitudes were identified. When a particular topic was being discussed for the first time, the researcher would pay attention to the attitudes that the participants portrayed towards

it, especially the negative attitudes, including counting how much of this was occurring in the postings in the subject. This involved things such as the tone used, the language and whether they were for or against the proposed HIV prevention behavior. Then this behaviour would be observed over a certain period of time depending on the lifespan of the discussion on that topic. Towards the end of the project, these topics were revived in a different form to find out what the attitudes were. For example, in this analysis it was found out that there were certain people who were negative about everything that was suggested as a method to fight HIV/AIDS. The frequency at which these negative attitudes appeared in each issue discussed was calculated. It was interesting to note that towards the end of the study, these negative voices decreased and eventually faded out by the time the study ended. Whenever someone posted a negative message about HIV prevention, other participants would quickly respond and to some extend offer counselling to these people, an example is shown in this posting "You really need to get a grip, you sound like you are angry at life, at everybody. There is no need trashing down all the efforts people are trying to fight HIV, especially if you are not providing an alternative. My suggestion is, if you don't have anything helpful to say then don't say anything at all, you need help buddy!" Therefore it was not far-fetched to suggest that the decline in negative attitude was due to the interactions in this forum.

Another example was a discussion on 'HIV testing', in this topic, a keyword that appeared most frequently in the postings was 'scary' describing how people felt about testing for HIV. The usage of this word was most prevalent in the first four to five months of the project and was found in about 90% of the postings on this issue. However, it was observed that in the last three months of the project, the frequency of this word had significantly dropped to about 38%, see Figure 3.

Figure 3. Coding results for HIV testing

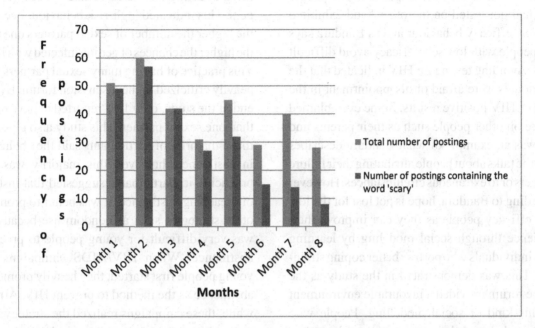

DISCUSSION

Behaviour, especially sexual behaviour should be at the centre of any HIV/AIDS prevention strategy. Global HIV Prevention WorkingGroup (2008) states that "wider delivery of effective behavior change strategies is central to reversing the global HIV epidemic." (pp4). In this study, knowing one's HIV status was regarded as a very important step in promoting HIV/AIDS prevention behaviour. At the beginning of the study, 77% of participants indicated that they knew their HIV status, with 23% saying they had not tested. By the end of the study, the number of people who knew their status had increased to 92%. This showed a significant increase in the number of people who had tested. These new people who had tested during the course of the study cited encouragement from the discussion forum as the main reason they went to test. This clearly indicated that the use of the forum had an impact on the behaviour of the participants in this regard. The number of females, who tested, still remained higher than that of men. There are various reasons that have been advanced to explain

why more women test for HIV compared to men such as women's susceptibility to various diseases which leads to them having to take an HIV test and pregnancy since it is a requirement for every pregnant woman to test for HIV.

In this study, people who had not tested for HIV cited fear as the main reason for not testing as they felt they were not capable of handling the situation if the results came back positive. According to Bandura's theory of social learning, this kind of people is regarded to have a low sense of efficacy. He describes self-efficacy as an "individual's perception of his or her capability to deal effectively with a situation and a sense of perceived control over a situation" (Bandura 1977, pp150). He says people with a strong sense of efficacy are often prepared to face challenges head on and trust their ability to deal with the consequences of any action they take and are not afraid to be disappointed. This is reflective of the people in the study who had tested for HIV. These people admitted that taking an initiative to test for HIV was very scary but this was something that implied taking responsibility for their own lives therefore making that difficult decision to test was very important. The people who had not tested on the other hand exhibited low self-efficacy behaviour and as Bandura says that people with low self-efficacy avoid difficult tasks. Avoiding testing for HIV indicated that the individuals were afraid of disappointment in the form of HIV positive results. Some even blamed failure on other people such as their parents and that was an example of what Bandura describes when he talks about people attributing their failure to others or to extraneous circumstances. However according to Bandura, hope is not lost for the low self- efficacy people as they can improve their resilience through social modeling by learning from individuals who portray better coping strategies. This was demonstrated in the study as the online forum provided a favourable environment for this kind of social modelling. People who had tested shared their experiences of how they went about the testing and acknowledging that it was a difficult thing to do, in this way they did not make themselves look super- human so others could identify with them. People who had tested for HIV cited support from their family and friends as the main thing that helped them to go through the process. So it was important for the low self- efficacy people to learn from their peers the strategies that could help them go through the testing. Bandura says collective efficacy can also assist those who are still lagging, which means in this study, if all the people who had not tested could come together with a common goal to test then they could give each other courage to do it. However, Bandura says the most effective change can happen with individual-level self - efficacy, therefore more effort should be put in encouraging stimulus that promote self-efficacy.

The number of sexual partners is an issue that is currently headlining most HIV/AIDS campaigns because it has been realized that having more than one sexual partner is one of the main contributing factors to the spread of HIV infection. In this study, 33% of the participants indicated that they had more than one sexual partner with 3% indicating

that they had as many as more than five sexual partners. This indicated high-risk behaviour because the higher the number of sexual partners one has, the higher the chances of getting infected with HIV. This practice of having many sexual partners was heavily criticized in the discussion forum. By the end of the study, only 11% reported to have more than one sexual partner. This study also reported that a majority of participants said they believed in abstinence, however, this majority was not practicing it. Participants suggested that instead of preaching abstinence, it was better to promote other strategies such as condom use because it was very difficult for young people to practice abstinence. When HIV/AIDS campaigns for young people first started, they heavily promoted abstinence as the method to prevent HIV. After a while, these campaigns realized the strategy was not working as young people were already having sex, so this strategy was improved to include other methods, giving birth to the famous Abstinence, Be faithful, Condomize (ABC) slogan. Condom use was reported to have increased in this study. However, participants indicated high usage of condoms at the beginning of a sexual relationship and a decline as the relationship progresses. NACA (2005) reported similar findings whereby there was a high percentage of people who used condoms in the productive age of 15 to 49 and this condom use was higher at the first time of sexual intercourse; from then this use declined. Bandura identifies three types of social modeling, and the one exhibited in this study was prestige modeling whereby individuals portrayed behaviour that was admirable both culturally and health wise. In this particular project specifically, role models were those students who had tested for HIV and practiced abstinence or had one sexual partner and practiced condom use.

Recommendations

Peer to peer learning has been credited to be very effective in educational settings; therefore HIV/

AIDS campaigns can adapt the use of these tools in the fight against the scourge. This study indicated that young people responded positively to advice from their colleagues which led to positive behavior changes. The anonymous nature of the forum used in this project provided freedom for participants to openly discuss issues, share their fears and life experiences that they may not be comfortable to discuss in face to face interactions. The discussions in the forum served a great role in providing peer counseling and support to other members to encourage them to adopt HIV/AIDS prevention behaviors. The behaviour that young people portray has a bearing on whether we are indeed moving towards an HIV free generation or not. HIV/AIDS is a problem that has crippled many developmental efforts in developing countries because a lot of financial resources are pumped into prevention strategies and providing better health care for those already infected. The use of platforms such as the one described in this study is very cost effective because it utilizes resources that are already available. This study recommends that countries tap more into the many services that computer technologies offer most of which do not come with additional costs as this can relieve the financial burden that usually characterize other strategies such as campaigns, rallies, workshops and many others.

FUTURE RESEARCH

Adopting HIV/AIDS intervention strategies such as the one presented in this chapter at a larger scale will require systematic planning and implementation to ensure that as many young people as possible benefit from the initiatives. Thus, future studies need to look at policy reforms that would ensure sufficient access of resources to young people and a commitment by governments and other stakeholders to consciously utilize technologies to educate young people about HIV/AIDS. One of the main criticisms laid against ICTs is that their use exacerbates the gap between the rich and the poor in societies. In order for healthcare provision to avoid this pitfall, it has to ensure that technologies are used to improve health for the less privileged. Studies have shown that HIV/AIDS is more prevalent among the poor and vulnerable (Drimie, 2002; Spiegel, 2004; Abbot et al, 2005) and as Chetley 2006 says, ICTs should be used as tools to advance equitable healthcare. Therefore, sound policies need to be in place to ensure that resources are provided even in the most remote areas so that young people in these locations are not left behind.

CONCLUSION

Overall, participants in this study indicated significant behaviour changes in regard to HIV/AIDS which were attributed to the use of the online forum. The interactions in the forum assisted to discourage behaviours that were detrimental to the fight against HIV/AIDS while promoting those behaviours that were regarded desirable. Singhal & Rogers (1999) say that information provided through entertainment format such as the discussion forum in this study, should not just be for information sake, but should be able to instigate observable behavioural changes. The findings of this study suggest that engaging social media in dealing with HIV/AIDS issues among young people is a positive step towards winning the fight against this disease. The entertainment nature of ICT tools is endearing to young people which stimulate them to participate more, therefore, utilizing these platforms to promote HIV/AIDS prevention behaviour can yield positive results.

REFERENCES

Abbot, J., Lenka, M., Lerotholi, P. J., Mahao, M., & Sechaba, M. (2005). Vulnerability, and HIV/AIDS mainstreaming in Lesotho: Livelihoods recovery through agriculture program and secure the child. South Africa-Lesotho, Cooperative for Assistance and Relief Everywhere, Inc. (CARE).

Adeyemi, A. A. (2004, March). *A Study on the use of Information Systems to Prevent HIV/AIDS in Lagos*. Paper presented at the Information and Communication Technologies in Healthcare Development 3rd Virtual Conference in Internet. New York, NY.

Affrinovator. (2011). *Upsurge in facebook and social media activity from African youth*. Retrieved January 5, 2013, from http://www.movements.org/blog/entry/upsurge-in-facebook-and-social-media-activityfrom-african-youth/

Altamirano, A. (2011). *Why is real-time so appealing?* Retrieved August 21, 2012, from http://www.altamirano.org/socialmedia/why-is-real-time-so-appealing/

Bandura, A. (1973). *Aggression: A social learning analysis*. Englewood Cliffs, NJ: Prentice Hall.

Bandura, A. (1977). *Social learning theory*. Englewood Cliffs, NJ: Prentice Hall.

Bouman, M. P. (1998). *The turtle and the peacock: Collaboration for social change*. Wageningen Agricultural University.

Chetley, A. (2006). *Improving health, connecting people: The role of ICTs in the health sector of developing countries*. InfoDev.

Christoper, A. (2004). *Tracing the evolution of social software*. Retrieved August 21, 2012, from http://www.lifewithalacrity.com/2004/10/tracing_the_evo.html

Coleman, P., & Meyer, R. C. (1990). *Entertainment for social change*. Baltimore, MD: John Hopkins University Center for Communication Programs.

Corlazzoli, V. (2013). *Assessing impact with media content analysis*. Retrieved September 6, 2013 from http://dmeforpeace.org/discuss/assessing-impact-media-content-analysis

Drimie, S. (2002). *The Impact of HIV/AIDS on Rural Households and Land Issues in Southern and Eastern Africa*. Retrieved February 2, 2013, from http://ftp.fao.org/docrep/nonfao/ad696e/ad696e00.pdf

Edwards, A. (2009). *Engestrom's Developmental Work Research: Research as provoking change*. Retrieved August 21, 2011, from http://education.monash.edu.au/research/seminars/show.php?id=443&archive=tue

Gerster Consulting. (2008). *ICT in Africa: Boosting Economic Growth and Poverty Reduction*. Paper presented at the 10th meeting of the Africa partnership forum. Tokyo, Japan.

Global HIV Prevention Working Group. (2008). *Behavior Change and HIV Prevention: Reconsiderations for the 21st Century*. Retrieved August 23, 2011, from http://www.globalhivprevention.org/pdfs/PWG_behavior%20report_FINAL.pdf

Kwankam, Y. S., & Ntomambang, N. N. (n.d.). *Information Technology in Africa: A proactive approach and the prospects of leapfrogging decades in the development process*. Retrieved August 21, 2011, from http://www.isoc.org/inet97/proceedings/B7/B7_1.HTM

National AIDS Coordinating Agency (NACA). (2005). *Botswana AIDS impact survey II*. Retrieved August 10, 2011, from http://unbotswana.org.bw/undp/documents/final_popular_report_feb06.pdf

Nations, D. (2011). *What is social networking? Social networking explained*. Academic Press.

Ogungbure, A. A. (2011). The possibilities of technological development in Africa: An evaluation of the role of culture. *The Journal of Pan African Studies, 14*(3).

Samie, N. (2011, October 19). *Social media popular with South African youth*. Voice of America.

Spiegel, P. B. (2004). HIV/AIDS among conflict-affected and displaced populations: Dispelling myths and taking action. *Disasters, 28*(3), 322–339. doi:10.1111/j.0361-3666.2004.00261.x PMID:15344944

United Nations Fund for Population Activities (UNFPA). (n.d.). *Young people: The greatest hope for turning the tide*. Retrieved July 22, 2012, from http://www.unfpa.org/hiv/people.htm

Wavecrest Computing. (2009). *Social networking or social not-working?* Retrieved August 3, 2011, from http://www.wavecrest.net/editorial/include/SocialNetworking_SocialNotworking.pdf

ADDITIONAL READING

ACHAP. (2004). *National review on AIDS/HIV education*. Botswana: Ministry of Health.

Adebohun, D., & Klindera, K. (2004, July). *Assessment of the effects of youth participation in HIV/AIDS and sexual health programming on the youth themselves: Results from qualitative study of youth leaders in Botswana and South Africa*. Paper presented at the International Conference on AIDS, Gaborone, Botswana.

Adigun, M. O. Ojo, S.O., Emuoyibofarhe, O.J., & Dehinbo, J. (2006, June). eHealthcare management: A partnership and collaboration model in developing countries. *Proceedings of the 1ˢᵗ all African Science and Technology Diffusion Conference (p*p68-77).

Anderson, G. F., Frogner, B. K., Johns, R. A., & Reinhardt, U. E. (2006). Health care spending and use of information technology in OECD countries. *Health Affairs, 25*(3), 819–831. doi:10.1377/hlthaff.25.3.819 PMID:16684749

Barnet, T., & Whiteside, A. (2002). *AIDS in the twenty-first century: Disease and globalization*. New York: Palgrave MacMillian. doi:10.1057/9780230599208

Bates, D. W., & Gawande, A. A. (2003). Improving safety with information technology. *The New England Journal of Medicine, 348*(25), 2526–2534. doi:10.1056/NEJMsa020847 PMID:12815139

Cutler, D. M., Rosen, A. B., & Vijan, S. (2006). The value of medical spending in the United States, 1960-2000. *The New England Journal of Medicine, 355*(9), 920–927. doi:10.1056/NEJMsa054744 PMID:16943404

Daniels, N., Bryant, J., Castano, R. A., Dantes, O. G., Khan, K. S., & Pannarunotha, S. (2000). Benchmarks of fairness for health care reform: A policy tool for developing countries. *Bulletin of the World Health Organization, 78*(6). PMID:10916911

Geers, B., & Page, S. (2007). *ICT for mitigating HIV/AIDS in Southern Africa. Swedish Program for ICT in Developing Regions*. SPIDER.

Jablonski, C. (2011, May 26). Five hot trends in healthcare technologies. *Emerging Tech*.

Jimenez, J. (2013, June 21). *Health Care's New Frontier*. Retrieved, June 30, from http://www.project-syndicate.org/commentary/improving-access-to-health-care-in-developing-countries-by-joseph-jimenez

Kizito, B. J., & Suhonen, J. (2011). Survey on ICT for HIV/AIDS preventive education: Are the teenagers forgotten in developing countries? *Journal of Emerging Trends in Computing and Information Science, 2*(6), 263–275.

Klapper, T. (1960). *The effects of mass communication.* New York: Free press.

Kotenko, J. (2013). The doctor will see you now: How the internet and social media are changing healthcare. Digital Trends. Retrieved May 13, 2013, from http://www.digitaltrends.com/social-media/the-internet-and-healthcare/

Lloyd, C. (2013). The stigmatization of problem drug users: A narrative literature review. *Drugs Education Prevention & Policy, 20*(2), 85–95. doi:10.3109/09687637.2012.743506

Mobile technologies, social media ignite HIV prevention revolution in Africa. Infectious Disease News, June 2011. Retrieved March 7, 2013, from http://www.healio.com/infectious-disease/hiv-aids/news/print/infectious-disease-news/%7B2b6d4ea7-1be2-43cb-8738-143fb2eccc9d%7D/mobile-technologies-social-media-ignite-hiv-prevention-revolution-in-africa

Nordqvist, J. (2013, May 21). Greatest Global Health Challenge Providing Healthcare in Developing Countries. *Medical News Today.*

Peters, D. H., Garg, A., Bloom, G., Walker, D. G., Brieger, W. R., & Rahman, M. H. (2008). Poverty and access to health care in developing countries. *Annals of the New York Academy of Sciences, 1136*(1), 161–171. doi:10.1196/annals.1425.011 PMID:17954679

Richard, F. (1999). *The politics of health in Europe.* Manchester: Manchester University Press.

Rosenfeld, S., & Mendelson, D. (2004). *Health information technology policy: Legislative and regulatory progress in 2003 and prospects for the future.* Washington, DC: Health Strategies Consultancy.

Russell, A. (2013). *7-Step Guide to Social Media Success in Healthcare ~ HootSuite University Lecture Series. Media.* Retrieved March 10, 2013 from http://blog.hootsuite.com/smc-7-steps-social-media-success-healthcare/

Shah, M., & Ambalam, S. (2004, July). *Knowledge of HIV/AIDS prevention and transmission among tenth and twelfth grade students in Delhi, India.* International Conference on AIDS. Evanston, United States.

Sorensen, T., Rivett, U., & Fortuin, J. (2008). A review of ICT systems for HIV/AIDS and anti-retroviral treatment management in South Africa. *Telecare., 14*(1), 37–41. doi:10.1258/jtt.2007.070502 PMID:18318928

Tan, J. (2011). Developments in healthcare information systems and technologies: Models and methods. Canada

Texts aim to fight AIDS in Kenya: A new mobile phone text message service. (2007). Retrieved May 12, from http://news.bbc.co.uk/1/hi/technology/4054475.stm

Thielst, C. B. (2010). *Social media in healthcare: Connect, communicate and collaborate.* College of Healthcare Executives.

Thomas, V. (2009). Health care in developing countries- Need for finance, education or both? *Calcutta Medical Journal, 7*(1), e1.

Tolly, K., & Cell, H.A. (2009). Innovative use of cell phone technology for HIV/AIDS behaviour change communications: 3 pilot projects. *Cellphones4HIV.*

Young, D.A. (2000, April). *Medical research, technology and improved healthcare.* Paper presented at the 25th Anniversary AAAS Colloquium on Science and Technology Policy, Washington, DC.

KEY TERMS AND DEFINITIONS

Discussion Forum: Online platform used to communicate and share information.

Formative Evaluation: Assessment of a situation before introducing an intervention.

HIV Testing: Finding out whether one has HIV or not.

HIV/AIDS Prevention Behavior: Practices that ensure safety against contacting HIV.

Intervention: Strategy used to cause change in an existing situation.

Mass Media: Media reaching many people at a time, specifically radio and television.

Social Learning Theory: A theory that holds that people learn by imitating behavior of others especially if the behavior is believed to be exemplary.

Social Media: Interactive communication through online technologies.

Summative Evaluation: Assessment of a situation after introducing an intervention.

Section 4
Challenges and Issues

This section focuses on the various challenges and issues facing the use of social media and mobile technologies in healthcare.

Chapter 16
Personal Health in My Pocket:
Challenges, Opportunities, and Future Research Directions in Mobile Personal Health Records

Helen Monkman
University of Victoria, Canada

Andre Kushniruk
University of Victoria, Canada

Elizabeth Borycki
University of Victoria, Canada

ABSTRACT

Consumers' access to their health records is increasing, and one of the ways they can gain access and potentially contribute to their records is by using a mobile Personal Health Record (mPHR). mPHRs emerged as a combination of mHealth and Personal Health Records (PHRs). Despite the current shortage of evidence supporting mPHR use, these systems are already being deployed, and examples of currently available mPHRs are provided. mPHRs have an array of potential uses and different target user groups, but there are also several challenges impeding their success. The physical constraints of mobile devices, health literacy, and usability all create obstacles for mPHRs. However, mPHRs create opportunities due to the affordances of mobile devices and the potential to integrate consumer mHealth applications. The challenges and opportunities of these nascent systems are outlined in this chapter, as they inform research topics with respect to mPHRs.

INTRODUCTION

There are a number of important changes occurring in healthcare today. Perhaps foremost among these is a greater move towards involvement and empowerment of consumers (i.e., citizens

and patients) in the self-management of their health. Indeed, over the past decade the concept of consumer access to their records has moved from a pilot in the late 1990's (Cimino, Patel, & Kushniruk, 2002), when electronic access by consumers to their health data via the worldwide

DOI: 10.4018/978-1-4666-6150-9.ch016

web (WWW) was being explored, to the current access by millions of patients and citizens to their own institutional health data today over the Internet (Halamka, Mandl & Tang, 2007; Protti, 2008). This movement has stemmed from a desire of consumers to have access to their own data, with the first manifestation of this appearing as the "stand-alone Personal Health Record (PHR)" (Tang, Ash, Bates, Overhage & Sage, 2006). This movement has included access by patients to health data contained in their own PHRs and it has also included a move towards increased access to their own data stored in hospital and even national databases. The objective of this chapter is to introduce the reader to the concept of mPHRs, provide examples of these systems, outline potential users and use environments, and discuss the challenges, opportunities and directions for future research.

What is a PHR?

According to the Medical Library Association (MLA) / National Library of Medicine (NLM) Joint Electronic Personal Health Record Task Force, a PHR is

a private, secure application through which an individual may access, manage, and share his or her health information. The PHR can include information that is entered by the consumer and/ or data from other sources such as pharmacies, labs, and health care providers. The PHR may or may not include information from the electronic health record (EHR) that is maintained by the health care provider and is not synonymous with the EHR (Jones, Shipman, Plaut & Selden, 2010, p. 244).

In the past decade, several models for providing consumers with personal health have emerged. PHRs are available in three basic types based on their connectivity or integration with other health information systems. PHRs under the sole control

of the consumer and which do not connect with any other health information systems are called stand-alone PHRs (Tang et al., 2006). In contrast, tethered PHRs allow patients to access their own personal information contained in their health provider's health information system (Tang et al., 2006). For example, the Epic health information system (used by many hospitals in the United States) has included in many implementations a component called MyChart that allows patients to access parts of their electronic record remotely. Interoperable PHRs are ideal, because they allow a variety of different health information systems to exchange data and thus, offer the most financial benefits (Kaelber & Pan, 2008) and utility (Tang et al., 2006). Yet another model for consideration are national portals, which allow citizens read-only access to their health data that is interconnected across regions and even nationally. This approach has emerged over the past ten years and examples include the Sundhed.dk patient portal in Denmark, which allows all Danish citizens to access their own health data over the Internet (Protti, 2008).

What is mHealth?

Concurrent with the trend towards PHRs has been a staggering increase in the use of mHealth applications (i.e., health applications running on mobile devices). mHealth is the use of mobile devices for healthcare, or "mobile computing, medical sensor, and communications technologies for health care" (Istepanian, Jovanov, & Zhang, 2004, p. 405). mHealth is revolutionizing the way health data is collected and how healthcare is delivered. A multitude of mHealth applications are available to clinicians and consumers. Consumer mHealth applications are a distinct subset of mHealth applications designed for use by health consumers, or laypeople, rather than healthcare professionals. Consumer mHealth applications have been developed for health promotion (e.g., exercise applications) and monitoring physical activities (e.g., pedometers), as well as more advanced applications used in conjunction with healthcare providers to monitor vital signs, such as heart rate and sleeping patterns (Househ, Borycki, Kushniruk, & Alofaysan, 2012). The devices used for such applications have varied, but cell phones, smartphones, and tablets are currently the most prevalent. Moreover, because mobile devices are becoming increasingly affordable, consumer mHealth applications are becoming viable options for facilitating healthcare in traditionally underserved populations.

What is an mPHR?

A mobile Personal Health Record (mPHR) is a Personal Health Record (PHR) integrated with a consumer mHealth application or mobile platform (See Figure 1). An mPHR is distinct from other consumer mHealth applications because it is in-

tegrated with the user's health records. Further, an mPHR can serve multiple purposes whereas a consumer mHealth application typically only serves a single purpose. Thus, an mPHR can be considered to be multiple integrated consumer mHealth applications, as well as a consumer mHealth application in and of itself. mPHRs are a potential forum for amalgamating various types of health information (e.g., allergies, family history, advanced directives, laboratory reports). The information in an mPHR therefore can be generated both by healthcare providers and consumers, within healthcare settings (e.g., hospital, clinic, laboratory) and also in naturalistic environments (e.g., consumer's home, workplace). Ideally, mPHRs are gateways to health information entered by healthcare providers, as well as repositories of complementary health information added by consumers. As is true for PHRs,

Figure 1. The mPHR

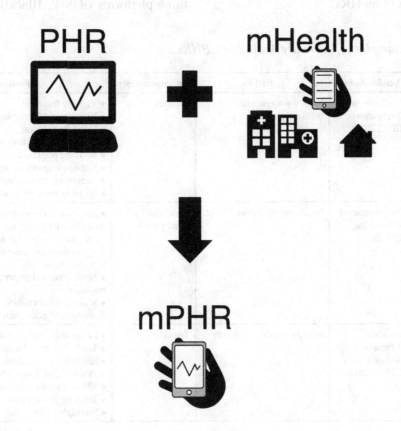

283

mPHRs are often comprised of tools to facilitate self-management by helping consumers adhere to individualized care plans, graph their symptoms, collect physiological data, receive tailored instructions or motivational feedback, use decision aids, and receive reminders (Pagliari, Detmer & Singleton, 2007). Ideally, every mPHR should be customized to the user's specific needs, in order to streamline the user's experience and increase efficiency. Thus, an mPHR can be envisioned as a collection of independent consumer mHealth applications as component modules, or as a single application that amalgamates disparate applications with health information. Given that they have only been deployed recently, there is a dearth of research on mPHRs. However, consumer mHealth applications have been more extensively studied. If mPHRs are viewed as compositions of consumer mHealth applications integrated with electronic patient record information, evidence from these domains can be leveraged to inform the design and development of mPHRs.

Examples of mPHRs

A number of experiments have allowed healthcare providers to access to health data using mobile devices since 2000. For example at Columbia University the PalmCIS application was created that allowed healthcare providers to access patient records using smartphones (Chen, Medonca, McKnight, Stetson, Lei, & Cimino, 2003). Since then, this approach has taken off and mobile interfaces have been developed not only for healthcare providers, but also for consumers to access their health records (i.e., mPHRs) (see Table 1 for examples).

To date, the primary functions of mPHRs are oriented around accessing ones personal health information. In a comparison of 19 stand-alone mPHR applications, Kharrazi, Chisholm, Van-Nasdale, and Thompson (2012) found that the functionality available in mPHRs was highly variable. These authors evaluated mPHRs from three platforms (iOS™, BlackBerry®, and An-

Table 1. Three Examples of Currently Available mPHRs

mPHR Name	Vendor Name	URL	Interoperability	Features
MyChart	Epic Systems Corporation (EPIC, 2013)	http://www.epic.com/software-phr.php	Tethered	• Viewing test results. • Viewing and scheduling appointments. • Uploading photos. • Updating medications and allergies. • Refilling prescriptions. • Filling out questionnaires. • Accessing chronic disease summaries. • Securely messaging providers.
motionPHR	Communication Software Inc. (CSI, 2013)	http://motionphr.com	Stand-alone or Interoperable	• Entering and storing information on medications, allergies, conditions, procedures, test results, advance directives & organ donation, emergency contact, and immunizations. • Medication and prescription refill reminders. • Managing information for multiple consumers (e.g., a family).
HealthTrak	University of Pittsburgh Medical Center (UPMC, 2013)	https://myupmc.upmc.com	Tethered	• Requesting appointments. • Tracking current health issues. • Renewing prescriptions. • eVisit digital house calls. • Viewing medical records. • Tracking medications. • Messaging providers.

droid™) and they ranged in price from no cost to $9.99. Kharrazi and colleagues evaluated PHRs' functionality by using 10 data elements (problems/conditions, procedures, medications, providers, allergies, labs, immunizations, family history, emergency contact, and insurance) and four features (import/export, images, in case of emergency feature, and password) as indices.

Kharrazi and colleagues' comparison may be valid for the current landscape of mPHRs, which are in their infancy and primarily stand-alone systems; however, as with PHRs, the value of mPHRs is affected by the extent of their integration with other health information systems, or mPHR interoperability. That is, the usefulness of mPHRs increases with the number of health information systems it can exchange information with, from stand-alone, to tethered, and finally to interoperable. As described, mPHRs may be used to store, maintain and manage a variety of different personal health information as well as

offer other features (see Figure 2a). In addition to containing information entered by healthcare professionals, in many circumstances it may be valuable to have consumers enter monitoring data into their mPHRs (see Figure 2b and c).

Depiction of possible mPHR information and features (a), potential mPHR data collected by consumers (b), mPHR blood pressure graph example (c).

WHO ARE mPHR USERS?

Identifying the needs and preferences of the users is an imperative process for any system that is designed, developed and deployed and mPHRs are no exception. It is estimated that approximately one in every seven people are currently using smartphones (Nmawston, 2012) and users may want to have access to their records via their smartphones. Although consumers are the primary

Figure 2. Example of an mPHR

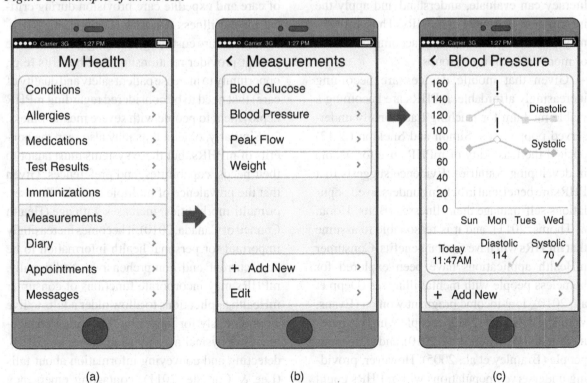

(a)   (b)   (c)

users of mPHRs healthcare providers and caregivers may also access consumers' mPHRs. Providers have a distinct set of user and information needs with respect to mPHRs. Thus, the provider-facing component of mobile personal health applications should be designed differently to accommodate these users. For example, providers may need automatic notifications when consumers have hit critical thresholds of specific values consumers are monitoring. These notifications will help providers gauge whether consumers need more support or changes to their medication and management plans. However, it is important that mPHRs avoid inundating providers with daily information that is not indicative of a problem; providers will likely find more value in reviewing the general trends and being notified of episodes that require their attention. Alternatively, caregivers may only need access to certain types of information (e.g., appointments, medication allergies). Health consumers and caregivers often have limited, or no, clinical understanding, it is imperative that mPHRs are designed such that users with limited health literacy can evaluate, understand and apply the information contained in mPHRs. Thus, mPHRs may need changes in design to accommodate two or more different user groups.

Given that mobile devices are becoming increasingly affordable, mPHRs are becoming a viable medium for reaching traditionally underserved populations. Simon and Sneldon (2012) posited the feasibility of mPHRs use for people in developing countries. Evidence suggests that PHRs are beneficial in helping underserved populations self-manage their illnesses (Botts, Horan & Thoms, 2011), and it is reasonable to assume that mPHRs will have similar benefits. Consumer mHealth applications have been explored for homeless people with mental illnesses (Depp et al., 2010), low-income pregnant women (Evans, Wallace, & Snider, 2012), people who live in remote areas (Proudfoot et al., 2010), and indigenous people (Bramley et al., 2005). However, providing underserved populations with mPHRs could

introduce the risk of theft of the mobile device, especially for consumers living in shelters (Depp et al., 2010). Mobile devices are gradually becoming less alluring to thieves, as they become more common and stolen devices can be deactivated and rendered unusable by anyone other than the owner. However, users might sell their devices, if they are in stressful financial situations. As mobile devices continue to become pervasive and affordable, loss of devices due to theft or sale will likely diminish. Thus, it is plausible that mPHRs will enable a broad range of previously underserved health consumers to access and share their health records.

Although there is vast potential reach for mPHRs, the unique needs of the different users groups must also be considered. For example, users with severe mental illness may feel that mPHRs with the capability of delivering interventions increase the physical and emotional distance between them and their providers (Depp et al., 2010). However, mPHRs designed for users with severe mental illness could also increase the continuity of care and expedite care provision during critical mental illness episodes (Depp et al., 2010). Thus, there are costs (e.g., creating distance in the patient-provider relationship) and benefits (e.g., opportunity to increase patient safety and quality of care) that need to be considered regarding mPHR deployment to people with severe mental illness.

Similarly, older adults may also reap the benefits of mPHRs, but these systems must adapt to their needs, capabilities, and preferences. Given that the prevalence of multiple chronic illnesses, or multi-morbidities, increases with age (Health Council of Canada, 2010), it becomes increasingly important for personal health information to be kept current and comprehensive. Additionally, mPHRs may incorporate functions of consumer mHealth applications to allow older adults to live autonomously for longer by facilitating engagement in physical activity (Sunwoo et al., 2010), detecting and conveying information about falls (Lee & Carlisle, 2011), contacting emergency assistance, as well as tracking dementia patients when they wander (e.g., Miskelly, 2005). However, older adults appear to have more challenges learning how to successfully use mobile devices (Kurniawan, Mahmud, & Nugroho, 2006). Further, given generational differences (Leung, McGrenere, & Graf, 2011) as well as perceptual, cognitive and motor changes associated with aging, special design considerations (e.g., Leung et al., 2012) are imperative for mPHRs to accommodate elderly peoples' needs and capabilities.

In addition to the aforementioned groups of users, consumers may have specific reasons for needing mPHRs. For example, people who travel often may benefit from having mPHRs. Also, consumers with specific illnesses or conditions may also find having mPHRs worthwhile. Studies have found that consumers are receptive to using consumer mHealth applications for mental health (Depp et al., 2010; Proudfoot et al., 2010), recovery after kidney transplantation (McGillicuddy et al., 2013), and managing asthma (Cleland, Caldow, & Ryan, 2007). Further, mPHRs with these functions could facilitate early identification of problems and improve continuity of care (e.g., Cleland et al., 2007). As mPHRs integrate functions such as those previously mentioned, it is reasonable to assume there will be a demand for mPHRs from frequent travellers and users with specific health conditions.

Although mPHRs may be valuable for a variety of different user groups, each of these groups has unique needs that need to be identified and addressed in the respective mPHR designs. It is not prudent to assume that a single mPHR solution will be suitable for all different types of users. To identify their specific needs, preferences and usability challenges, target consumers should be included in the design process. Further, these investigations can also be used to reveal what functionality is most important to specific types of users and what contexts they are likely to use mPHRs in.

WHERE AND WHERE ARE mPHRs USED?

One of the main advantages of mPHRs is that they can be used almost anytime, anywhere. For example, users who travel or move frequently may find mPHRs particularly valuable. However, this ubiquity also presents novel design challenges. For example, privacy may present as an issue in certain circumstances. Historically, to enter personal health information, users logged-in from the privacy of their own homes, but mPHRs may send messages and reminders to users without any sensitivity or regard to the particular context the user is in. As such, if messages were sent to the consumer at an inopportune time (e.g., in a meeting, on a busy commuter bus) bystanders could potentially read sensitive information.

Although their constant availability is appealing, there will inevitably be fluctuations in mPHR use, as a reflection of a user's health status at a given time. Depp and colleagues (2010) argued that is unreasonable to expect participants to partake in mobile interventions for an infinite duration. Users' participation may decrease over time and/ or become more sporadic, which is referred to as "fatigue effects" (Shiffman, Stone, & Hufford, 2008). Thus, instead of continuous intervention delivery, a more flexible approach that identifies critical periods and increases the frequency of intervention events during windows of opportunity should be developed (Depp et al., 2010). Similarly, mPHRs should identify critical time points for intervention delivery. For example, if a user is not ready to quit smoking currently, but indicates that she might be ready to consider it in a few months, the mPHR could store this response and query the consumer again after the indicated time has elapsed. Further, mPHRs should also give users the opportunity to participate in or withdraw from interventions as they see fit.

mPHRs have inherent possibilities for delivering tailored health information when users and providers need it most. That is, the delivery of information that is suited to the users' levels of health literacy can be triggered by specific events (e.g., disease diagnosis, pregnancy) to educate consumers when they are facing new health challenges or experiences and perhaps when they are most in need of credible, personalized, health information. For example, if an mPHR is populated with a positive pregnancy test, it could prompt the user to ask if she would like to receive information related to prenatal care and could activate a pregnancy module. Furthermore, in emergency situations, context-aware mPHRs could also make important health information (e.g., allergies, medications, pre-existing conditions) available to providers upon user arrival at the hospital and automatically notify to the user's emergency contact or caregiver. Thus, mPHRs have the potential to effectively deliver information to consumers and providers in such a way that will foster patient safety.

CHALLENGES FOR mPHRs

In addition to some of the advantages and disadvantages of mPHRs due to their nearly limitless use cases, there are a variety of other challenges that deploying these new systems to consumers present.

Constraints of Mobile Devices

Mobile devices have unique affordances and constraints that differ from computers. In order to optimize the human-mobile device system, designers must capitalize on the affordances and minimize the limitations by using human factors methods to evaluate design solutions. Understandably, the screen size of mobile devices plays a critical factor in mPHR design whereby the conciseness of content on smaller screens is imperative. Given that users understood significantly less content read on a phone-sized screen than on a desktop computer

(Singh, Sumeeth, & Miller, 2011), limited display size increases the demand for succinct, actionable information in mPHRs. Additionally, text data may be more difficult to input due smaller keyboards and interacting with graphic user interface elements (e.g., menus, buttons) may be more challenging and error prone as a result of the limited screen size of mobile devices. Thus, the physical constraints of mobile devices generate a unique set of problems for mPHRs.

Health Literacy

Another challenge relevant to all consumer health information systems is making information appropriate for people with limited health literacy. The World Health Organization (WHO) endorses Nutbeam's (1998) definition of health literacy, which states that health literacy "represents the cognitive and social skills which determine the motivation and ability of individuals to gain access to, understand and use information in ways which promote and maintain good health" (p. 357). Consumers with limited health literacy present a challenge for healthcare. The Canadian Council on Learning (2008) argued that "without adequate health-literacy skills, ill-informed decisions may be taken, health conditions may go unchecked or worsen, questions may go unasked or remain unanswered, accidents may happen and people may get lost in the health-care system" (p. 5). Thus, it is not surprising that people with limited health literacy are more likely to report low health statuses (Canadian Council on Learning, 2008) and are prone to worse health outcomes (DeWalt, Berkman, Sheridan, Lohr, & Pignone, 2004).

The health literacy challenge cannot merely be reduced into increasing consumers' health literacy levels, as lowering the demands on health literacy is an equally important goal. Baker (2006) argued that health literacy is a combination of both the consumers' capabilities and the health literacy related demands of the healthcare system. Unlike the majority of health information systems, those designed for consumers are unusual because consumers often have limited or no health care experience (Segall et al., 2011). Thus, to optimize the value mPHRs, it is imperative that the demands mPHRs impose on consumers are aligned with the users' levels of health literacy.

Usability

Although mPHRs are being deployed rapidly and they have the potential to exceed the value of PHRs, mPHRs are inherently unique from their PHR counterparts due the medium they are delivered on (i.e., mobile devices). However, all of the possible opportunities associated with mPHRs, require research from a human factors perspective to confirm that consumers consider them useful and usable.

One of the most difficult problems facing mPHRs designers is creating an efficient user experience. First, the more seamlessly added functionality can be built directly into mobile devices and alleviate the need for additional external medical devices, the more likely these devices will be available (not forgotten or misplaced) when users need them. Second, as mPHRs develop and provide more diverse functions and inevitably become more complex, a simple, efficient means of using these systems must be preserved. Thus, a balance between complexity and ease of use must be achieved. Although mPHRs have considerable potential, consumers' adoption of mPHRs relies on their usability.

Several evaluation methods are available to identify usability issues and thus generate design solutions to make systems easier to use (Jaspers, 2009). Many of these methods are relevant for evaluating mPHRs, yet they remain to be applied. Resources that could inform usability focused user-centred design include Kushniruk (2002) and Årsand and Demiris (2008). Årsand and Demiris' (2008) provided advice for using these methods and when specific methods are most useful. Further, a resource focused on designing

for users with limited health literacy is *Health Literacy Online* (U.S. Department of Health and Human Services, 2010). Årsand and colleagues' (2012) provided the following suggestions based on their research of consumer mHealth applications that could inform the design of mPHRs: whenever possible, data should be transferred automatically; user interfaces should be visual and motivational; effort exerted to use the system should be minimized and benefits from use should be maximized; and systems should be dynamic and adaptable.

Usability testing is considered the gold standard of usability evaluation methods because it identifies problems that typical users encounter and it is a promising method for evaluating mPHRs. Usability testing has been recognized as a valuable method for investigating usability problems in health information systems for well over a decade (Kushniruk, Patel, & Cimino, 1997). Despite that these methods have been used to investigate PHRs (e.g., Haggstrom et al., 2011; Segall et al., 2011) and mobile Web sites and applications (e.g., Nielsen & Budiu, 2013), to date, no usability testing of mPHRs was found.

An important research consideration for mPHRs are the physical settings for usability testing. mPHRs should be subjected to usability testing with different levels of naturalism, in order to reveal all of the potential usability problems. That is, mPHR usability testing may begin in a laboratory setting to identify obvious problems with the system, but additional testing should be conducted with mPHRs "in-situ" or in naturalistic environments. Due to the complexity of healthcare environments, this "in-situ" evaluation approach for health information systems is being promoted for identifying problems that may not be revealed due to the over simplified context of laboratory settings (Kushniruk, Borycki, Kuwata, & Kannry, 2011). Similarly, many issues that users encounter in specific contexts may go undetected if mPHR evaluation is limited to the confines of the laboratory. Thus, mPHRs could benefit from "in-situ" usability testing to identify problems that only occur in particular contexts, in users' day-to-day lives and activities; however, given the nearly limitless contexts in which mPHRs could be used, new data collection methods (e.g., the snippit technique developed by Brandt, Weiss, and Klemmer, 2007) may warrant exploration.

Challenges associated with usability testing of mPHRs also include mobile screen recording and inferring users' attention. Currently, mobile screen recording is less than robust, but the software is continuously improving. Inexpensive mobile screen recording applications exist, but they have limitations (e.g., brief maximum recording length, beta versions). Fortunately, there are alternative methods to collect data of users interacting with mobile devices. Presently, the most vigorous and reliable methods available for mobile screen recording are tethering or mirroring the mobile device under investigation to a computer and recording the computer screen. This can be accomplished with software such as Ashot (Sourceforge, 2013) for Android™, and Reflector (Squirrels, 2013) for iOS™ devices. Unlike screen recordings of computers, where users' attention may be inferred from the location of the cursor, there is no cursor on mobile devices so it is more important to have both screen recordings and scene camera recordings for mobile usability testing. One potential method for supplementing traditional usability test data for mPHR evaluations is collecting eye-tracking data. This technique has demonstrated utility in detecting usability problems in eBook readers (Siegenthaler, Wurtz, & Groner, 2010). Cheng (2011) argued for using both head-mounted (i.e., portable) and stationary (i.e., remote) eye-trackers to collect data for mobile device usability evaluations. It is expected that screen recording will become increasingly reliable and eye-tracking data may become increasingly viable for mobile usability tests such as those conducted on mPHRs.

In addition to usability testing, usability inspection methods (e.g., heuristic evaluation, cognitive walkthrough) may improve mPHR design through usability expert analyses. Heuristic evaluation is a popular usability inspection method because it is informal, rapid, inexpensive, and relatively easy to perform and it may be useful for investigating mPHRs. Given its advantages, it is not surprising that heuristic evaluation has been used to investigate PHRs (e.g., Monkman & Kushniruk, 2013b) and consumer mHealth applications (Monkman & Kushniruk, 2013a). Further, Monkman and Kushniruk's (2013a) method may be a viable option for identifying both usability and health literacy issues in mPHRs, given that their heuristics originate from evidence synthesized by the U.S. Department of Health and Human Services (2010).

There are undoubtedly challenges associated with mPHRs and usability evaluation of mPHRs; however, there are a variety of potential benefits to mPHRs over PHRs accessed traditionally on full sized computers. Some of the opportunities that mPHRs have yet to capitalize on will be outlined.

OPPORTUNITIES OF mPHRs

Despite the challenges associated with mPHRs, these systems introduce a wide range of new opportunities. Combining the advantages of PHR technology with mobile devices is beginning to be explored and promises even greater patient and citizen (i.e., consumer) access to their health data than was previously possible, through access to PHRs via smartphones, tablets, cell phones and other emerging pervasive computing devices that are wearable and portable (Bardram, Mihailidis, & Wan, 2007). Further, mobile device users, especially generations X and Y (i.e., born after 1965), are very receptive to the idea of accessing their health information using their mobile devices (Keckley, & Hoffman, 2010). Thus, the move towards mPHRs is an exciting trend that is likely to help promote health and ultimately empower healthcare consumers.

Leveraging the Affordances of Mobile Devices

mPHRs create unique opportunities for information to be delivered to consumers, as well as for consumers to enter data into their records. People have changed the method and frequency of their communication and information sharing as a result of the advent and proliferation of mobile devices. Short message service (SMS or text messages) for synchronous or asynchronous communication between individuals has rapidly increased in use, and many people prefer receiving text messages to phone calls (Smith, 2011). In addition to the propensity of users to text, text messaging is an appealing form of health communication for several other reasons. First, text messages can be asynchronous, the user decides whether or not, and when she will respond to a text message. Second, health topics are often sensitive in nature and texting provides a discreet way of health information exchange. Third, texting is often a relatively inexpensive way of communicating and likely entails minimal adaptation from existing paper-based materials. Given these potential advantages, it may be useful to explore text messaging as a method of information delivery and data entry into mPHRs.

With respect to information delivery, many mobile devices have Text-To-Speech (TTS), a development that could enhance the output of mPHRs. TTS generators convert written text into spoken language. Many mobile devices come equipped with TTS generators, which merely have to be activated. TTS generators have become increasingly more natural sounding and thus, are an appealing complementary method of delivering health information to people who may have challenges reading it (e.g., if the information is not in the user's native tongue, users with limited health literacy). Similarly, multimedia messaging system (MMS) (i.e., photograph and movie messages) and video clips also provide opportunities to increase understanding and enhance data entry accuracy. For example, Vargas, Robles, Harris and Radford (2010) found that reducing the amount of reading (i.e., by showing native language video clips) and writing (i.e., by providing questions with multiple choice answers) required by users with limited health literacy facilitated accurate reporting (Vargas et al., 2010). Thus, audio and audiovisual materials are viable complementary modes of delivering information through mPHRs to improve user comprehension and data entry accuracy.

Mobile devices are equipped with microphones, which create opportunities for both interacting and perhaps eventually entering data into mPHRs. Currently, touch (i.e., finger or stylus contact with the screen) is the predominant method for user interaction with smartphones and tablets. However, multi-touch gestures (e.g., pinch-to-zoom) broaden the number of commands available. Nielsen and Budiu (2012) provided an insightful comparison between mouse and fingers as inputs devices. Due to the limited size of keyboards on mobile devices, it important to limit the extent of typing required for all types of interaction (e.g., searching terms, booking appointments) with mPHRs. Typing can be reduced through strategies such as auto-complete, selection wheels, and more recently voice commands. Given the recent influx in the use of natural language user interaction (e.g., Siri for iOS™), and the increasing robustness of these systems, in the near future, users may simply speak into the microphone of their mobile devices perform mPHR tasks (e.g., find lab results, schedule appointments). Voice commands are a promising mode of interaction for users who can talk but have limited dexterity.

Thus, natural language interaction should be explored with respect to how it can benefit mPHRs (e.g., data entry) and mPHR users.

Other recent advances in mobile device interaction may also benefit mPHRs. Specifically, the use of front facing cameras which track the eyes allow users to interact with onscreen information using their focal attention. For example, the Samsung GALAXY S4® enables users to scroll up or down by focusing their gaze on upper or lower portions of the screen. Similar techniques are also in early development for iOS™ devices (Pino & Kavasidis, 2012). The feasibility of blinking gestures to serve as button-clicks has also been explored (Miluzzo, Wang, & Campbell, 2010). Additionally, simply by swiping a hand in the air above the sensor, the Samsung GALAXY S4® allows users to check the display status, scroll through pages, browse forward and backward, and answer calls (Samsung, 2013). Eye movements and hand gestures for interacting with mPHRs is promising for users who have physical impairments, or limited fine motor skills, but whose gross motor and/or eye control is preserved.

Mobile devices are typically equipped with accelerometers and gyroscopes, which users' physical movements of a device (e.g., tilt, twist, rotate) to be translated into inputs. Initial exploration of this method of interaction has yielded evidence that gesture based mobile games have potential for engaging older adults in range of motion exercises (Sunwoo et al., 2010). Thus, it is reasonable to assume that accelerometers and gyroscopes could be valuable for such purposes as they are relevant to mPHRs.

A variety of possibilities are created because mPHRs are accessed through mobile devices. Some of these opportunities include delivering information to consumers through SMS, MMS, and TTS, as well as allowing consumers to enter information and interact with mPHRs through voice commands, gestures, eye movements and physically manipulating the mobile device.

Integrating Functionality from Consumer mHealth Applications

There is currently sparse evidence linking mPHR use to improved patient outcomes; however, the evidence is mounting in support using consumer mHealth applications for an array of purposes. Multiple independent consumer mHealth applications could demonstrate value if effectively incorporated into mPHRs. Further, given the commonalities between consumer mHealth applications and mPHRs, insight from research in the previous domain can be used to inform the latter.

Perhaps one of the most promising purposes for PHRs and mPHRs alike, as well as one of the most popular research topics for consumer mHealth applications, is the potential utility of scaffolding self-management and monitoring in people with chronic illnesses. Chronic illnesses (e.g., arthritis, cancer, chronic obstructive pulmonary disease, diabetes, heart disease, high blood pressure) cannot be cured and often occur in conjunction with other chronic illnesses. Management of chronic illnesses may benefit from frequent (i.e., several times a day) consumer reports of health and wellbeing (e.g., peak flow measurements, sleep quality). As consumers who have mobile devices are rarely without them, they are ideal for the collection of real-time personal health data and the delivery of information to facilitate self-management. In a review by Holtz and Lauckner (2012), trends of improved self-efficacy, hemoglobin A1c, and self-management behaviors were found in the studies of consumer mHealth applications for supporting diabetics. Given their demonstrated effectiveness, it is likely that mPHRs will adopt functionality to facilitate self-management of diabetes and other chronic illnesses.

If incorporated into mPHRs, other potential functionality that may benefit users include offering preliminary screening tools, providing educational resources, and facilitating access to healthcare services. These features have been already developed as independent consumer mHealth applications. For example, preliminary screening tools for hearing, vision, and sleep apnea are available (see Pope, Silva, & Almeyda, 2010). Preliminary screenings may be a rapid, cost-effective way to determine whether more robust, traditional screening methods are necessary. Additionally, the Detroit Medical Center (DMC) currently offers two consumer mHealth application educational resources aimed to educate parents and pregnant women (DMC, 2013). Both the DMC ER Wait Times application (DMC, 2013) and the Alberta Health Services (AHS, 2013) smartphone applications were launched to expedite access to emergency services by providing users with local hospital wait times, phone numbers, and directions. The AHS application also offers information about other nearby healthcare facilities, programs, services, and immunization clinics. By offering consumers different types of consumer mHealth applications, the DMC and AHS seek to engage and educate consumers, as well as help their users make better use of emergency services in critical situations. iTriage is a consumer mHealth application that has recently been integrated with Microsoft's HealthVault PHR (Microsoft, 2013). Several million patients previously used iTriage to view information on symptoms, procedures, medications, diseases, facilities, and healthcare providers. By integrating this application with Microsoft HealthVault, users of iTriage can also now view their records (stored on HealthVault) when using the iPhone application (Microsoft, 2013). It is expected that this trend for integrating consumer health applications with PHRs will continue and lead to greater usage of mPHRs by the general population.

mPHRs may a help extend the length of time older adults can live independently, by increasing physical activity, and providing alerts and information in case of emergency. Consumer mHealth applications have shown limited success for tracking dementia patients (Miskelly, 2005).

However, using mobile devices to detect falls (e.g., Lee & Carlisle, 2011; Zhang, Wang, Liu, & Hou, 2006) and automatically contact emergency services (Sposaro, & Tyson, 2009) have shown promise and could be beneficial if incorporated into mPHRs. Consumer mHealth applications for fall detection and tracking are both ineffective, if the consumer is not wearing the mobile device at the time of the event (i.e., fall, or wandering). This may be exacerbated by some consumers' reluctance against carrying the mobile device continuously due to its size and weight (e.g., Miskelly, 2005) or simply forgetting to carry the device. Thus, it may be prudent to explore compact wearable devices that are more comfortable and less likely to be forgotten. Despite these potential limitations, developing mPHRs that can detect falls, contact the user's emergency contact and/ or emergency services, as well as provide crucial health information upon arrival at the hospital have potential value.

From a telehealth perspective, mPHRs are very encouraging (Simon & Seldon, 2012). Telehealth aims to "maintain or improve the health of people outside the normal healthcare infrastructure" (Simon & Sneldon, 2012, p. 125). The University of Pittsburgh Medical Center offers an eVisit service that enables consumers to interact with their healthcare providers remotely, in real-time, which may be very valuable for users who have difficulty commuting to healthcare facilities due to the distance or mobility challenges (UPMC, 2013). Additionally, mPHRs may overcome data collection limitations. Specifically, Simon and Sneldon (2012) identified three key limitations of collecting biosensor information restricted to traditional healthcare facilities (e.g., clinics, hospitals) that could be overcome by mPHR monitoring in naturalistic, daily environments. Specifically, the limitations to monitoring solely within healthcare facilities are:

1. Failure to sample rare events.

2. Failure to measure physiological responses during normal periods of activity, rest, and sleep.

3. Brief periods of monitoring cannot capture rhythmic variations in physiological signals (Simon & Sneldon, 2012, p. 126).

Home telemonitoring, or collecting a consumer's physiological and/or biological data while at home and transferring the data to remotely located providers, overcomes some of these limitations, but mobile monitoring offers consumers even more flexibility and freedom. Evidence has shown that home telemonitoring improved clinical outcomes for diabetes, asthma, and hypertension (Paré, Moqadem, Pineau, & St-Hilaire, 2010). As biosensors (i.e., devices that collect physiological and/or biological data) become increasingly compact and portable, it is increasingly possible to monitor consumers beyond the confines of the home, in any location through mPHRs. Although mPHRs exhibit potential for monitoring, few available mPHRs are currently equipped with monitoring capabilities, and furthermore, no research was found identifying the benefits and challenges of mPHR monitoring.

A variety of biosensors are available that work in conjunction with mobile devices and the data they collect include: heart rate, pulse, blood oxygen saturation, blood glucose, temperature, and weight. Another recently developed biosensor is a phone case embedded with electrodes that works as a single lead electrocardiogram (ECG) (Lau et al., 2013). The developers of this mobile ECG suggest that it will facilitate large-scale community screenings to detect atrial fibrillation (Lau et al., 2013). Using mobile devices to collect continuous physiological information, which can be stored in an mPHR, is a valuable approach to providing baseline or prototypical consumer data that can used for comparison during healthcare events (e.g., diagnosis of chronic illness, acute injury). In addition to monitoring physiological data, it may be beneficial to use mPHRs to deliver questionnaires and monitor consumers' self-reported health status. Bielle and colleagues (2004) found some success administering quality-of-life questionnaires remotely to cancer inpatients, which led them to posit that this method could result in earlier detection of suffering and improved intervention timing. Thus, mPHRs may soon enable the collection and storage of physiological, biological, and self-reported health statuses, to facilitate care provision.

mPHRs may soon follow the lead of consumer mHealth applications as meands of delivering interventions. Mobile interventions have the potential to mitigate obstacles associated with "accessing, sustaining and benefiting from clinic-based services" (Depp et al., 2010, p. 2). Evidence suggests that mobile interventions may be viable options for health promotion to help users adopt healthy behaviours. Specifically, several studies supported using consumer mHealth applications to help consumers lose weight (Kubota, Fujita, & Hatano, 2004; Patrick et al., 2009; Wang, Kogashiwa, Ohta, & Kira, 2002), increase physical activity (Consolvo, Everitt, Smith, & Landay, 2006; Hurling et al., 2007), quit smoking (Bramley et al., 2005; Free et al., 2009; Free et al., 2011; Lazev, Vidrine, Arduino, & Gritz, 2004; Obermayer, Riley, Asif, & Jean-Mary, 2004; Rodgers et al., 2005; Vidrine, Arduino, & Gritz, 2006a; Vidrine, Arduino, Lazev, & Gritz, 2006b), as well as reduce drug use (Freedman, Lester, McNamara, Milby, & Schumacher, 2006) and alcohol consumption (Collins, Kashdan, & Gollnisch, 2003; Wilkins, Casswell, Barnes, & Pledger, 2003). In addition to health promotion, mobile interventions have been investigated for medication adherence (Brath et al., 2013), mental illness (Depp et al., 2010), and prenatal beliefs and behaviour (Evans et al., 2012). mPHRs could benefit from offering interventions such as these to consumers and allowing them to opt in (and out) of these programs at their discretion.

Perhaps unsurprisingly, most consumer mHealth applications have been developed to serve a single, isolated purpose (e.g., monitoring blood glucose). However, many individuals have an array of different conditions or needs that mPHRs have the potential to meet and further, these needs may vary over time. Depending on their unique condition(s), consumers may require a variety of specialized mobile applications to serve their individual health needs. Indeed, an mPHR has the potential to satiate user needs by providing a selection of tools that can be tailored to the individual and adapt to their changing needs over time. Furthermore, this type of mPHR is destined to provide a more comprehensive perspective of the user's health. However, added functionality is typically associated with added complexity making them more difficult to use; this obstacle must be overcome in order for mPHRs to reach their potential.

FUTURE RESEARCH DIRECTIONS FOR mPHRs

This next generation of PHRs delivered through mobile devices, or mPHRs, is expected to enable a new set of complementary capabilities for consumers to participate in their health and carry their health information wherever they go. Despite the vast potential of mPHRs, and their availability, there is currently very limited evidence to support their use. Throughout this chapter, different potential users, use contexts, and various opportunities and challenges associated with mPHRs were presented. All of the topics identified here require investigation.

Investigations should be devoted to identifying different types of target users' and their distinct characteristics and needs. It is encouraged that new studies aim to explore the needs of different potential mPHR user groups, what functions they want and will use, as well as where and when mPHRs will be used. Some conjunctures were made about how mPHRs could be valuable for different types of users; however, the needs of

these groups may differ and should be investigated before and during development (i.e., adopt a user-centred, iterative, design process). It is unlikely that a single mPHR solution will meet the distinct needs and preferences of different user groups, or even the same user over time. Therefore, it is important to explore the different characteristics (e.g., age, illnesses) of mPHRs users and how their needs vary. Additionally, communicating with users who have different levels of health literacy should also be considered to ensure the information is understandable and to increase the accuracy of the data in the mPHR. Thus, flexible mPHRs, that can accommodate different user needs initially, as well as their evolving knowledge and skills over time, should be explored.

The advantages and disadvantages of having ubiquitous personal health records (i.e., mPHRs) should also be explored. That is, where and when mPHRs can demonstrate the most utility, and in what situations are they less useful or potentially problematic (e.g., compromising privacy) should be examined.

Several challenges associated with mPHR use require further attention. Not only are there the physical constraints associated with mobile devices, but consumers' levels of health literacy, and usability evaluation are issues that require investigation to reveal effective strategies to ameliorate these potential obstacles. Although the tools for collecting usability test data are becoming increasingly robust, there are still challenges associated with testing mPHRs "in situ". However, given their nearly limitless use environments, it is imperative to test these systems beyond the confines of the laboratory, to reveal usability problems that only arise in real world situations. A wide range of scenarios where users access their health records using mPHRs are possible and new usability challenges are likely to arise given this unprecedented accessibility. Further, users are not static and their needs may change over time; therefore, mPHRs should be designed to adapt to users' evolving needs.

Despite the challenges associated with mPHRs, there are many inherent opportunities created through these systems. New ways of delivering (e.g., TTS, MMS), entering (e.g., SMS, speech recognition), health information, as well as new methods of interacting (e.g., eye tracking) with mPHRs warrant exploration. These new methods may contribute to overcoming health literacy challenges, as well as difficulty entering data into an mPHR.

Although the features and functionality of mPHRs is generally limited at the moment, it is reasonable to expect the number of mPHR functions available will increase. Given the current expansion and success of consumer mHealth applications that could complement the information in mPHRs, it is anticipated that many of these functions will soon become integrated and offered through mPHRs. Some of the anticipated benefits of incorporating consumer mHealth applications into mPHRs include facilitating self-management of chronic illnesses, providing educational resources, pre-screening for health problems, expediting service delivery, monitoring conditions, complementing care for older adults, and delivering interventions. Further, the timing of information and how interventions are delivered are also important considerations for mPHRs, in order to maximize their opportunity for success. Moreover, whether mPHR use is actually related to user empowerment, enhanced understanding and participation, as well as improved self-management has yet to be empirically supported.

CONCLUSION

In this chapter, examples of currently available mPHRs were described and speculations were made regarding the potential users and use contexts of mPHRs. mPHRs are emergent consumer health information systems and there are a variety of different directions mPHRs may take in the future. Additionally, some of the challenges and opportunities regarding mPHR development, which constitute some of the future research directions, were discussed. Although PHRs are rapidly expanding into the mHealth environment, there is a dearth of research evidence supporting their use. Furthermore, most mPHRs currently available have limited value, because they are stand-alone systems (i.e., not integrated with a consumer's electronic health record) and/or do not offer tools that can be tailored to each user to foster health promotion and facilitate illness management. Thus, we anticipate that as mPHRs mature, more research will be focused on their efficacy, as well as how to integrate them with other health information systems and consumer mHealth applications to maximize their utility.

Given that mPHRs have recently been developed, it is not surprising that there is an array of topics requiring research. Future studies should aim to reveal how to optimize mPHRs by overcoming the obstacles and capitalizing on the opportunities inherent to mPHRs. Usability evaluation for mPHRs is critical to increase the likelihood of their adoption. That is, a successful mPHR will leverage the benefits of mPHRs and ensure that it can be used quickly and easily. mPHRs are bound to include more functionality to better serve their users and hopefully exchange information with other information systems. As these systems evolve, one of the biggest challenges facing mPHR designers is to conceal their complexity and provide a streamlined user experience.

REFERENCES

AHS. (2013). *Alberta Health Services*. Retrieved October 17, 2013 from www.albertahealthservices.ca/mobile.asp

Årsand, E., & Demiris, G. (2008). User-centered methods for designing patient-centric self-help tools. *Informatics for Health & Social Care, 33*(3), 158–169. doi:10.1080/17538150802457562 PMID:18850399

Årsand, E., Frøisland, D. H., Skrøvseth, S. O., Chomutare, T., Tatara, N., Hartvigsen, G., & Tufano, J. T. (2012). Mobile health applications to assist patients with diabetes: Lessons learned and design implications. *Journal of Diabetes Science and Technology, 6*(5), 1197–1206. doi:10.1177/193229681200600525 PMID:23063047

Baker, D. W. (2006). The meaning and the measure of health literacy. *Journal of General Internal Medicine, 21*(8), 878–883. doi:10.1111/j.1525-1497.2006.00540.x PMID:16881951

Bardram, J., Mihailidis, A., & Wan, D. (Eds.), *Pervasive Computing in Healthcare.* New York: CRC Press.

Bielli, E., Carminati, F., La Capra, S., Lina, M., Brunelli, C., & Tamburini, M. (2004). A wireless health outcomes monitoring system (WHOMS), Development and field testing with cancer patients using mobile phones. *BMC Medical Informatics and Decision Making, 4*(1), 7–7. doi:10.1186/1472-6947-4-7 PMID:15196308

Botts, N. E., Horan, T. A., & Thoms, B. P. (2011). HealthATM: Personal health cyberinfrastructure for underserved populations. *American Journal of Preventive Medicine, 40*(5), S115–S122. doi:10.1016/j.amepre.2011.01.016 PMID:21521584

Bramley, D., Riddell, T., Whittaker, R., Corbett, T., Lin, R., Wills, M., & Rodgers, A. (2005). Smoking cessation using mobile phone text messaging is as effective in Maori as non-Maori. *The New Zealand Medical Journal, 118*(1216), U1494. PMID:15937529

Brandt J. Weiss N. Klemmer S. R. (2007). txt 4 l8r: Lowering the burden for diary studies under mobile conditions. In Proceedings of CHI'07 Extended Abstracts on Human Factors in Computing Systems (pp. 2303-2308). ACM. 10.1145/1240866.1240998

Brath, H., Morak, J., Kästenbauer, T., Modre-Osprian, R., Strohner-Kästenbauer, H., Schwarz, M., & Schreier, G. (2013). Mobile health (mHealth) based medication adherence measurement – A pilot trial using electronic blisters in diabetes patients. *British Journal of Clinical Pharmacology, 76*, 47–55. doi:10.1111/bcp.12184 PMID:24007452

Canadian Council on Learning. (2008). *Health Literacy in Canada: A Healthy Understanding.* Retrieved March 17, 2013, from http://www.ccl-cca.ca/pdfs/HealthLiteracy/HealthLiteracyReportFeb2008E.pdf

Chen, E., Medonca, E., McKnight, L., Stetson, P., Lei, J., & Cimino, J. (2003). PalmCIS: A wireless handheld application for satisfying clinician information needs. *Journal of the American Medical Informatics Association, 11*(1), 19–28. doi:10.1197/jamia.M1387 PMID:14527976

Cheng S. (2011). The research framework of eye-tracking based mobile device usability evaluation. In Proceedings of the 1st International Workshop on Pervasive Eye Tracking & Mobile Eye-Based Interaction (pp. 21-26). ACM. 10.1145/2029956.2029964

Cimino, J. J., Patel, V. L., & Kushniruk, A. W. (2002). The patient clinical information system (PatCIS), Technical solutions for and experiences with giving patients access to their electronic medical records. *International Journal of Medical Informatics, 68*(1-3), 113–127. doi:10.1016/S1386-5056(02)00070-9 PMID:12467796

Cleland, J., Caldow, J., & Ryan, D. (2007). A qualitative study of the attitudes of patients and staff to the use of mobile phone technology for recording and gathering asthma data. *Journal of Telemedicine and Telecare, 13*(2), 85–89. doi:10.1258/135763307780096230 PMID:17359572

Collins, R. L., Kashdan, T. B., & Gollnisch, G. (2003). The feasibility of using cellular phones to collect ecological momentary assessment data: Application to alcohol consumption. *Experimental and Clinical Psychopharmacology, 11*(1), 73–78. doi:10.1037/1064-1297.11.1.73 PMID:12622345

Consolvo, S., Everitt, K., Smith, I., & Landay, J. (2006). *Design requirements for technologies that encourage physical activity.* doi:10.1145/1124772.1124840

CSI. (2013). *motionPHR*. Retrieved October 8, 2013, from http://motionphr.com/

Depp, C. A., Mausbach, B., Granholm, E., Cardenas, V., Ben-Zeev, D., Patterson, T. L., & Jeste, D. V. (2010). Mobile interventions for severe mental illness: Design and preliminary data from three approaches. *The Journal of Nervous and Mental Disease, 198*(10), 715–721. doi:10.1097/NMD.0b013e3181f49ea3 PMID:20921861

DeWalt, D. A., Berkman, N. D., Sheridan, S., Lohr, K. N., & Pignone, M. P. (2004). Literacy and health outcomes: A systematic review of the literature. *Journal of General Internal Medicine, 19*(12), 1228–1239. doi:10.1111/j.1525-1497.2004.40153.x PMID:15610334

DMC. (2013). *Detroit Medical Center*. Retrieved October 17, 2013, from www.dmc.org/apps

Epic. (2013). *Epic Systems Corporation: Mobile Applications and Portals*. Retrieved October 8, 2013, from http://www.epic.com/software-phr.php

Evans, W. D., Wallace, J. L., & Snider, J. (2012). Pilot evaluation of the text4baby mobile health program. *BMC Public Health, 12*(1), 1031. doi:10.1186/1471-2458-12-1031 PMID:23181985

Free, C., Roberts, I., Knight, R., Robertson, S., Whittaker, R., Edwards, P., & Kenward, M. G. (2011). Smoking cessation support delivered via mobile phone text messaging (txt2stop), A single-blind, randomised trial. *Lancet, 378*(9785), 49–55. doi:10.1016/S0140-6736(11)60701-0 PMID:21722952

Free, C., Whittaker, R., Knight, R., Abramsky, T., Rodgers, A., & Roberts, I. G. (2009). Txt2stop: A pilot randomised controlled trial of mobile phone-based smoking cessation support. *Tobacco Control, 18*(2), 88–91. doi:10.1136/tc.2008.026146 PMID:19318534

Freedman, M. J., Lester, K. M., McNamara, C., Milby, J. B., & Schumacher, J. E. (2006). Cell phones for ecological momentary assessment with cocaine-addicted homeless patients in treatment. *Journal of Substance Abuse Treatment, 30*(2), 105–111. doi:10.1016/j.jsat.2005.10.005 PMID:16490673

Haggstrom, D. A., Saleem, J. J., Russ, A. L., Jones, J., Russell, S. A., & Chumbler, N. R. (2011). Lessons learned from usability testing of the VA's personal health record. *Journal of the American Medical Informatics Association, 18*(Suppl 1), i13–i17. doi:10.1136/amiajnl-2010-000082 PMID:21984604

Halamka, J., Mandl, K., & Tang, P. (2007). Early experiences with personal health records. *Journal of the American Medical Informatics Association, 15*(1), 1–7. doi:10.1197/jamia.M2562 PMID:17947615

Health Council of Canada. (2010). *Helping patients help themselves: Are Canadians with chronic conditions getting the support they need to manage their health?* Toronto, Canada: Health Council of Canada.

Holtz, B., & Lauckner, C. (2012). Diabetes management via mobile phones: A systematic review. *Telemedicine Journal and e-Health, 18*(3), 175–184. doi:10.1089/tmj.2011.0119 PMID:22356525

Househ, M., Borycki, E., Kushniruk, A., & Alofaysan, S. (2012). mHealth: A passing fad or here to stay? In Telemedicine and E-health Services, Policies, and Applications: Advancements and Developments. Hershey, PA: IGI Global.

Hurling, R., Catt, M., Boni, M. D., Fairley, B. W., Hurst, T., Murray, P., & Sodhi, J. S. (2007). Using internet and mobile phone technology to deliver an automated physical activity program: Randomized controlled trial. *Journal of Medical Internet Research, 9*(2), e7. doi:10.2196/jmir.9.2.e7 PMID:17478409

Istepanian, R. S. H., Jovanov, E., & Zhang, Y. T. (2004). Guest editorial introduction to the special section on M-health: Beyond seamless mobility and global wireless health-care connectivity. *IEEE Transactions on Information Technology in Biomedicine, 8*(4), 405–414. doi:10.1109/TITB.2004.840019 PMID:15615031

Jaspers, M. W. M. (2009). A comparison of usability methods for testing interactive health technologies: Methodological aspects and empirical evidence. *International Journal of Medical Informatics, 78*(5), 340–353. doi:10.1016/j.ijmedinf.2008.10.002 PMID:19046928

Jones, D. A., Shipman, J. P., Plaut, D. A., & Selden, C. R. (2010). Characteristics of personal health records: Findings of the medical library association/national library of medicine joint electronic personal health record task force. *Journal of the Medical Library Association: JMLA, 98*(3), 243–249. doi:10.3163/1536-5050.98.3.013 PMID:20648259

Kaelber, D., & Pan, E. C. (2008). The value of personal health record (PHR) systems. In *Proceedings of AMIA Annual Symposium*. American Medical Informatics Association.

Keckley, P. H., & Hoffman, M. (2010). *2010 Survey of Health Care Consumers: Key Findings, Strategic Implications*. Deloitte Center for Health Solutions. Retrieved October 10, 2013, from http://www.deloitte.com/assets/Dcom-UnitedStates/Local%20Assets/Documents/US_CHS_2010SurveyofHealthCareConsumers_050310.pdf

Kharrazi, H., Chisholm, R., VanNasdale, D., & Thompson, B. (2012). Mobile personal health records: An evaluation of features and functionality. *International Journal of Medical Informatics, 81*(9), 579–593. doi:10.1016/j.ijmedinf.2012.04.007 PMID:22809779

Kubota, A., Fujita, M., & Hatano, Y. (2004). Development and effects of a health promotion program utilizing the mail function of mobile phones. *Japanese Journal of Public Health, 51*(10), 862. PMID:15565995

Kurniawan, S., Mahmud, M., & Nugroho, Y. (2006). *A study of the use of mobile phones by older persons*. doi:10.1145/1125451.1125641

Kushniruk, A. (2002). Evaluation in the design of health information systems: Application of approaches emerging from usability engineering. *Computers in Biology and Medicine, 32*(3), 141–149. doi:10.1016/S0010-4825(02)00011-2 PMID:11922931

Kushniruk, A. W., Borycki, E. M., Kuwata, S., & Kannry, J. (2011). Emerging approaches to usability evaluation of health information systems: Towards in-situ analysis of complex healthcare systems and environments. *Studies in Health Technology and Informatics, 169*, 915. PMID:21893879

Kushniruk, A. W., Patel, V. L., & Cimino, J. J. (1997). Usability testing in medical informatics: Cognitive approaches to evaluation of information systems and user interfaces. In *Proceedings of the AMIA Annual Fall Symposium* (pp. 218). American Medical Informatics Association.

Lau, J. K., Lowres, N., Neubeck, L., Brieger, D. B., Sy, R. W., Galloway, C. D., & Freedman, S. B. (2013). iPhone ECG application for community screening to detect silent atrial fibrillation: A novel technology to prevent stroke. *International Journal of Cardiology, 165*(1), 193–194. doi:10.1016/j.ijcard.2013.01.220 PMID:23465249

Lazev, A., Vidrine, D., Arduino, R., & Gritz, E. (2004). Increasing access to smoking cessation treatment in a low-income, HIV-positive population: The feasibility of using cellular telephones. *Nicotine & Tobacco Research: Official Journal of the Society for Research on Nicotine and Tobacco, 6*(2), 281–286. doi:10.1080/14622200410001676314 PMID:15203801

Lee, R. Y. W., & Carlisle, A. J. (2011). Detection of falls using accelerometers and mobile phone technology. *Age and Ageing, 40*(6), 690–696. doi:10.1093/ageing/afr050 PMID:21596711

Leung, R., McGrenere, J., & Graf, P. (2011). Age-related differences in the initial usability of mobile device icons. *Behaviour & Information Technology, 30*(5), 629–642. doi:10.1080/01449290903171308

Leung, R., Tang, C., Haddad, S., Mcgrenere, J., Graf, P., & Ingriany, V. (2012). How older adults learn to use mobile devices: Survey and field investigations. *ACM Transactions on Accessible Computing, 4*(3), 1–33. doi:10.1145/2399193.2399195

McGillicuddy, J. W., Weiland, A. K., Frenzel, R. M., Mueller, M., Brunner-Jackson, B. M., Taber, D. J., & Treiber, F. A. (2013). Patient attitudes toward mobile phone-based health monitoring: Questionnaire study among kidney transplant recipients. *Journal of Medical Internet Research, 15*(1), e6. doi:10.2196/jmir.2284 PMID:23305649

Microsoft. (2013). *Microsoft HealthVault Personal Health Record Goes Mobile in 2012 with iTriage.* Retrieved October 8, 2013, from http://www.prweb.com/releases/2011/12/prweb9064141.htm

Miluzzo, E., Wang, T., & Campbell, A. (2010). *EyePhone: Activating mobile phones with your eyes.* doi:10.1145/1851322.1851328

Miskelly, F. (2005). Electronic tracking of patients with dementia and wandering using mobile phone technology. *Age and Ageing, 34*(5), 497–499. doi:10.1093/ageing/afi145 PMID:16107453

Monkman, H., & Kushniruk, A. W. (2013a). A Health Literacy and Usability Heuristic Evaluation of a Mobile Consumer Health Application. *Studies in Health Technology and Informatics, 192*, 724. PMID:23920652

Monkman, H., & Kushniruk, A. W. (2013b). Applying Usability Methods to Identify Health Literacy Issues: An Example Using a Personal Health Record. *Studies in Health Technology and Informatics, 183*, 179–185. PMID:23388278

Nielsen, J., & Budiu, R. (2012). *Mobile usability*. Pearson Education.

Nmawston. (2012, October 17). Worldwide smartphone population tops 1 billion in Q3 2012. *Strategy Analytics*.

Nutbeam, D. (1998). Health promotion glossary. *Health Promotion International, 13*(4), 349–364. doi:10.1093/heapro/13.4.349

Obermayer, J. L., Riley, W. T., Asif, O., & Jean-Mary, J. (2004). College smoking-cessation using cell phone text messaging. *Journal of American College Health, 53*(2), 71–78. doi:10.3200/JACH.53.2.71-78 PMID:15495883

Pagliari, C., Detmer, D., & Singleton, P. (2007). Potential of electronic personal health records. *BMJ (Clinical Research Ed.), 335*(7615), 330–333. doi:10.1136/bmj.39279.482963.AD PMID:17703042

Paré, G., Moqadem, K., Pineau, G., & St-Hilaire, C. (2010). Clinical effects of home telemonitoring in the context of diabetes, asthma, heart failure and hypertension: A systematic review. *Journal of Medical Internet Research, 12*(2), e21. doi:10.2196/jmir.1357 PMID:20554500

Patrick, K., Raab, F., Adams, M. A., Dillon, L., Zabinski, M., Rock, C. L., & Norman, G. J. (2009). A text message-based intervention for weight loss: Randomized controlled trial. *Journal of Medical Internet Research, 11*(1), e1. doi:10.2196/jmir.1100 PMID:19141433

Pino, C., & Kavasidis, I. (2012). Improving mobile device interaction by eye tracking analysis. In *Proceedings of Computer Science and Information Systems (FedCSIS), 2012 Federated Conference on* (pp. 1199-1202). IEEE.

Pope, L., Silva, P., & Almeyda, R. (2010). i-Phone applications for the modern day otolaryngologist. *Clinical Otolaryngology: Official Journal of ENT-UK. Official Journal of Netherlands Society for Oto-Rhino-Laryngology & Cervico-Facial Surgery, 35*(4), 350. doi:10.1111/j.1749-4486.2010.02170.x

Protti, D. (2008). A comparison of how Canada, England and Demark are managing their electronic health record journeys. In *Human, Social and Organizational Aspects of Healthcare Information Systems*. Hershey, PA: IGI Global. doi:10.4018/978-1-59904-792-8.ch012

Proudfoot, J., Parker, G., Hadzi Pavlovic, D., Manicavasagar, V., Adler, E., & Whitton, A. (2010). Community attitudes to the appropriation of mobile phones for monitoring and managing depression, anxiety, and stress. *Journal of Medical Internet Research, 12*(5), e64. doi:10.2196/jmir.1475 PMID:21169174

Rodgers, A., Corbett, T., Bramley, D., Riddell, T., Wills, M., Lin, R., & Jones, M. (2005). Do u smoke after txt? Results of a randomised trial of smoking cessation using mobile phone text messaging. *Tobacco Control, 14*(4), 255–261. doi:10.1136/tc.2005.011577 PMID:16046689

Samsung. (2013). How do I use Air Gestures to control my Samsung Galaxy S® 4? In *How to Guides*. Retrieved, November 1, 2013, from http://www.samsung.com/us/support/howtoguide/N0000003/10141/120552

Segall, N., Saville, J. G., L'Engle, P., Carlson, B., Wright, M. C., Schulman, K., & Tcheng, J. E. (2011). Usability evaluation of a personal health record. In *Proceedings of AMIA Annual Symposium*. American Medical Informatics Association.

Shiffman, S., Stone, A. A., & Hufford, M. R. (2008). Ecological momentary assessment. *Annual Review of Clinical Psychology, 4*(1), 1–32. doi:10.1146/annurev.clinpsy.3.022806.091415 PMID:18509902

Siegenthaler, E., Wurtz, P., & Groner, R. (2010). Improving the usability of e-book readers. *Journal of Usability Studies, 6*(1), 25–38.

Simon, S. K., & Seldon, H. L. (2012). Personal health records: Mobile biosensors and smartphones for developing countries. *Studies in Health Technology and Informatics, 182*, 125. PMID:23138087

Singh, R. I., Sumeeth, M., & Miller, J. (2011). Evaluating the Readability of Privacy Policies in Mobile Environments. *International Journal of Mobile Human Computer Interaction, 3*(1), 55–78. doi:10.4018/jmhci.2011010104

Smith, A. (2011, September 19). *Americans and text messaging*. Pew Internet & American Life Project: A Project of the Pew Research Center. Retrieved from http://www.pewinternet.org/~/media//Files/Reports/2011/Americans%20and%20Text%20Messaging.pdf

Sourceforge. (2013). *Android Screenshots and Screen Capture*. Retrieved November 8, 2013, from http://sourceforge.net/projects/ashot/

Sposaro, F., & Tyson, G. (2009). iFall: An Android application for fall monitoring and response. In Proceedings of Engineering in Medicine and Biology Society, (pp. 6119-6122). IEEE.

Squirrels. (2013). Reflector. In *Products*. Retrieved November 8, 2013, from http://www.airsquirrels.com/reflector/

Sunwoo, J., Yuen, W., Lutteroth, C., & Wünsche, B. (2010). Mobile games for elderly healthcare. In *Proceedings of the 11th International Conference of the NZ Chapter of the ACM Special Interest Group on Human-Computer Interaction* (pp. 73-76). ACM.

Tang, P. C., Ash, J. S., Bates, D. W., Overhage, J. M., & Sands, D. Z. (2006). Personal health records: Definitions, benefits, and strategies for overcoming barriers to adoption. *Journal of the American Medical Informatics Association, 13*(2), 121–126. doi:10.1197/jamia.M2025 PMID:16357345

UPMC. (2013). *HealthTrak: Your health online – and on your schedule*. Retrieved November 2, 2013, from https://myupmc.upmc.com/

U.S. Department of Health and Human Services. (2010). *Health literacy online: A guide to writing and designing easy-to-use health Web sites*. Retrieved July 4, 2013, from http://www.health.gov/healthliteracyonline/

Vargas, P. A., Robles, E., Harris, J., & Radford, P. (2010). Using information technology to reduce asthma disparities in underserved populations: A pilot study. *The Journal of Asthma: Official Journal of the Association for the Care of Asthma, 47*(8), 889–894. doi:10.3109/02770903.2010.497887 PMID:20846082

Vidrine, D. J., Arduino, R. C., & Gritz, E. R. (2006a). Impact of a cell phone intervention on mediating mechanisms of smoking cessation in individuals living with HIV/AIDS. *Nicotine & Tobacco Research: Official Journal of the Society for Research on Nicotine and Tobacco, 8*(1), S103–S108. doi:10.1080/14622200601039451 PMID:17491177

Vidrine, D. J., Arduino, R. C., Lazev, A. B., & Gritz, E. R. (2006b). A randomized trial of a proactive cellular telephone intervention for smokers living with HIV/AIDS. *AIDS (London, England)*, *20*(2), 253–260. doi:10.1097/01. aids.0000198094.23691.58 PMID:16511419

Wang, D., Kogashiwa, M., Ohta, S., & Kira, S. (2002). Validity and reliability of a dietary assessment method: The application of a digital camera with a mobile phone card attachment. *Journal of Nutritional Science and Vitaminology*, *48*(6), 498–504. doi:10.3177/jnsv.48.498 PMID:12775117

Wilkins, C., Casswell, S., Barnes, H. M., & Pledger, M. (2003). A pilot study of a computer assisted cell phone interview (CACI) methodology to survey respondents in households without telephones about alcohol use. *Drug and Alcohol Review*, *22*(2), 221–225. doi:10.1080/09595230100100651 PMID:12850908

Zhang, T., Wang, J., Liu, P., & Hou, J. (2006). Fall detection by embedding an accelerometer in cellphone and using KFD algorithm. *International Journal of Computer Science and Network Security*, *6*(10), 277–284.

KEY TERMS AND DEFINITIONS

Consumer mHealth Application: A program for use by laypeople to educate and/or monitor and/or manage health information delivered on mobile platforms (e.g., smartphones, tablets).

Electronic Health Record (EHR): An integrated, longitudinal patient record curated by healthcare providers that is electronically stored and accessed.

Health Information System (HIS): An electronic system that enables the acquisition, storage, management and sharing of health information (e.g., laboratory reports, prescriptions, immunizations) for different health-related purposes (e.g., disease surveillance, clinical decision-making, development of management plans).

Health Literacy: The ability for consumers to find, acquire, and understand health information and use this information to guide health-related decisions.

Mobile Health (mHealth): The use of mobile platforms (e.g., smartphones, tablets) to deliver health information systems.

Mobile Personal Health Record (mPHR): A Personal Health Record (PHR) integrated with a consumer mHealth application or mobile platform.

Personal Health Record (PHR): A record accessed and/or curated by consumers' containing their own clinical health information.

Telehealth: Healthcare delivery or data collection conducted remotely, beyond the confines of traditional clinical environments (e.g., hospitals, primary care facilities).

Usability: The ease and efficiency with which a tool can be used to accomplish a given task.

Chapter 17
Mobile Health Technology in the US:
Current Status and Unrealized Scope

Tridib Bandyopadhyay
Kennesaw State University, USA

Bahman Zadeh
Kennesaw State University, USA

ABSTRACT

ICT technologies like the Internet, mobile telephony, and other enabled handheld gadgets have penetrated our lives in an unprecedentedly disruptive fashion. Explosive computing and communicating power with ever-decreasing price of service over the passage of time have been the hallmark of this success. The success of these technologies has been effectively appropriated in many business processes and systems including the banking sector and the social media applications. However, in spite of having stupendous potential in the healthcare sector, especially in providing access to service for patients in rural and difficult-to-reach areas, very limited ICT appropriation has been witnessed. The authors explain the current extent of ICT penetration and seek reasons for such lackluster inclusion of ICT and mobile technology in the healthcare sector. They use the TAM model to identify the critical factors of technology adoption, and use such understandings to help readers understand the barriers of adoption of ICT and mobile technologies in the healthcare sector. The authors also provide indicative guidelines about how such barriers may be overcome, and widespread adoption and deployment of these technologies can be made possible in the healthcare sector, yielding benefits to large sections of population in the US.

INTRODUCTION

One of the much voiced concerns today is that the amount of money spent on healthcare services is quickly getting out of control. In the United States, the Health and Human Service Department

estimates that the cost of healthcare will reach 19.5 percent of Gross Domestic Product by 2017 (Keehan et al., 2008). It is of general understanding that among other measures, Information and Communication Technology (henceforth ICT) artifacts and systems can play a significant role

DOI: 10.4018/978-1-4666-6150-9.ch017

in bringing efficiency to the current healthcare system and cut down costs of service at multiple levels. For a vast country like US, where population is distributed over large areas, information and communication technologies, especially m-health technologies can be of critical impact in terms of increased efficiency, cost effectiveness and reduced time lag between the need and access of services.

According to a study conducted by Pricewater-houseCoopers' Health Research Institute (2010), one-third of the surveyed clinicians believed that their assessments were not based on complete information and they could greatly benefit from access to more health information. These clinicians also believed that acquiring more accurate and relevant health information in real-time would speed up their decision process. Further, the study found that up to 30% of clinicians believed that remote monitoring technology would substantially increase their productivity by reducing travel and other costs of inefficiency. Similar studies have confirmed that health technologies, such as remote patient monitoring systems would likely improve patient health and cut organization's costs by major proportions. For example, Wu et al., 2010 demonstrate that such systems have helped some patients manage their diabetes by measuring capillary blood glucose daily and compare the result with the measurements conducted by physicians.

Many ICT applications, such as mobile banking and social networks have demonstrated the explosive potential that these technologies have to offer and continue to receive massive institutional support and deployment. Unfortunately the public and private healthcare organizations including the insurance providers have not pushed much for adoption of these technologies. As a result, impactful absorption of ICT has not been replicated in the healthcare industry. Many have asked whether or not our society is open to accepting and adopting another technology to increase efficiency and improve quality of life at the expense of being ubiquitously intertwined

with the basic constituent and wellness of our very being! General concerns like the above, unknown risks from of a new technology including those of security and privacy concerns around inadequate handling of personal healthcare data have caused stakeholders to be conservative in general, and zealously guarded in those cases where sensitive data could travel over unpropriety channels including wireless networks.

Institutional supports aside, there is an additional factor that remains central to deriving value out of an implemented technology in an organizational set up. A technology is only as good as the value it brings through utilization and use. Implementation of a great technology is valuable only when users at various levels of an organization fully and effectively accept and utilize the technology in the business processes. There are numerous examples of great technologies that are implemented in organizations but are not used effectively by the end users. For instance, the cloud-based patient monitoring technology is not likely to generate expected value unless the user groups viz. the patients and clinicians accept and utilize the technology to their designed level of implementation.

In this chapter, we ask why adoption of mobile based Information and Communication Technology (ICT) by healthcare organizations has been so slow. Further, we attempt to identify the barriers that organizations must overcome to accelerate adoption of mobile technology in healthcare sector. We analyze the dichotomy between technologically viable, theoretically sound and empirically supported usefulness of ICT, and the reality of lackluster adoption of m-health technologies in the healthcare industries of US, and tease out the barriers of adoption. Once these barriers are understood and analyzed, an appropriate framework of policies, initiatives and legal provisions can be ensured. When that happens, m-health technology initiatives can facilitate widespread adoption and acceptance, leading to great benefits to our society.

BACKGROUND OF M-HEALTH

Before we explore mHealth and its current status, we take a look at the background and development of mobile technology and its widespread diffusion in our daily life.

Growth of Mobile Technology

Since 1940s, when the first radiotelephone technology was introduced, companies like Bell and AT&T have been making significant improvements in the level of service, reliability and capabilities of their mobile networks on a regular basis. By the early 1970s, Bell System had introduced a system known as Improved Mobile Telephone Service or IMTS. Later, the first IMTS based analog phone systems, called Cellular systems, were introduced to the public. These systems could provide large coverage by dividing the area into smaller areas called 'cells'. Great numbers of

low power transmitters and receivers were placed to provide service to distant areas. The first generation of mobile telephone technology, known as 1G, was introduced in early 80s which was followed by faster and much improved 2G, 3G, and 4G technologies in quick succession. Latest technologies such as the High Speed Packet Access (HSPA) and LTE use Internet instead of the Public Switching Telephone Networks (PSTN), and are capable of downlink rate of 100Mbps and uplink rates up to 50 Mbps. This is in sharp contrast to the diffident first generation wireless telephone technology 1G that was only capable to handle speeds up to 1.9Kbps (Pathuru Raj et al, 2010).

The later advancements in the wireless telephone technology coincided with the arrival of smaller wireless portable computers such as tablet computers, and smart phones. Consequently, mobile technologies like smart phones became synonymous with wireless communication technology. Thus converged mobile technologies have

Figure 1. Mobile Internet access market. (Adapted from PricewaterhouseCoopers Entertainment and Media Outlook, 2010–2014). Fees paid for mobile Internet access by mobile users in the U.S. (Rates for 2013 and 2014 are projections).

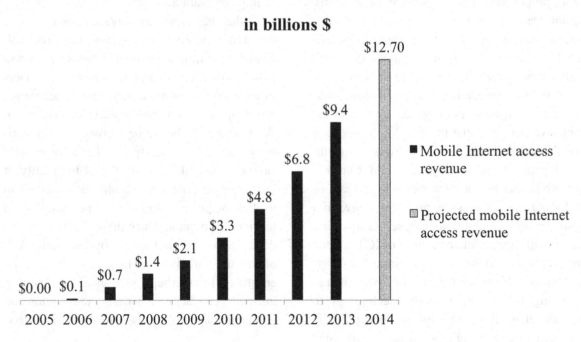

witnessed tremendous growth (Figure 2) in variety of industries including the healthcare industry (Stanford, 2002).

Mobile phones have now permeated our lives in ways that no other technology has ever been successful. Shipment of smart phones has grown to approximately to1 billion units worldwide in 2013! Some analysts argue that smart phones will dominate all of the mobile phone market in most of the developed countries by the end of 2017(Eddy, 2013). In what follows, we expand on some of the factors that are recognized to have contributed to this explosive growth:

Handset Subsidies in Smart Phone Based Service Contracts

Some of this growth is contributed to device subsidies given by wireless network providers. New smart phones are more sophisticated and more powerful than ever and their features and capabilities are increasingly more numerous. Companies such as Apple and Samsung regularly release new phones with more powerful processors. To make these phones more affordable for consumers, many wireless carriers extend steep subsidies in return for long-term service contracts. This strategy has contributed to the growth of smartphones in countries like the United States. According to the Nielsen Company report (2013), close to 96% of mobile users in the U.S subscribe to a data plan and on average pay $96 a month for their service. On the other hand, in countries like Russia and India where the average cost of a data plan is considerably higher than the average mobile phone bill, consumers have gravitated more towards prepaid plans. For example, in India, only 57% of mobile users subscribed to a data plan. In these countries fewer consumers have adopted smart phones primarily because they cannot afford the upfront cost of the device.

Figure 2. Global ICT trends and broadband penetration from 2008 to 2013. (Adapted from World Tele-communication/ICT Indicators database 2013 prepared by ITU).

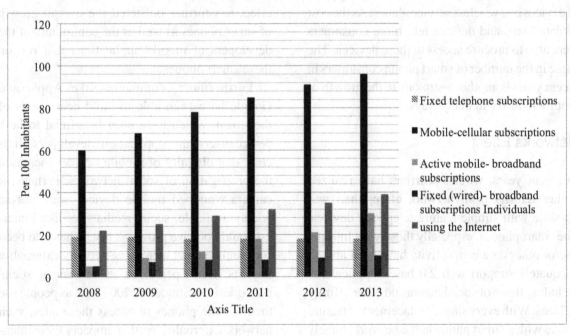

Figure 3. Mobile-cellular subscriptions per 100 inhabitants from 2003 to 2013. (Adapted from World Telecommunication/ICT Indicators database).

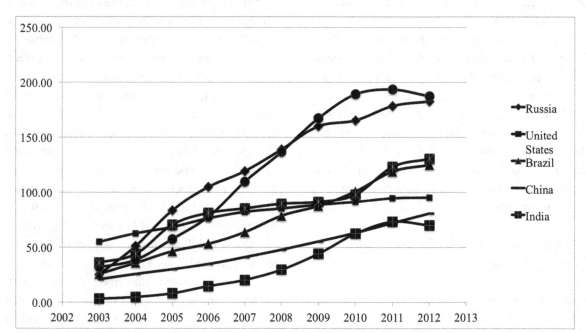

Falling Prices

Another important factor to the growth of mobile phones in the last decade has been the falling price of devices and wireless service planes. As the cost of data plans and devices fell, more consumers were able to procure access to these devices. The surge in the number of smart phone consumers in recent years is another testimony to the growth of mobile industry in many ways.

Networks Effect

In recent years, wireless carriers have realized higher returns from network effect than was possible with simple feature telephone devices. The smart phones, especially those with Internet and/or other data connectivity have been able to adequately support web 2.0 based applications including those of social media and other affinity villages. With every single replacement of feature phone with a smart phone in the network, hugely

accelerated network effect has been experienced by the provider; thereby increasing the value of their product and their ability to subsidize smart handsets on phone contracts. The cumulative effect has further bolstered the overall growth of smart phones as well as the community of the developers of mobile applications that run on these smart phones.

Furthermore, companies like Apple and Google have been able to build ecosystems of their own, which have been beneficial to both device users and application developers. It is clear that ubiquity of mobile devices increased the propagation of social networks. Perhaps, if camera equipped mobile devices were not so widely available, social media sites like Pinterest could not have grown as fast. It has also been substantiated that increasing network externality impacts users' perceived usefulness of social network sites (Strader al, 2007) and as people use their mobile phones to access these sites, such network externality further impacts their intention to adopt these devices as well. Although it is difficult to exactly determine whether social networks are imparting growth to mobile devices or the growth of more powerful mobile devices is causing explosive growth of social media, a sense of cumulatively positive network effect is quite apparent - further validating research which shows that as a technology becomes instrumental to real-time interaction with other users, it becomes more positively sensitive to the effects of network externality (Van et al, 2007).

Defining mHealth

Mobile Health or mHealth can be defined as use of mobile information and communication technologies to support the practice of medicine and increase access to affordable health related services by making delivery of these services more efficient and cost effective. Mobile Health is revolutionizing healthcare delivery particularly where distance separates consumers from clinicians (Angaran, 1999). It encompasses technologies that enable remote patient monitoring, Short Message Service (SMS) messaging, and mobile applications that drive active health participation by patients and practitioners.

Healthcare and Distance Health Service Delivery

In the last several years, there has been a wave of debate on how to reform the U.S. healthcare system. The advancements in medicine and rising costs of an aging population are some of the factors that have made the current healthcare system approaching levels that are difficult to sustain in a viable manner. According to a study conducted by World Health Organization (2011), when people were asked to identify some of the benefits that practitioners at their organization are getting from use of mHealth technology, 79% pointed to easier access to patient health data. Table 1 is a list of some other benefits pointed by these respondents.

Some of the critics of the current healthcare system in the U.S. have argued that healthcare reform must go beyond just insurance reform. For example, Michael Porter argues that restructuring the care delivery system is a critical component of a comprehensive healthcare reform strategy and it can only be achieved when more people have access to primary and preventive care. The first step in achieving an efficient value-based delivery system is to make health information more readily available. Without having access to sufficient treat-

Table 1. Perceived usefulness of mobile technology by clinicians

Benefits	Percent
Enhanced accessibility to patient data.	80%
Made it possible to access patient information remotely.	70%
Enhanced access to patient reference information.	69%
Made it possible to manipulate information from device enter/modify patient information using device.	45%
Enhanced patient safety.	38%
Made clinical decision support tools more accessible.	37%
Decreased number of devices used by clinicians.	33%
Can't Identify any.	2%

ment outcomes and results data, health providers are less likely to be able to improve the treatment outcomes and make the system more efficient or cost effective. He also argues that the medical data must be assessed from the beginning to the end of treatment process so that the degree of health and sustainability of recovery can be assessed more accurately (Porter, 2009). Considering that more patients spend large portion of their recovery at their own house, data collection and true measurement of health outcomes can rely on mobile ICT that support such processes.

For more than a decade researchers have argued that mobile communication devises have the potential to improve delivery of healthcare services to distanced areas (Angaran, 1999). But use of communication technology in health goes even further back. For years, practitioners have utilized terrestrial phone systems to communicate with their patients. However, the invention of the Internet disrupted many organizations, including healthcare organizations. The disruption was mainly due to the fact that the Internet made access to information more affordable. The effect of this disruption was felt by some industries more than others. For example, most individual travel agents have been driven out of business by intermediary online travel websites, since they no longer have any insider's information that an average traveler can find on their own. However, the healthcare sector was not greatly impacted by the emergence of new ICT innovations. In fact, despite some extraordinary interruptions in sectors such as banking and finance industry, healthcare organization never felt obligated to spend resources on research and development of ICT in order stay competitive.

The limited diffusion of ICT in healthcare, mostly as a result of government regulations or encouragement from health insurance companies, has proved to be very beneficial to clinicians of healthcare organizations as well as the patients treated by these organizations. In addition, improvement in sharing and accessing patient infor-

mation makes it possible for patients to receive services that once could only be obtained face to face in a clinical setting. When more information is available, physicians diagnose, track, and manage diseases more effectively and efficiently. For example, remote patient monitoring technology can constantly monitor patient's heart rate even after the patient leaves hospital. This is extremely helpful in continuous monitoring of health status of these patients and help their recovery process beyond hospital settings. Further, rising healthcare cost in recent years has increased the need for in-home clinical care services. As an effort to control cost, clinicians are more inclined to utilize remote patient monitoring services and release patients form hospitals early and continue the treatment processes from a distance. This has further caused remote health delivery systems to takes center stage of considerations. Some of the health related services made possible by mobile ICT are:

- Monitoring patients remotely.
- Supporting treatment and diagnosis process.
- Improving public education and public awareness.
- Improving communication and education for healthcare workers.
- Tracking illness and epidemic eruption.
- Colleting patient medical data remotely.

Diffusion of Mobile Devices with High Potential for m-Health Application:

In recent years, Mobile manufactures have been expanding in terms of their capabilities including processing power approaching the capability of low end computers. Coupled with lower prices and flexible contracts that we have discussed earlier, mobile phones are becoming an essential part of people's daily life. These small, interconnected computers are integrated seamlessly around us and provide extremely useful services to our information needs and current situation (Stojanovic, 2009).

The new context-aware mobile phone is a new concept that has gained much traction in recent years. The idea is to provide remote caller of the phone information on the current status of the phone user (Siewiorek et al., 2003). Buoyant with wide diffusion of affordable smart phones, context-aware mobile applications are revolutionizing many industries. For example, these mobile applications now can provide search results based on a user's geographical location, making it much more useful to the user. Since these phones collect data from the changing environment of the user in a continuous fashion, information thus collected can be utilized to assess the physiological conditions of the users and provide help when needed.

According to the McDonough and Doucette's model of collaborative (McDonough & Doucette, 2001) working relationship in healthcare, the continuity of care in a patient-centered health care is critical (McCarthey, Schafermeyer, & Plake, 2012). Lately, the advent of social media and other Web 2.0 applications has improved the continuity of care in the U.S. As such the continuity of care is categorized into three types: Informational links, Disease management, and Relational (McCarthey, Schafermeyer, & Plake, 2012). Social media has helped patients with chronic diseases to collaborate online and find other patients who suffer from similar condition. These networks provide a support platform for patients and their family. Furthermore, the Web 2.0 applications have made the interdisciplinary teamwork among clinicians more efficient.

Lessons from Healthcare in the Emerging Markets

Emerging markets in India and South Africa have made significant improvements by making healthcare more accessible for their citizens in recent years. Emerging markets in general struggle to provide basic health care for all their citizens. Some of the difficulties that these countries face stem from lack of infrastructure necessary for building a modern healthcare system. Interestingly, this has motivated entrepreneurs and innovators in these countries to come up with innovative ways to use the existing technologies in order to compensate for the lack of infrastructure. This has resulted in many compelling innovations in the area of healthcare delivery in emerging markets. These innovators have also been able to take advantage of the lack of regulatory oversight and freely experiment new ways of delivering healthcare. Unlike U.S, where layers of oversight approve and monitor introduction and use of new technologies in delivering healthcare services preclude procedural shortcuts and wide experimentations, the freedom and flexibility in the emerging markets enabled innovators in those markets to innovate much faster and bring new innovations quickly to the market.

The utilization of telecommunication and information technologies to deliver healthcare, also known as Telemedicine, has proved to save life in many developing countries. Consider the countries where existing mobile networks have been used to deliver healthcare to far-flung areas. One good example of using telemedicine to improve the quality of pediatric care is Somalia, where more than two decades of internecine war resulted in significant shortage in healthcare facilities. Reaching remote locations and providing care for ill children was challenging. Clinicians decided to use the existing mobile infrastructure to provide clinical healthcare services. The examination of Somalian case clearly shows that use of telemedicine served as a life saving intervention. All physicians involved in the study that examined the use of telemedicine in Somalia believed that the telemedicine played a significant role in improving health in the country during the time of the study 2010 to 2011. For example, According to the World Health Report (2013) the respiratory tract infections dropped from 75% to 45% and the complicated malnutrition dropped from 86% to

40%. More significantly, adverse outcomes such as death in pediatric wards decreased by 30% during this period.

CURRENT STATUS OF M-HEALTH IN USA

In this section we will assess issues, factors, and challenges involved in adoption of mHealth technology and identify factors that have encumbered adoption of m-health by patients and health organizations.

Innovation in Mobile Technology and mHealth

A holistic understanding of innovation in mHealth requires us to consider the discontinuous as well as the rapid cycles of incremental IS innovation of the Internet. On one hand, we have witnessed how the Internet has drastically changed the way that information systems are developed and deployed in our daily life. Internet computing has also transformed itself by changing the software development methods and information system services over time (Lyytinen & Rose, 2003). On the other, we see how rapidly cycling between innovation and production - mobile technology, especially the smart phone - has created one of the fastest growing industries and has become one most significant contributor to the global economy. It is of little surprise that in this confluence between the mobile and Internet technologies, we repose our expectation of future ICT revolutions around those of m-health technologies that have the potential to benefit our lives in significant ways! However, the innovations in mobile technology in particular and ICT in general have not impacted the healthcare sector in the same way that they have been able to do so on other sectors of the economy. One ponders, why? The answer to this obvious question is however not easy!

It is clear that the healthcare sector has not been able to create and capture ICT value as rapidly as other sectors like banking or finance, yet research on barriers to innovation in mHealth has been limited. In order capture the true value of mobile technology, health sector must be able to innovate and disseminate new technology. There are many reasons for a sluggish innovation trend in mHealth. For one, health care professionals and not ICT specialists manage the dissemination of new ICT technologies and execute related R&D efforts in health care. We don't expect R&D departments that mostly focus on medical research to come up with new ways to use mobile technology to deliver healthcare. Moreover, medical community in general looks for hard data to support the benefits of a new technology. Given their training and practice, it is much easier for them to measure efficacy of a new treatment than to show improvement in health outcome as a result of using an ICT technology. The healthcare system is a large complex system and quantifying value driven from a new ICT system is very difficult because of obvious overlaps with many other variables in health delivery system. For a community that demands impervious proof before any attempt to use it, it is very difficult to adopt a mobile technology whose direct benefits are not as documented as medical research or whose benefits accrue differently across sectors and usage patterns. ICT is very different from most healthcare technologies and demands different knowledge sets for proper appreciation and assimilation, which also appears to have hindered innovation in mobile healthcare. In a closed system like healthcare, even a large-scale R&D is not enough to capture true value of new technologies (Chesbrough, 2003). We feel that a new model is necessary to meet today's challenges in terms of managing ICT innovation in healthcare.

The healthcare sector in the U.S can benefit from methods and approaches that enable open innovations. Open innovation has been successfully used by organizations like P&G and 3M to move the mindset of their decision makers from traditional inward-focused approach to networked innovation (Tidd & Bessant, 2009). For example, the mHealth summit provides a stage to technology leaders from the government, private sector, researchers, and mobile technology companies to engage in collaboration and find new ways to use wireless technology to improve health outcomes and generate new paradigms in health care delivery. In what follows, we provide a brief introduction to the principles of open innovation by Chesbrough that may benefit the readers to understand the barriers of adoption of m-health technologies, which we cover in a later stage of the chapter.

Open innovation is considered as a vital instrument for inventing and benefiting from technology and it is based on the simple idea that neither all smart employees work for one single organization nor all required capabilities are available in every organization. The fundamental concept of open innovation suggests that organizations must be able to use in-house as well as external ideas and capabilities to advance their technology with the help of formal and informal relations in the form of alliances and networks. Extant innovation models are not equipped to answer today's' challenges in advanced nations such as USA, argues Chesbrough (Chesbrough, 2003). He further points that merely having strong R&D is not going to be enough anymore and propounds six principles to describe an open innovation model:

1. It is wrong to assume all the intelligent people work in your organization.
2. Without internal R&D, it is difficult to extract value from an idea that is coming from outside.
3. It is preferred to have a superior business model than to get to market first.
4. To succeed, your firm must make the best use of external and internal ideas.
5. Value your intellectual property and buy those that benefit your business model.

6. Grow R&D's role to encompass knowledge brokering, in addition to knowledge generation.

Well-founded R&D has been a reliable solution to improve existing products and processes in the healthcare sector for large enterprises. There is no denying of the fact that the medical community in general, and pharmaceutical companies in particular greatly benefit from having a rigid structure that supports their strong R&D establishments. The direct impact that their innovations bring on the aspects of medicine and healthcare of the patient make them imperative to maintain strict control in every aspect of their operations. Unfortunately, this structure is not efficient in finding innovative ways to use ICT to improve healthcare delivery. These existing R&D structures are not agile to counter threats from disruptive innovations either. Healthcare organizations must find new ways to internalize external ICT innovations, which are mostly created by small technology startups, and operationalize such combined innovations with their might of deep pocket and long range of influence. However, an agile, discontinuous innovation often requires new mindsets in order to experience a successful take off and a new, expanded market to thrive.

Innovation Networks for Healthcare

We all have used the word network loosely at some point. The word network is usually synonymous with collaboration, openness, and interaction with others. We may consider our friends and work colleagues constituting networks. While these all may be true for rudimentary understandings, from social science perspective though, the word *network* has a precise meaning. Commonly, a network is defined as a complex, interconnected group or systems that may impose additional constrains and present additional opportunities to its members. Understanding network is very important in business and social interactions since it links diverse and autonomous entities together and provide the necessary protocols to collaborate and share knowledge. High-technology firms may use knowledge networks to collaborate and access each other's resources through direct and indirect relationships. When these knowledge networks are used to stimulate new ideas, we call them innovation networks.

In today's fast changing environment, it is very difficult for a firm to bring an idea to market without utilizing an innovation network. Innovation networks could help a firm to assemble and deploy new knowledge, provide access to diverse and matching knowledge sets, mitigate risk by sharing information, and finally provide access to new markets and technologies. Additionally, an innovation network may go beyond assembling and deploying knowledge. For example, the process of creating innovation networks, by itself, is proven to be very valuable for an organization by opening up potential unseen territories (Tidd & Bessant, 2009). Thus, creating and being part of an effective innovation network is generally known to be beneficial.

On the other hand, there could be costly consequences in not participating in an innovation network. Innovation is a risky proposition because it often involves deploying scarce resources on projects that might not succeed. Innovation networks can help organizations spread the risk between the network entities and thus extend the range of ideas that might be tried. Health organizations that do not use networking to help their innovation are likely to find themselves more vulnerable to risks involved in developing and deploying mobile-based health delivery systems. These firms are also less likely to invest on ICT related R&D in their core strength.

There are many examples of the ways in which innovation networks have helped innovation process. The following case of China is one example of using open innovation in order to improve development of new technologies. Importing external technology is not without challenges, but leverag-

ing domestic research and development (R&D) could be done in conjunction with employment of external ideas. Health organizations may look at China as an example of using external innovation to develop internal technology capabilities. China has been developing its technology capabilities by having a strategy for utilizing external innovations. Even though the technological gap between advanced countries and developing countries will always exist, having a strategy like the above has helped China to close those gaps in different stages of acquiring technology. For example, the government of China has played a role in setting up an intermediary organization called Quasi-external Innovation Network to help its industries to domesticize foreign innovations and later improve the effective development of technology in China (Wu, X., Gu, & Wei, 2008).

Similarly, healthcare organizations can greatly benefit from innovation networks since they do not have the structure necessary for fostering ICT innovations- a type of innovation that demands distinctive managerial skills that allows enough agility and flexibility so that new ideas can blossom (Riddle, 2008). By networking with other IT organizations, healthcare organizations can respond to change in the technological environment. Through cooperative efforts in developing R&D capability, healthcare organizations can respond to changes in ICT and sustain themselves through a continuous stream of innovation.

Where the innovations are complex and multifaceted and the costs are high, a well-governed innovation network is a great instrument for obtaining new innovations, ideas and testing them with minimum commitments. For example, a large US healthcare group located in the southeast has established a long-standing relationship with the College of Health and Human Services of a large university in Atlanta Metro. The partnership has produced number of network externalities which benefit both parties and generated a win-win scenario. The extent of value which could have never been achieved through traditional market models such as acquisition or integration is characteristic of the benefits that accrue from successful innovation networks. Here, both entities focus on what they do the best and freely share resources that may be beneficial to the other.

A more interesting fact of the above network is that the number of collaborative innovation projects between these entities has increased over time. As both entities are able to increase or decrease the number of nodes/partners in each of their networks, an innovation network is quite elastic in nature. For instance, the health organization has been able to expand and enrich its innovation network by establishing new relationships with other technical and business departments in the same university and expand the horizon of the innovation network to include cost effective experimentations on acquisition and implementation of health information technology and mobile health technology acceptance issues among stakeholders in their supply chain. In this example, the relationship started with a high degree of formalization but through continued relationship over multiple innovation projects between the health organization and the university faculty, a strong, expanding innovation network emerged. This is a great example of a scenario where benefit of sharing infrastructure and standards has more than compensated the expense of network maintenance while the innovation network has grown considerably in size and scope from where it originally started.

Fundamentals of Technology Adoption

This section examines the affective, psychographic, attributive and situational bearings that comprehensively affect technology adoption in organizations including sectors of healthcare, viz.:

- Characteristics of the mHealth technology.

- Characteristics, beliefs and perceptions of the individuals involved in the process leading to adoption of mHealth.
- Organizational and other situational environment in which mHealth is adopted.

We first look at the prominent frameworks and models and use them to understand the perceptions that shape individual's attitudes since those attitudes determine future behaviors such as the intention to adopt and use a technology. We examine the Theory of Planned Behavior (TPB) leading to the Technology Acceptance Model (TAM). These models have helped other industries such as banking and finance to grow their mobile-based services and products. While we explain these influential models, we also provide definitions for important terminologies used in the chapter:

Origins of the Technology Acceptance Model

Two most important studies that shape our understanding of technology adoption are the Theory of Planned Behavior (TPB) – a seminal work by Ajzen (1991) and the Technology Acceptance Model (TAM) by Davis (1989) shown in Figure 4. Researchers have empirically tested hybridized and consolidated variants of TAM and TPB models to predict user adoption of information technology applications in various organizational workplaces including healthcare settings. For example, researchers used the model to examine physician acceptance of telemedicine technology and found that physician's intention to use telemedicine mainly depends on perceived usefulness of the technology (Hu et al., 1999).

The increasing level of online communication and higher involvement of critical information has led to higher level of uncertainty among technology users. Consequently, many research-

Figure 4. Technology acceptance model

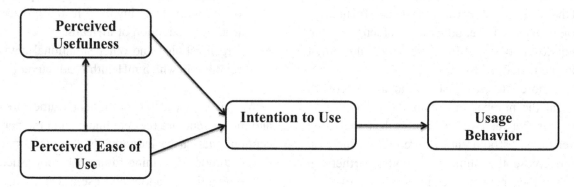

ers have advocated the consideration of perceived trust and perceived risk elements to describe the user acceptance of a new technology (Pavlou, 2003). Venkatesh and his colleagues evaluated a majority of competing models and generated the Unified Theory of Acceptance and Use of Technology (UTAUT). The model has received more attention in recent years since it has been validated with original data. The new model also considers variables such as: gender, age, experience, and voluntariness of use. Interestingly, this model outperformed the eight individual models, which are the original constituents of UTAUT (Venkatesh, Morris, & Davis, 2003)!

Evaluating the Adoption of Mobile Technology in Healthcare

Researchers have also attempted to investigate the predictors and antecedents of technology acceptance within the healthcare environment. For example, Chau and Hu (2002) focus on the effects of preliminary trust on user's adoption of mobile technology and conclude that integration of information technology into the process of healthcare delivery presents both technological and managerial challenges. One of the important findings of this study indicates that structural assurance and information quality directly affect users' initial sense of trust. This in turn impacts the perceived usefulness of technology – leading

to its final acceptance (Mayer, Davis, & Schoorman, 1995). Moreover, similar research dealing with cloud based mobile monitoring devices in somewhat related areas of application, e.g., mobile banking, exhort us to enhance our understanding of the trust issues raised during adoption of mobile health monitoring systems such as bed-fall detection or prevention systems.

Lapointe and Rivard (2005) point to the balance of power between groups such as patients and clinicians during implementation of a new technology, which demonstrates inherent complexity of technology adoption in a healthcare value chain. Results from their study show that physicians fear loss of control over their job at multiple levels and thus exhibit resistance towards adopting e-Health technologies. Similarly, other researchers have argued that users of a new technology perceive risk due to the lack of control and uncertainties involved in the new technology. Researchers suggest that end user's perception of lack of control over potentially uncertain modalities of information transactions in e-health technologies increase their perception of risk, which in turn tends to decrease trust to a given e-health technology (Pavlou, 2003). Further, these researchers also argue that increase in perception of risk increases resistance to change, thereby hindering users' intention to use a technology in the first place. In line with such understandings, our own research (not explained or cited here) explains "the need for control" as a significant variable of influence that directly corresponds to perceived usefulness and ease of use of m-health technology.

Solutions and Recommendations

The lessons learned from healthcare delivery in emerging markets have showed us that a more innovative health delivery system is not common but not unachievable. In this chapter we explained how mobile technology has penetrated many industries including the healthcare sector in recent years. We have shown how members of value delivery chain in healthcare system should be cognizant of these recent achievements and make an effort to champion adoption of mobile technologies in healthcare delivery. We have pointed out the inadequacy of innovations healthcare and showed how the sector lagged behind almost every other industry in terms of effective adoption of the mobile technology. Having explained the problems that plague innovations in the delivery of healthcare, we suggest that health organizations utilize innovation networks to link with young ICT firms, universities, and government agencies and incorporate their diverse knowledge and skills to innovate or incorporate new technologies in the way they do things. We further note that one obstacle in changing the trajectory to innovation network is the traditional paradigm of allocating organizational resources only in hard R&D arrangements. Healthcare organizations must alter their organizational mindset, be flexible and open to other approaches in innovation because traditional R&D investments are ineffective against threats from disruptive innovations. Finally, we emphasize that in order to successfully deploy a mobile-based health delivery system, every member of the health value delivery chain must fully adopt the purchased or developed technology and be willing to utilize it effectively. This is also the reason why we suggest organizations to spend resources on understanding and measuring user experience with technology mediated healthcare delivery. We suggest that these organizations start by one of the dominant technology adoption models such as TAM and later train the model to make it more relevant to the incoming technology that they would use for delivery of the healthcare services. It is critical that health organizations define long term strategies for finding, establishing, and maintaining relationships that lead to effective innovation networks. Only this can ensure our long terms success in terms of a technology integrated efficient healthcare system.

CONCLUSION

In this chapter we examined the current status of mobile health technology including issues involved in acceptance of mobile ICT in healthcare. We examined why and how the clinician's attitude and perception of a new technology is critical in accepting ICT in healthcare. We discussed a growing literature on extant Technology Acceptance Model (TAM) which highlights importance of attitudinal factors when it comes to accepting a healthcare technology by all different stakeholders of an organization. We examined how factors such as perceived usefulness and perceived ease of use influence physicians' intention to use a mobile health technology. In addition to these factors, we also examined the role of the need for control and perceived trust in adoption and utilization of health information technologies. We found that issues related to trust and control over various aspect of a health information technology play a significant role in successful adoption of mobile health technology. We evaluated some of the barriers in adoption of a mobile health technology and recommended that healthcare organizations should collaborate with outside organizations in order to develop and nurture new ideas that may further help adoption of ICT in healthcare delivery to remote and distant areas.

REFERENCES

Ajzen, I. (1991). The theory of planned behavior. *Organizational Behavior and Human Decision Processes*, *50*(2), 179–211. doi:10.1016/0749-5978(91)90020-T

Angaran, D. M. (1999). Telemedicine and Telepharmacy: Current status and future implications. *American Journal of Health-System Pharmacy*, *56*(14), 405–426. PMID:10428449

Chau, P. Y. K., & Hu, P. J. H. (2002). Investigating healthcare professionals' decisions to accept telemedicine technology: An empirical test of competing theories. *Information & Management*, *39*(4), 297–311. doi:10.1016/S0378-7206(01)00098-2

Chesbrough, H. (2003). *Open Innovation: The New Imperative for Creating and Profiting From Technology*. Harvard Business School Press.

Davis, F. D. (1989). Perceived usefulness, perceived ease of use, and user acceptance of information technology. *MIS Quart*, *13*(3), 319–340. doi:10.2307/249008

Eddy, N. (2013). Smartphones Power Strong Growth in Mobile Phone Sales: IDC. *Eweek*, 6.

Hu, P. J., Chau, P. K., Liu Sheng, O. R., & Kar Yan, T. (1999). Examining the Technology Acceptance Model Using Physician Acceptance of Telemedicine Technology. *Journal of Management Information Systems*, *16*(2), 91–112.

Keehan, S., Sisko, A., Truffer, C., Smith, S., Cowan, C., Poisal, J., & Clemens, M. (2008). Health spending projections through 2017: The baby-boom generation is coming to medicare. *Health Affairs*, *27*(2), 145–155. doi:10.1377/hlthaff.27.2.w145 PMID:18303038

Lapointe, L., & Rivard, S. (2005). A multilevel model of resistance to information technology implementation. *MIS Quart*, *29*(3), 461–491.

Lyytinen, K., & Rose, G. M. (2003). Disruptive information system innovation: The case of internet computing. *Information Systems Journal*, *13*(4), 301–330. doi:10.1046/j.1365-2575.2003.00155.x

Mayer, R. C., Davis, J. H., & Schoorman, F. D. (1995). An integrative model of organizational trust. *Academy of Management Review*, *20*(3), 709–734.

McCarthy, R. L., Kenneth, W., Schafermeyer, K., & Plake, S. (2012). *Introduction to Health Care Delivery: A Primer for Pharmacists*. Sudbury, MA: Jones & Bartlett Learning.

McDonough, R. P., & Doucette, W. R. (2001). Developing CWRs between pharmacists and physicians. *Journal of the American Pharmaceutical Association*, (41): 682–692.

Nielson Company. (2013). *The Mobile Consumer: A Global Snapshot*. Retrieved from http://www.nielsen.com/content/dam/corporate/us/en/reports-downloads/2013 Reports/Mobile-Consumer-Report-2013.pdf

Pathuru Raj, D., Ravichandiran, C. C., & Vaithiyanathan, D. R. (2010). A Comparison and SWOT Analysis of Towards 4G Technologies: 802.16e and 3GPP-LTE. *International Journal on Computer Science & Engineering*, *2*(2), 109–114.

Pavlou, P. A. (2003). Consumer Acceptance of Electronic Commerce: Integrating Trust and Risk with the Technology Acceptance Model. *International Journal of Electronic Commerce*, *7*(3), 101.

Porter, M. E. (2009). A Strategy for Health Care Reform - Toward a Value-Based System. *The New England Journal of Medicine*, *361*(2), 109–112. doi:10.1056/NEJMp0904131 PMID:19494209

Price Waterhouse Coopers. (2010). *Healthcare unwired: New business models delivering care anywhere*. Retrieved from http://www.pwc.com/us/en/health-industries/publications/healthcare-unwired.jhtml

Report, W. H. (2013). *Research for Universal Health Coverage*. World Health Organization.

Riddle, D. I. (2008). *Managing service innovation*. CMC Service-Growth Consultants Inc.

Siewiorek, D. Smailagic, Furukawa, A., Krause, A., Moraveji, N., Reiger, K., & Shaffer, J. (2003). Sensay: A context-aware mobile phone. In *Proceedings of the 7th IEEE International Symposium on Wearable Computers*. IEEE.

Stanford, V. (2002). Pervasive Health Care Applications Face Tough Security Challenges. *IEEE Pervasive Computing / IEEE Computer Society [and] IEEE Communications Society, 1*(2), 8–12. doi:10.1109/MPRV.2002.1012332

Stojanovic, D. (2009). *Context-aware Mobile and Ubiquitous Computing for Enhanced Usability: Adaptive Technologies and Applications*. Hershey, PA: Information Science. doi:10.4018/978-1-60566-290-9

Strader, T. J., Ramaswarni, S. N., & Houle, P. (2007). Perceived Network Externalities and Communication Technology Acceptance. *European Journal of Information Systems, 16*(1), 54–65. doi:10.1057/palgrave.ejis.3000657

Tidd, J., & Bessant, J. (2009). *Managing innovation: Integrating technological, market and organizational change*. Academic Press.

Utterback, J. M. (1994). *Mastering the Dynamics of Innovation*. Harvard Business School Press.

Utterback, J. M., & Acee, H. J. (2005). Disruptive Technologies: An Expanded View. *International Journal of Innovation Management, 9*(1), 1–17. doi:10.1142/S1363919605001162

Van, S. C., Ilie, V., Lou, H., & Stafford, T. (2007). Perceived critical mass and the adoption of a communication technology. *European Journal of Information Systems*. doi: doi:10.1057/palgrave.ejis.3000680

Venkatesh, V., Morris, M., & Davis, F. D. (2003). User acceptance of information technology: Toward a unified view. *Management Information Systems Quarterly, 27*(3), 425.

Vital Wave Consulting. (2009). *mHealth for Development: The Opportunity of Mobile Technology for Healthcare in the Developing World*. United Nations Foundation, Vodafone Foundation.

World Health Organization. (2011). *Mhealth: New Horizons for Health Through Mobile Technologies*. Retrieved from http://www.himss.org/content/files/Code%20491%20-%20mHealth-New%20horizons%20for%20health%20through%20mobile%20technologies_WHO_2011.pdf

Wu, L., Forbes, A., Griffiths, P., Milligan, P., & While, A. A. (2010). Telephone follow-up to improve glycaemic control in patients with type 2 diabetes: Systematic review and meta-analysis of controlled trials. *Diabetic Medicine, 27*(11), 1217–1225. doi:10.1111/j.1464-5491.2010.03113.x PMID:20950378

Wu, X., Gu, Z., & Wei, Z. (2008). The construction of innovation networks and the development of technological capabilities of industrial clusters in China. *International Journal of Innovation and Technology Management, 5*(2), 179–199. doi:10.1142/S0219877008001321

ADDITIONAL READING

Bhattacherjee, A., & Hikmet, N. (2007). Physicians' resistance toward healthcare information technology: A theoretical model and empirical test. *European Journal of Information Systems, 16*(6), 725–737. doi:10.1057/palgrave.ejis.3000717

Chandra, S. Srivastava, C.S., Theng, Y. (2010). Evaluating the Role of Trust in Consumer Adoption of Mobile Payment Systems: An Empirical Analysis. *Communications Of AIS, 27*561-588.

Conway & Steward. (1998). Mapping Innovation Networks. *International Journal of Innovation Management, 2*(2), 165–196.

Curry, S. J. (2007). EHealth research and health-care delivery: Beyond intervention effectiveness. *American Journal of Preventive Medicine, 32*(5), 127–130. doi:10.1016/j.amepre.2007.01.026 PMID:17466817

Davis, F. D. (1989). Perceived usefulness, perceived ease of use, and user acceptance of information technology. *MIS Quart, 13*(3), 319–340. doi:10.2307/249008

Dixon, B. E. (2007). A roadmap for the adoption of eHealth. *e-Service Journal, 5*(3), 3–13.

Hargadon, A. (2003). *How Breakthrough Happens.* Harvard Business School Press.

José Manuel Ortega, E., & María Victoria Román, G. (2011). Explaining physicians' acceptance of EHCR systems: An extension of TAM with trust and risk factors. *Computers in Human Behavior, 27*(1), 319–332. doi:10.1016/j.chb.2010.08.010

Koenig-Lewis, N., Palmer, A., & Moll, A. (2010). Predicting young consumers' take up of mobile banking services. *International Journal of Bank Marketing, 28*(5), 410–432. doi:10.1108/02652321011064917

Lapointe, L., & Rivard, S. (2005). A multilevel model of resistance to information technology implementation. *MIS Quart, 29*(3), 461–491.

Levine, R. J. (1986). *Ethics and Regulation of Clinical Research* (2nd ed., pp. 80–82). Baltimore: Urban and Schwarzenberg.

Lishan, X., Ching Chiuan, Y., Leanne, C., Hock Chuan, C., Bee Choo, T., Say Beng, T., & Mahesh, C. (2008). An exploratory study of ageing women's perception on access to health informatics via a mobile phone-based intervention. *International Journal of Medical Informatics.*

Pavlou, P. A. (2003). Consumer Acceptance of Electronic Commerce: Integrating Trust and Risk with the Technology Acceptance Model. *International Journal of Electronic Commerce, 7*(3), 101.

Riemenschneider, C. K., Hardgrave, B. C., & Davis, F. D. (2002). Explaining Software Developer Acceptance of Methodologies: A Comparison of Five Theoretical Models. *IEEE Transactions on Software Engineering, 28*(12), 1135–1145. doi:10.1109/TSE.2002.1158287

Ross, S., Todd, J., Moore, L., Beaty, B., Wittevrongel, L., & Lin, C. (2005). Expectations of patients and physicians regarding patient-accessible medical records. *Journal of Medical Internet Research, 7*(2), e13. doi:10.2196/jmir.7.2.e13 PMID:15914460

Sachs, A. G., & Cassel, C. K. (1990). Biomedical research involving older human subjects. *Law, Medicine & Health Care, 18*(3), 234–243. PMID:2122133

Stachura, M. E., & Khasanshina, E. V. (2007). *Telehomecare and remote monitoring: An outcomes overview.* The Advanced Medical Technology Association.

Suh, B., & Han, I. (2003). The impact of customer trust and perception of security control on the acceptance of electronic commerce. *International Journal of Electronics and Communications, 7*(3), 135–161.

Venkatesh, V., Morris, M., & Davis, F. D. (2003). User acceptance of information technology: Toward a unified view. *Management Information Systems Quarterly, 27*(3), 425.

Venkatesh, V., Speier, C., & Morris, M. G. (2002). User acceptance enablers in individual decision making about technology: toward an integrated model. *Decision Sciences, 33*(2), 297–316. doi:10.1111/j.1540-5915.2002.tb01646.x

KEY TERMS AND DEFINITIONS

An Innovation Network: An external network that enables and facilitate the move to more open innovation.

mHealth: Use of mobile information and communication technologies to support the practice of medicine and provide healthcare in a cost-efficient manner.

Mobile Information Communication Technology or Mobile ICT: Study of impacts that proliferation of mobile phones, computers, tablet, and smartphones have on other sectors of economy such as healthcare and education.

Open Innovation: A new way of looking at innovation. It states that firms can share risks and

rewards involved in investments in new ideas by collaborating and building innovation networks.

Remote Patient Monitoring: Any technology that enables monitoring of patients and transfer of health related data from and to a distanced location.

Technology Acceptance Model or TAM: Theory that explains how potential users of a particular technology come to accept and use a technology. Two most important factors of TAM are perceived usefulness and perceived ease-of-use. These two elements can greatly influence adoption of technology.

Technology Adoption: The process of accepting and utilizing a technology by users of that technology.

322

Compilation of References

Aanensen, D., Huntley, D., Feil, E., Al-Own, F., & Spratt, B. (2009). EpiCollect: Linking smartphones to web applications for epidemiology, ecology and community data collection. *PLoS ONE*, *4*(9), e6968. doi:10.1371/journal.pone.0006968 PMID:19756138

AARP Public Policy Institute. (2011). *Valuing the invaluable: 2011 update the growing contributions and costs of family caregiving*. Retrieved July 13, 2012 from http://www.aarp.org/relationships/caregiving/info-07-2011/valuing-the-invaluable.html

Aase, L., Goldman. D., Gould, M., Noseworthy, J., & Timimi, F. (2012). *Bringing the Social-media Revolution to Health Care*. Mayo Clinic Center for Social-Media.

Abbot, J., Lenka, M., Lerotholi, P. J., Mahao, M., & Sechaba, M. (2005). Vulnerability, and HIV/AIDS mainstreaming in Lesotho: Livelihoods recovery through agriculture program and secure the child. South Africa-Lesotho, Cooperative for Assistance and Relief Everywhere, Inc. (CARE).

Abbott, P., & Coenen, A. (2008). Globalisation and advances in information and communication technologies: The impact of nursing and health. *Nursing Outlook*, *56*(5), 238–246, 246.e2. doi:10.1016/j.outlook.2008.06.009 PMID:18922277

Ackerman, M. S. (1998). Augmenting organizational memory: A field study of answer garden. *ACM Transactions on Information Systems*, *16*(3), 203–224. doi:10.1145/290159.290160

ACN. (2013a). *Continuing Professional Development*. Retrieved 23 July 2013, from http://www.nursing.edu.au/CPDh

ACN. (2013b). *External CPD providers*. Retrieved 23 July, from http://www.nursing.edu.au/CPDh

Adams, N., Stubbs, V., & Woods, V. (2005). Psychological barriers to Internet usage among older adults in the U.K. *Medical Informatics and the Internet in Medicine*, *30*(1), 3–17. doi:10.1080/14639230500066876 PMID:16036626

Adams, S. A. (2010a). Blog-based applications and health information: Two case studies that illustrate important questions for Consumer Health Informatics (CHI) research. *International Journal of Medical Informatics*, *79*(6), e89–e96. doi:10.1016/j.ijmedinf.2008.06.009 PMID:18701344

Adams, S. A. (2010b). Revisiting the on-line health information reliability debate in the wake of web 2.0: an inter-disciplinary literature and website review. *International Journal of Medical Informatics*, *79*(6), 391–400. doi:10.1016/j.ijmedinf.2010.01.006 PMID:20188623

Adeyemi, A. A. (2004, March). *A Study on the use of Information Systems to Prevent HIV/AIDS in Lagos*. Paper presented at the Information and Communication Technologies in Healthcare Development 3rd Virtual Conference in Internet. New York, NY.

Administration on Aging. (2011). *Supporting family caregivers through Title III of the OAA (Research Brief No. 5)*. Author.

Affrinovator. (2011). *Upsurge in facebook and social media activity from African youth*. Retrieved January 5, 2013, from http://www.movements.org/blog/entry/upsurge-in-facebook-and-social-media-activityfrom-african-youth/

Agency for Healthcare Research and Quality. (2011). Improving Consumer Health IT Application Development: Lessons from Other Industries--Background Report (AHRQ Publication No. 11-0065-EF). Rockville, MD: AHRQ.

AHIMA. (2007). *Statement on Quality Healthcare Data and Information.* Retrieved 10 Jan 2013, from http://library.ahima.org/xpedio/groups/public/documents/ahima/bok1_047492.pdf

AHPRA. (2013). *Australian Health Practitioner Regulation Agency Registration Standards.* Retrieved 24 July 2013, from http://www.ahpra.gov.au/Registration/Registration-Standards.aspx

AHS. (2013). *Alberta Health Services.* Retrieved October 17, 2013 from www.albertahealthservices.ca/mobile.asp

Ajzen, I. (1991). The theory of planned behavior. *Organizational Behavior and Human Decision Processes, 50*(2), 179–211. doi:10.1016/0749-5978(91)90020-T

Alali, H., & Salim, J. (2013). Virtual Communities of Practice Success Model to Support Knowledge Sharing behaviour in Healthcare Sector. *Procedia Technology, 11*(0), 176–183. doi:10.1016/j.protcy.2013.12.178

Albrecht, U. V., & Gonnermann, A. (2013). *Appreciem – Appropriate reporting of EbM content in electronic media.* Retrieved January 21, 2014 from http://www.appreciem-statement.org

Albrecht, U. V., von Jan, U., & Gonnermann, A. (2013). *Appropriate reporting of EbM content in electronic media – APPRECIEM.* Paper presented at Medicine 2.0 ´13. London, UK.

Albrecht, U. V., von Jan, U., Pramann, O., & Matthies, H. (2012). *I, app: Trustworthy medical apps.* Paper presented at T11 – Village of the Future – Pillar 5: Social and Policy Incentive Framework. Pisa, Italy.

Albrecht, U. V. (2013). Transparency of health-apps for trust and decision making. *Journal of Medical Internet Research, 15*(12), e277. doi:10.2196/jmir.2981 PMID:24449711

Albrecht, U. V., Matthies, H., & Pramann, O. (2012). Vertrauenswürdige Medical Apps. In H. Reiterer, & O. Deussen (Eds.), *Mensch & Computer 2012 – Workshopband: Interaktiv informiert – allgegenwärtig und allumfassend!?* (pp. 261–266). München: Oldenbourg Verlag.

Albrecht, U. V., von Jan, U., & Pramann, O. (2013). Standard reporting for medical apps. *Studies in Health Technology and Informatics, 190,* 201–203. PMID:23823422

Albrecht, U.-V., von Jan, U., Sedlacek, L., Groos, S., Suerbaum, S., & Vonberg, R.-P. (2013). Standardized, app-based disinfection of ipads in a clinical and nonclinical setting: Comparative analysis. *Journal of Medical Internet Research, 15*(8), e176. doi:10.2196/jmir.2643 PMID:23945468

AlGhamdi, K. M., & Moussa, N. A. (2012). Internet use by the public to search for health-related information. *International Journal of Medical Informatics, 81*(6), 363–373. doi:10.1016/j.ijmedinf.2011.12.004 PMID:22217800

Altamirano, A. (2011). *Why is real-time so appealing?* Retrieved August 21, 2012, from http://www.altamirano.org/socialmedia/why-is-real-time-so-appealing/

ALTC. (2008). *e-Portfolio use by university students in Australia: Informing excellence in policy and practice.* Australian E-Portfolio Project final Report. Retrieved 20 July 2011, from http://www.altc.edu.au/resources?text=Australian+E-Portfolio+Project

Altman, D., Moher, D., & Schulz, K. F. (2012). Improving the reporting of randomised trials: The CONSORT Statement and beyond. *Statistics in Medicine, 31*(25), 2985–2997. doi:10.1002/sim.5402 PMID:22903776

American National Standards Institute & Association For the Advancement of Medical Instrumentation. (2009). ANSI/AAMI HE75, 2009 Ed. - Human factors engineering - Design of medical devices. Arlington, VA: American National Standards Institute.

Anders, S., Woods, D. D., Patterson, E. S., & Schweikhart, S. (2008). Shifts in Functions of a New Technology over Time: An Analysis of Logged Electronic Intensive Care Unit Interventions. *Proceedings of the Human Factors and Ergonomics Society Annual Meeting, 52*(12), 870-874.

Andersen, N. B., & Söderqvist, T. (2012). *Social Media and Public Health Research* (Working Paper/Technical Report). Faculty of Science, University of Copenhagen.

Andersen, K. M., Medaglia, R., & Henriksen, H. Z. (2012). Social media in public health care: Impact domain propositions. *Government Information Quarterly, 29*(4), 462–469. doi:10.1016/j.giq.2012.07.004

Anders, S., Albert, R., Miller, A., Weinger, M. B., Doig, A. K., Behrens, M., & Agutter, J. (2012). Evaluation of an integrated graphical display to promote acute change detection in ICU patients. *International Journal of Medical Informatics, 81*(12), 842–851. doi:10.1016/j.ijmedinf.2012.04.004 PMID:22534099

Anders, S., Miller, A., Joseph, P., Fortenberry, T., Woods, M., Booker, R., & France, D. (2011). Blood product positive patient identification: Comparative simulation-based usability test of two commercial products. *Transfusion, 51*(11), 2311–2318. doi:10.1111/j.1537-2995.2011.03185.x PMID:21599676

Android. (2013). *Android application.* Retrieved March 4, 2013, from http://www.Android.com/

ANF. (2013). *Continuing Professional Education.* Retrieved 25 July 2013, from http://anf.org.au/pages/cpe

Angaran, D. M. (1999). Telemedicine and Telepharmacy: Current status and future implications. *American Journal of Health-System Pharmacy, 56*(14), 405–426. PMID:10428449

ANMAC. (2012). *Australian Nursing and Midwifery Accreditation Council Registered Nurse Accreditation Standards.* Retrieved 23 July 2013, from http://www.anmac.org.au/sites/default/files/documents/ANMAC_RN_Accreditation_Standards_2012.pdf

ANMC. (2006). *Australian Nursing and Midwifery Competency Standards for Nurses and Midwives.* Retrieved 26 February 2011, from http://www.nursingmidwiferyboard.gov.au/Codes-and-Guidelines.aspx

Arata, G. (2011). *#TwitterPA T3/2011: Mapping the Presence and Activities of the Italian Public Bodies on Twitter.* Retrieved December 29, 2013, from http://t.co/lC5lEKMFK0

Archambault, P. M., Van De Belt, T. H., Grajales, F. J., III, Eysenbach, G., & Aubin, K. (2012). *Wikis and Collaborative Writing Applications in Health Care: Preliminary Results of a Scoping Review.* iPROCEEDINGS Medicine 2.0 Boston. Retrieved from http://www.medicine20congress.com/ocs/index.php/med/med2012/paper/view/994

Archer, N., Keshavjee, K., Demers, C., & Lee, R. (2014). Online self-management interventions for chronically ill patients: Cognitive impairment and technology issues. *International Journal of Medical Informatics, 83*(4), 264–272. doi:10.1016/j.ijmedinf.2014.01.005 PMID:24507762

Arksey, H., & O'Malley, L. (2005). Scoping Studies: Towards a Methodological Framework. *International Journal of Social Research Methodology, 8*(1), 19–32. doi:10.1080/1364557032000119616

Armstrong, A., & Hagel, I. J. (1996). The Real Value of ON-LINE Communities. *Harvard Business Review, 74*(3), 134–141.

Armstrong, K., & Kendall, E. (2010). Translating knowledge into practice and policy: The role of knowledge networks in primary health care. *The Health Information Management Journal, 39*(2), 9–17. PMID:20577019

Armstrong, R. M. (2012). App. review-FoodSwitch. *The Medical Journal of Australia, 196*(3), 207. doi:10.5694/mja12.10203

Årsand, E., & Demiris, G. (2008). User-centered methods for designing patient-centric self-help tools. *Informatics for Health & Social Care, 33*(3), 158–169. doi:10.1080/17538150802457562 PMID:18850399

Årsand, E., Frøisland, D. H., Skrøvseth, S. O., Chomutare, T., Tatara, N., Hartvigsen, G., & Tufano, J. T. (2012). Mobile health applications to assist patients with diabetes: Lessons learned and design implications. *Journal of Diabetes Science and Technology, 6*(5), 1197–1206. doi:10.1177/193229681200600525 PMID:23063047

Audiweb. (2013). Online l'81% della popolazione italiana tra 11 e 74 anni. *Prima Comunicazione Online.* Retrieved July 28, 2013, from http://www.primaonline.it/2013/07/23/169869/online-l81-della-popolazione-italiana-tra-11-e-74-anni/

Ausburn, L., & Ausburn, F. (2004). Desktop Virtual Reality: A Powerful New Technology for Teaching and Research in Industrial Teacher Education. *Journal of Industrial Teacher Education, 41*(4), 33–58.

Australian Health Ministers' Conference. (2008). *National E-Health Strategy*. Author.

Australian Institute of Health and Welfare (AIHW). (2010). *Australia's health 2010. Australia's health series no. 12. Cat. no. AUS 122*. Canberra, Australia: AIHW.

Australian Institute of Health and Welfare (AIHW). (2012). *Risk factors contributing to chronic disease chronic disease, Cat. no. PHE 157*. Canberra, Australia: AIHW.

Avnet, L. (2013). Twitter could be useful in tracking disease outbreaks, study suggest. *Mashable*. Retrieved February 5, 2013, from http://www.huffingtonpost.com/2013/01/24/twitter-disease-outbreaks_n_2543495.html

Baghaei, N., Kimani, S., Freyne, J., Brindal, E., Berkovsky, S., & Smith, G. (2011). Engaging Families in Lifestyle Changes through Social Networking. *International Journal of Human-Computer Interaction, 27*(10), 971–990. doi:10.1080/10447318.2011.555315

Bail, K. D. (2003). Electronic tagging of people with dementia: Devices may be preferable to locked doors. *BMJ, 326*(7383), 281. doi:10.1136/bmj.326.7383.281 PMID:12560288

Baker, D. W. (2006). The meaning and the measure of health literacy. *Journal of General Internal Medicine, 21*(8), 878–883. doi:10.1111/j.1525-1497.2006.00540.x PMID:16881951

Bakken, S., Cimino, J. J., & Hripcsak, G. (2004). Promoting patient safety and enabling evidence-based practice through informatics. *Medical Care, 42*(2Suppl), II49–II56. PMID:14734942

Bandura, A. (1973). *Aggression: A social learning analysis*. Englewood Cliffs, NJ: Prentice Hall.

Bandura, A. (1977). *Social learning theory*. Englewood Cliffs, NJ: Prentice Hall.

Bardram, J., Mihailidis, A., & Wan, D. (Eds.), *Pervasive Computing in Healthcare*. New York: CRC Press.

Bardus, M. (2011). The Web 2.0 and Social Media Technologies for Pervasive Health Communication: Are They Effective? *Studies in Communication Sciences, 11*(1), 119–136.

Baroudi, J. J., Olson, M. H., & Ives, B. (1986). An empirical study of the impact of user involvement on system usage and information satisfaction. *Communications of the ACM, 29*(3), 232–238. doi:10.1145/5666.5669

Barton, A. J. (2012). The regulation of mobile health applications. *BMC Medicine, 10*(46). PMID:22569114

Bautista, C. (2013). Twitter can help health officials track outbreaks. *Mashable*. Retrieved March 5, 2013, from http://mashable.com/2013/01/24/twitter-can-track-disease-outbreaks/

Beck, R. S., Daughtridge, R., & Sloane, P. D. (2002). Physician-patient communication in the primary care office: A systematic review. *The Journal of the American Board of Family Practice, 15*(1), 25–38. PMID:11841136

Beer, M., Slack, F., & Armitt, G. (2005). Collaboration and teamwork: Immersion and presence in an online learning environment. *Information Systems Frontiers, 7*(1), 27–37. doi:10.1007/s10796-005-5336-9

Bell, L. M., Grundmeier, R., Localio, R., Zorc, J., Fiks, A. G., Zhang, X., & Guevara, J. P. (2010). Electronic health record-based decision support to improve asthma care: A cluster-randomized trial. *Pediatrics, 125*(4), e770–e777. doi:10.1542/peds.2009-1385 PMID:20231191

Bembridge, E., Levett-Jones, T., & Yeun-Sim Jeong, S. (2011). The transferability of information and communication technology skills from university to the workplace: A qualitative descriptive study. *Nurse Education Today, 31*(3), 245–252. doi:10.1016/j.nedt.2010.10.020 PMID:21093125

Bertot, J. C., Jaeger, P. T., & Grimes, J. M. (2010). Using ICTs to create a culture of trasparency: E-government and social media as openness and anti-corruption tools for societies. *Government Information Quarterly, 27*(3), 264–271. doi:10.1016/j.giq.2010.03.001

Bertot, J. C., Jaeger, P. T., & Hansen, D. (2012). The impact of policies on government on social media usage: Issues, challenges, and recommendations. *Government Information Quarterly*, *29*(1), 30–40. doi:10.1016/j.giq.2011.04.004

Bertulis, R., & Cheeseborough, J. (2008). The Royal College of Nursing's information needs survey of nurses and health professionals. *Health Information and Libraries Journal*, *25*(3), 186–197. doi:10.1111/j.1471-1842.2007.00755.x PMID:18796079

Bhaumik, S. (2013). BRICS nations agree to collaborate on research and public health challenges. *BMJ (Clinical Research Ed.)*, *346*, f369. PMID:23335476

Bielli, E., Carminati, F., La Capra, S., Lina, M., Brunelli, C., & Tamburini, M. (2004). A wireless health outcomes monitoring system (WHOMS), Development and field testing with cancer patients using mobile phones. *BMC Medical Informatics and Decision Making*, *4*(1), 7–7. doi:10.1186/1472-6947-4-7 PMID:15196308

Binks, M., van Mierlo, T., & Edwards, C.L. (2012). Relationships of the Psychological Influence of Food and Barriers to Lifestyle Change to Weight and Utilization of Online Weight Loss Tools. *The Open Medical Informatics Journal*, (6), 9-14.

Bjornland, D., Goh, E., Haanæs, K., Kainu, T., & Kennedy, S. (2012). *The Socio-Economic Impact of Mobile Health*. The Boston Consulting Group.

Bluetooth, S. I. G. (2007). *Specification of the Bluetooth system*. Core Version 1.1. 1 February 22, 2001.

Blumenthal, D. (2010). Launching HITECH. *The New England Journal of Medicine*, *362*(5), 382–385. doi:10.1056/NEJMp0912825 PMID:20042745

Bodenheimer, T., Wagner, E. H., & Grumbach, K. (2002). Improving primary care for patients with chronic illness. *Journal of the American Medical Association*, *288*(15), 1909–1914. doi:10.1001/jama.288.15.1909 PMID:12377092

BodHuin. T., & Totorella, M. (2003). Using grid technologies for web-enabling legacy systems. In *Proceedings of Eleventh Annual International Workshop on Software Technology and Engineering Practice (STEP'03)*, (pp. 186-195). STEP.

Boisvert, S. (2012). An enterprise look at mHealth. *Journal of Healthcare Risk Management*, *32*(2), 44–52. doi:10.1002/jhrm.21094 PMID:22996431

Bonsón, E., Torres, L., Royo, S., & Flores, F. (2012). Local e-goverment 2.0: Social media and corporate transparency in municipalities. *Government Information Quarterly*, *29*(2), 123–132. doi:10.1016/j.giq.2011.10.001

Booth, A., Sutton, A., & Falzon, L. (2003). Working together: Supporting projects through action learning. *Health Information and Libraries Journal*, *20*(4), 225–231. doi:10.1111/j.1471-1842.2003.00461.x PMID:14641495

Borycki, E. M., & Kushniruk, A. W. (2008). Where do Technology-Induced Errors Come From? Towards a Model for Conceptualizing and Diagnosing Errors Caused by Technology. In A. W. Kushniruk, & E. M. Borycki (Eds.), *Human, Social, and Organizational Aspects of Health Information Systems* (pp. 148–166). Hershey, PA: IGI Global. doi:10.4018/978-1-59904-792-8.ch009

Borycki, E., Foster, J., Sahama, T., Frisch, N., & Kushniruk, A. (2013). Developing national level informatics competencies for undergraduate nurses: Methodological approaches from Australia and Canada. *Studies in Health Technology and Informatics*, *183*, 345–349. PMID:23388312

Borycki, E., Kushniruk, A., Kuwata, S., & Watanabe, A. (2009). Simulations to assess medication administration systems. In B. Staudinger, V. Höss, & H. Ostermann (Eds.), *Nursing and clinical informatics: Socio-technical approaches* (pp. 144–159). Hershey, PA: Information Science Reference. doi:10.4018/978-1-60566-234-3.ch010

Botts, N. E., Horan, T. A., & Thoms, B. P. (2011). HealthATM: Personal health cyberinfrastructure for underserved populations. *American Journal of Preventive Medicine*, *40*(5), S115–S122. doi:10.1016/j.amepre.2011.01.016 PMID:21521584

Bouman, M. P. (1998). *The turtle and the peacock: Collaboration for social change*. Wageningen Agricultural University.

boyd, D. M., & Ellison, N. B. (2007). Social network sites: Definition, history and scholarship. *Journal of Computer-Mediated Communication, 13*(1), 210-230.

Bramley, D., Riddell, T., Whittaker, R., Corbett, T., Lin, R., Wills, M., & Rodgers, A. (2005). Smoking cessation using mobile phone text messaging is as effective in Maori as non-Maori. *The New Zealand Medical Journal*, *118*(1216), U1494. PMID:15937529

Brandt, C. L., Dalum, P., Skov-Ettrup, L., & Tolstrup, J. S. (2013). After all–It doesn't kill you to quit smoking: An explorative analysis of the blog in a smoking cessation intervention. *Scandinavian Journal of Public Health*, *41*(7), 655–661. doi:10.1177/1403494813489602 PMID:23696257

BrandtJ.WeissN.KlemmerS. R. (2007). txt 4 l8r: Lowering the burden for diary studies under mobile conditions. In Proceedings of CHI'07 Extended Abstracts on Human Factors in Computing Systems (pp. 2303-2308). ACM. 10.1145/1240866.1240998

Brath, H., Morak, J., Kästenbauer, T., Modre-Osprian, R., Strohner-Kästenbauer, H., Schwarz, M., & Schreier, G. (2013). Mobile health (mHealth) based medication adherence measurement – A pilot trial using electronic blisters in diabetes patients. *British Journal of Clinical Pharmacology*, *76*, 47–55. doi:10.1111/bcp.12184 PMID:24007452

Brooks, F., & Scott, P. (2006a). Exploring knowledge work and leadership in online midwifery communication. *Journal of Advanced Nursing*, *55*(4), 510–520. doi:10.1111/j.1365-2648.2006.03937.x PMID:16866846

Brooks, F., & Scott, P. (2006b). Knowledge work in nursing and midwifery: An evaluation through computer-mediated communication. *International Journal of Nursing Studies*, *43*(1), 83–97. doi:10.1016/j.ijnurstu.2005.02.003 PMID:16326164

Brown, M., & Muchira, R. (2004). Investigating the Relationship between Internet Privacy Concerns and Online Purchase Behavior. *Journal of Electronic Commerce Research*, *5*(1), 62–70.

Brownstein, C. A., Brownstein, J. S., Williams, D. S., Wicks, P., & Heywood, J. A. (2009). The power of social networking in medicine. *Nature Biotechnology*, *27*, 888–890. doi:10.1038/nbt1009-888 PMID:19816437

Brunetto, Y., Farr-Wharton, R., & Shacklock, K. (2012). Communication, Training, wellbeing and commitment across generations. *Nursing Outlook*, *60*(1), 7–15. doi:10.1016/j.outlook.2011.04.004 PMID:21703652

Bryer, T. (2010). Across the great divide: Social media and networking for citizens engagement. In J. H. Svara, & J. Denhardt (Eds.), *Connected communities, local government as partners in citizens engagement and community building* (pp. 73-79). Retrieved March 10, 2011, from http://www.tlgconference.org/communitycon-nectionswhitepaper.pdf

Buijink, A. W., Visser, B. J., & Marshall, L. (2013). Medical apps for smartphones: Lack of evidence undermines quality and safety. *Evidence-Based Medicine*, *18*(3), 90–92. doi:10.1136/eb-2012-100885 PMID:22923708

Burgess, J., Bruns, A., & Hjort, L. (2013). Emerging methods for digital research: An introduction. *Journal of Broadcasting & Electronic Media*, *57*(1), 1–3. doi:10.1080/08838151.2012.761706

Burns, J. (2012). The Next Frontier: Patient Engagement. *Managed Care*. Retrieved from http://www.managed-caremag.com/archives/1206/1206.engagement.html

Byron, P., Albury, K., & Evers, C. (2013). It would be weird to have that on Facebook: Young people's use of social media and the risk of sharing sexual health information. *Reproductive Health Matters*, *21*(41), 35–44. doi:10.1016/S0968-8080(13)41686-5 PMID:23684185

California Environmental Health Investigation Branch. (2012). California Environmental Health Tracking Program. *Environmental Health Investigation Branch*. Retrieved June 4, 2012, from http://www.ehib.org/project.jsp?project_key=EHSS01

Camarinha-Matos, L. M., & Afsarmanesh, H. (2011). *Collaborative Ecosystems in Ageing Support*. Paper presented at PRO-VE'11. São Paulo, Brazil.

Canadian Council on Learning. (2008). *Health Literacy in Canada: A Healthy Understanding*. Retrieved March 17, 2013, from http://www.ccl-cca.ca/pdfs/HealthLiteracy/HealthLiteracyReportFeb2008E.pdf

Carpenter, D. M., Elstad, E. A., Blalock, S. J., & Devellis, R. F. (2014). Conflicting Medication Information: Prevalence, Sources, and Relationship to Medication Adherence. *Journal of Health Communication*, *19*(1), 67–81. doi:10.1080/10810730.2013.798380 PMID:24015878

Casaló, L. V., Flavián, C., & Guinalíu, M. (2010). Determinants of the intention to participate in firm-hosted online travel communities and effects on consumer behavioral intentions. *Tourism Management*, *31*(6), 898–911. doi:10.1016/j.tourman.2010.04.007

Cayzer, S. (2004). Semantic blogging and decentralized knowledge management. *Communications of the ACM*, *47*(12), 47–52. doi:10.1145/1035134.1035164

Celcom. (2012). Celcom focuses on innovative mobile healthcare solutions. *Celcom*. Retrieved July 8, 2012, from http://www.theborneopost.com/2012/06/08/celcom-focuses-on-innovative-mobile-healthcare-solutions/

Censis –Forum per la Ricerca Biomedica. (2012). *Quale futuro per il rapporto medico paziente nella nuova sanità?* Retrieved June 28, 2013, from http://www.sanita.ilsole24ore.com/art/dibattiti-e-idee/2012-10-02/informazione-temi-sanitari-internet-130026.php

Censis-Ucsi. (2011). *I media tra crisi e personali nell'era digitale*. Retrieved July 10, 2013, from http://www.censis.it/17?shadow_pubblicazione=112567

Censis-Ucsi. (2013). *L'evoluzione digitale della specie*. Retrieved December 20, 2013, from http://www.censis.it/17?shadow_pubblicazione=120563

Center for Connected Health Policy. (2013). *What is telehealth?* Retrieved July 27, 2013 from http://cchpca.org/

Center for Disease Control and Prevention (CDC). (2012). *CDC'S Guide to Writing for Social Media*. Retrieved July 10, 2013, from http://www.cdc.gov/socialmedia/tools/guidelines/pdf/guidetowritingforsocialmedia.pdf

Centers for Medicare & Medicaid Services. (2013). *Medicare program - general information*. Retrieved July 12, 2013, from http://www.cms.gov/

Centres for Disease Control and Prevention. (2010). *National environmental public health tracking network*. Center for Disease Control and Prevention. Retrieved June 5, 2012, from http://ephtracking.cdc.gov/showLocationLanding.action

Chang, H. H., & Chuang, S.-S. (2011). Social capital and individual motivations on knowledge sharing: Participant involvement as a moderator. *Information & Management*, *48*(1), 9–18. doi:10.1016/j.im.2010.11.001

Charness, N., & Boot, W. R. (2009). Aging and information technology use: Potential and barriers. *Current Directions in Psychological Science*, *18*(5), 253–258. doi:10.1111/j.1467-8721.2009.01647.x

Chau, P. Y. K., & Hu, P. J. H. (2002). Investigating healthcare professionals' decisions to accept telemedicine technology: An empirical test of competing theories. *Information & Management*, *39*(4), 297–311. doi:10.1016/S0378-7206(01)00098-2

Chen, C. J., & Hung, S. W. (2010). To give or to receive? Factors influencing members' knowledge sharing and community promotion in professional virtual communities. *Information & Management*, *47*(4), 226–236. doi:10.1016/j.im.2010.03.001

Chen, E., Medonca, E., McKnight, L., Stetson, P., Lei, J., & Cimino, J. (2003). PalmCIS: A wireless handheld application for satisfying clinician information needs. *Journal of the American Medical Informatics Association*, *11*(1), 19–28. doi:10.1197/jamia.M1387 PMID:14527976

ChengS. (2011). The research framework of eye-tracking based mobile device usability evaluation. In Proceedings of the 1st International Workshop on Pervasive Eye Tracking & Mobile Eye-Based Interaction (pp. 21-26). ACM. 10.1145/2029956.2029964

Chen, I. Y. L. (2007). The factors influencing members' continuance intentions in professional virtual communities—A longitudinal study. *Journal of Information Science*, *33*(4), 451. doi:10.1177/0165551506075323

Chen, I.Y.L., & Chen, N.S., & Kinshuk. (2009). Examining the Factors Influencing Participants' Knowledge Sharing Behavior in Virtual Learning Communities. *Journal of Educational Technology & Society, 12*(1), 134–148.

Chen, Y. F., Madan, J., Welton, N., Yahaya, I., Aveyard, P., & Bauld, L. et al. (2012). Effectiveness and cost-effectiveness of computer and other electronic aids for smoking cessation: A systematic review and network meta-analysis. *Health Technology Assessment, 16*(38). doi: doi:10.3310/hta16380 PMID:23046909

Chesbrough, H. (2003). *Open Innovation: The New Imperative for Creating and Profiting From Technology.* Harvard Business School Press.

Chetley, A. (2006). *Improving health, connecting people: The role of ICTs in the health sector of developing countries.* InfoDev.

Cheung, C. M. K., & Lee, M. K. O. (2009). Understanding the sustainability of a virtual community: Model development and empirical test. *Journal of Information Science, 35*(3), 279–298. doi:10.1177/0165551508099088

Chhablani, J., Kaja, S., & Shah, V. (2012). Smartphones in ophthalmology. *Indian Journal of Ophthalmology, 60*(2), 127–131. doi:10.4103/0301-4738.94054 PMID:22446908

Chiu, C. M., Hsu, M. H., & Wang, E. T. G. (2006). Understanding knowledge sharing in virtual communities: An integration of social capital and social cognitive theories. *Decision Support Systems, 42*(3), 1872–1888. doi:10.1016/j.dss.2006.04.001

Choi, S. Y., Kang, Y. S., & Lee, H. (2008). The effects of socio-technical enablers on knowledge sharing: an exploratory examination. *Journal of Information Science, 34*(5), 742–754. doi:10.1177/0165551507087710

Chou, W., Hunt, Y., Beckjord, E., Moser, R., & Hesse, B. (2009). Social media use in the United States: implications for health communication. *Journal of Medical Internet Research, 11*(4), 48. doi:10.2196/jmir.1249 PMID:19945947

Christoper, A. (2004). *Tracing the evolution of social software.* Retrieved August 21, 2012, from http://www.lifewithalacrity.com/2004/10/tracing_the_evo.html

Chunara, R., Andrews, J. R., & Brownstein, J. S. (2012). Social and news media enable estimation of epidemiological patterns early in the 2010 Haitian cholera outbreak. *The American Journal of Tropical Medicine and Hygiene, 86*(1), 39–45. doi:10.4269/ajtmh.2012.11-0597 PMID:22232449

Chute, C. G., Beck, S. A., Fisk, T. B., & Mohr, D. N. (2010). The Enterprise Data Trust at Mayo Clinic: A semantically integrated warehouse of biomedical data. *Journal of the American Medical Informatics Association, 17*(2), 131–135. doi:10.1136/jamia.2009.002691 PMID:20190054

Cimino, J. J., Patel, V. L., & Kushniruk, A. W. (2002). The patient clinical information system (PatCIS), Technical solutions for and experiences with giving patients access to their electronic medical records. *International Journal of Medical Informatics, 68*(1-3), 113–127. doi:10.1016/S1386-5056(02)00070-9 PMID:12467796

CINAHL ®. (n.d.). Retrieved 1 August 2012, from http://web.ebscohost.com/ehost/search/selectdb?sid=a54fae89-7491-46d4-953c-958345858902%40sessionmgr4&vid=1&hid=28

Clarke, A., Lewis, D., Cole, I., & Ringrose, L. (2005). A strategic approach to developing e learning capability for healthcare. *Health Information and Libraries Journal, 22*(2), 33–41. doi:10.1111/j.1470-3327.2005.00611.x PMID:16279974

Cleland, J., Caldow, J., & Ryan, D. (2007). A qualitative study of the attitudes of patients and staff to the use of mobile phone technology for recording and gathering asthma data. *Journal of Telemedicine and Telecare, 13*(2), 85–89. doi:10.1258/135763307780096230 PMID:17359572

Cline, R. J. W., & Haynes, K. M. (2001). Consumer health information seeking on the internet: The state of the art. *Health Education Research, 16*(6), 671–692. doi:10.1093/her/16.6.671 PMID:11780707

Coleman, K., Austin, B. T., Brach, C., & Wagner, E. H. (2009). Evidence on the Chronic Care Model in the new millennium. *Health Affairs, 28*(1), 75–85. doi:10.1377/hlthaff.28.1.75 PMID:19124857

Coleman, P., & Meyer, R. C. (1990). *Entertainment for social change.* Baltimore, MD: John Hopkins University Center for Communication Programs.

Colineau, N., & Paris, C. (2010). Talking about your health to strangers: Understanding the use of online social networks by patients. *New Review of Hypermedia and Multimedia*, *16*(1-2), 141–160. doi:10.1080/13614 568.2010.496131

Collins, R. L., Kashdan, T. B., & Gollnisch, G. (2003). The feasibility of using cellular phones to collect ecological momentary assessment data: Application to alcohol consumption. *Experimental and Clinical Psychopharmacology*, *11*(1), 73–78. doi:10.1037/1064-1297.11.1.73 PMID:12622345

Commonwealth Fund. (2005). *Issue brief: A look at working-age caregivers' roles, health concerns, and need for support*. Retrieved November 2, 2010, from http://www.commonwealthfunorg

ComtoisG.SalisburyJ. I.SunY. (2012). A smartphone-based platform for analyzing physiological audio signals. In Proceedings of Bioengineering Conference (NEBEC), 2012 38th Annual Northeast (pp. 69–70). IEEE. 10.1109/NEBC.2012.6206966

Comunello, F. (Ed.). (2012). *Networked Sociability and Individualism: Technology for Personal and Professional Relationships*. Hershey, PA: IGI Global.

Condon, B. (2013). The present state of presence in technology. *Nursing Science Quarterly*, *26*(1), 24–28. doi:10.1177/0894318412466738 PMID:23247344

Consolvo, S., Everitt, K., Smith, I., & Landay, J. (2006). *Design requirements for technologies that encourage physical activity*. doi:10.1145/1124772.1124840

CONSORT. (2010). *CONSORT Statement*. Retrieved January 21, 2014 from http://www.consort-statement.org/consort-statement/overview0/

Contini, F., & Lanzara, G. F. (2009). *ICT and innovation in the public sector: European studies in the making of e-government*. New York, NY: Palgrave.

Cook, R. I., Render, M., & Woods, D. D. (2000). Gaps in the continuity of care and progress on patient safety. *British Medical Journal*, *320*(7237), 791–794. doi:10.1136/bmj.320.7237.791 PMID:10720370

Corlazzoli, V. (2013). *Assessing impact with media content analysis*. Retrieved September 6, 2013 from http://dmeforpeace.org/discuss/assessing-impact-media-content-analysis

Correa, T., Willard Hinsley, A., & de Zúñiga, H. G. (2010). Who interacts on the Web? The intersection of users' personality and social media use. *Computers in Human Behavior*, *26*(2), 247–253. doi:10.1016/j.chb.2009.09.003

Cosenza, V. (2013). *Osservatorio Social Media in Italia e Facebook*. Retrieved July 10, 2013, from www.vincos.it

Croll, A. (2011). *Who Owns Your Data?* Retrieved 17 December, 2012, from http://mashable.com/2011/01/12/data-ownership/

CSI. (2013). *motionPHR*. Retrieved October 8, 2013, from http://motionphr.com/

CTIA. The Wireless Association. (2012). *Wireless Quick Facts: Year-End Figures*. Retrieved September 30, 2013, from http://www.ctia.org/advocacy/research/index.cfm/aid/10323

Cummings, E. (2008). *An investigation of the influence of an online patient diary on the health outcomes and experiences of people with chronic obstructive pulmonary disease (COPD) participating in a mentored self-management clinical controlled trial*. (PhD Thesis). University of Tasmania, Hobart, Australia.

Cummings, E., Borycki, E. M., & Roehrer, E. (2013). Issues and considerations for healthcare consumers using mobile applications. *Studies in Health Technology and Informatics*, *183*, 227–231. PMID:23388288

Cummings, E., Chau, S., & Turner, P. (2009). Assessing a Patient-Centered E-Health Approach to Chronic Disease Self-Management. In E. V. Wilson (Ed.), *Patient-Centered E-Health*. Hershey, PA: Medical Information Science Reference.

Cummings, E., Robinson, A., Courtney-Pratt, H., Cameron-Tucker, H., Wood-Baker, R., & Walters, E. et al. (2010). Pathways Home: Comparing Voluntary IT and Non-IT Users Participating in a Mentored Self-Management Project. *Studies in Health Technology and Informatics*, *160*, 23–27. PMID:20841643

Cummings, E., & Turner, P. (2007). Considerations for deploying web and mobile technologies to support the building of patient self-efficacy and self-management of chronic illness. In L. Al-Hakim (Ed.), *Web Mobile-Based Applications for Healthcare Management*. Hershey, PA: Idea Group, Inc. doi:10.4018/978-1-59140-658-7.ch011

Cummings, E., & Turner, P. (2010). Patients at the Centre: Methodological Considerations for Evaluating Evidence from Health Interventions Involving Patients use of Web-Based Information Systems. *The Open Medical Informatics Journal*, *4*, 188–194. PMID:21594007

Davis, F. D. (1989). Perceived usefulness, perceived ease of use, and user acceptance of information technology. *MIS Quart*, *13*(3), 319–340. doi:10.2307/249008

Davis, R. (2009). Exploring Possibilities: Virtual Reality in Nursing Research. *Research and Theory for Nursing Practice: An International Journal*, *23*(2), 133–147. doi:10.1891/1541-6577.23.2.133 PMID:19558028

de Jongh, T., Gurol-Urganci, I., Vodopivec-Jamsek, V., Car, J., & Atun, R. (2012). Mobile phone messaging for facilitating self-management of long-term illnesses. *Cochrane Database of Systematic Reviews*, *12*. doi:10.1002/14651858.CD007459.pub2 PMID:23235644

Dede, C. (2005). *Planning for Neomillennial Learning Styles: Implications for Investments in Technology and Faculty*. Retrieved 30 July 2013, from www.educause.edu/educatingthenetgen

DEEWR. (2008). *Digital education revolution: Overview*. Retrieved 20 June 2013, from http://www.digitaleducationrevolution.gov.au/about.htm

DeLone, W., & McLean, E. (1992). Information systems success: The quest for the dependent variable. *Information Systems Research*, *3*(1), 60–95. doi:10.1287/isre.3.1.60

Demiris, G., Afrin, L. B., Speedie, S., Courtney, K. L., Sondhi, M., Vimarlund, V., & Lynch, C. (2008). Patient-centered applications: Use of information technology to promote disease management and wellness. *Journal of the American Medical Informatics Association*, *15*(1), 8–13. doi:10.1197/jamia.M2492 PMID:17947617

Denecke, K., Krieck, M., Otrusina, L., Smrz, P., Dolog, P., Nejdl, W., & Velasco, E. (2013). How to Exploit Twitter & Co. for Public Health Monitoring? *Methods of Information in Medicine*. doi:10.3414/ME12-02-0010

Denecke, K., & Nejdl, W. (2009). How valuable is medical social media data? Content Analysis of the Medical Web. *Journal of Information Science*, *179*, 1870–1880. doi:10.1016/j.ins.2009.01.025

Denecke, K., & Soltani, N. (2013). The Burgeoning of Medical Social-Media Postings and the Need for Improved Natural Language Mapping Tools. In *Where Humans Meet Machines - Innovative Solutions for Knotty Natural-Language Problems*. Springer. doi:10.1007/978-1-4614-6934-6_2

Department of Environment. (2011). Air Pollutant Index Management System (APIMS). *Department of Environment Ministry of Natural Resources and Environment*. Retrieved June 5, 2011, from http://www.doe.gov.my/apims/

Department of Health New York. (2009). Glossary. *Department of Health*. Retrieved June 15, 2011, from http://www.health.ny.gov/environmental/public_health_tracking/about/glossary.htm

Depp, C. A., Mausbach, B., Granholm, E., Cardenas, V., Ben-Zeev, D., Patterson, T. L., & Jeste, D. V. (2010). Mobile interventions for severe mental illness: Design and preliminary data from three approaches. *The Journal of Nervous and Mental Disease*, *198*(10), 715–721. doi:10.1097/NMD.0b013e3181f49ea3 PMID:20921861

Detmer, D., Bloomrosen, M., Raymond, B., & Tang, P. (2008). Integrated Personal Health Records: Transformative Tools for Consumer-Centric Care. *BMC Medical Informatics and Decision Making*, *8*(45). PMID:18837999

DeWalt, D. A., Berkman, N. D., Sheridan, S., Lohr, K. N., & Pignone, M. P. (2004). Literacy and health outcomes: A systematic review of the literature. *Journal of General Internal Medicine*, *19*(12), 1228–1239. doi:10.1111/j.1525-1497.2004.40153.x PMID:15610334

Dexter, P. R., Perkins, S. M., Maharry, K. S., Jones, K., & McDonald, C. J. (2004). Inpatient computer-based standing orders vs physician reminders to increase influenza and pneumococcal vaccination rates: A randomized trial. *Journal of the American Medical Association*, 292(19), 2366–2371. doi:10.1001/jama.292.19.2366 PMID:15547164

Dickerson, S. S., Reinhart, A., Boemhke, M., & Akhu-Zaheya, L. (2011). Cancer as a Problem to Be Solved: Internet Use and Provider Communication by Men With Cancer. *Computers, Informatics, Nursing*, 29(7), 388–395. doi:10.1097/NCN.0b013e3181f9ddb1 PMID:20975535

Digital Scoreboard Agenda. (2012). *Life Online*. European Commission. Retrieved July 15, 2013, from https://ec.europa.eu/digital-agenda/sites/digital-agenda/files/scoreboard_life_online.pdf

DiPietro, M., Ferdig, R. E., Boyer, J., & Black, E. W. (2007). Towards a Framework for Understanding Electronic Educational Gaming. *Journal of Educational Multimedia and Hypermedia*, 16(3), 225–248.

Divall, P., Camosso-Stefinovic, J., & Baker, R. (2013). The use of personal digital assistants in clinical decision making by health care professionals: A systematic review. *Health Informatics Journal*, 19(1), 16–28. doi:10.1177/1460458212446761 PMID:23486823

DMC. (2013). *Detroit Medical Center*. Retrieved October 17, 2013, from www.dmc.org/apps

Docherty, C., Hoy, D., Topp, H., & Trinder, K. (2005). eLearning techniques supporting problem based learning in clinical simulation. *International Journal of Medical Informatics*, 74(7-8), 527–533. doi:10.1016/j.ijmedinf.2005.03.009 PMID:16043082

DoHA. (2013). *Welcome to eHealth.gov.au*. Retrieved 25 July, from http://www.ehealth.gov.au/internet/ehealth/publishing.nsf/Content/home

Dolan, P. L. (2014). *Health app. certificiation program halted*. Retrieved January 21, 2014 from http://exclusive.multibriefs.com/content/health-app-certification-program-halted

Doll, W. J., & Torkzadeh, G. (1991). The measurement of end-user computing satisfaction: Theoretical and methodological issues. *Management Information Systems Quarterly*, 15(1), 5–10. doi:10.2307/249429

Drimie, S. (2002). *The Impact of HIV/AIDS on Rural Households and Land Issues in Southern and Eastern Africa*. Retrieved February 2, 2013, from http://ftp.fao.org/docrep/nonfao/ad696e/ad696e00.pdf

Dubé, L., Bourhis, A., & Jacob, R. (2005). The impact of structuring characteristics on the launching of virtual communities of practice. *Journal of Organizational Change Management*, 18(2), 145–166. doi:10.1108/09534810510589570

Dumas, J. S., & Redish, J. (1999). *A practical guide to usability testing* (Rev. ed.). Norwood, NJ: Intellect Books.

Dutta, M. J. (2009). Health communication: trends and future directions. In J. C. Parker, & E. Thorson (Eds.), *Health communication in the new media landscape* (pp. 59–93). New York, NY: Springer Publishing Company.

Eddy, N. (2013). Smartphones Power Strong Growth in Mobile Phone Sales: IDC. *Eweek*, 6.

Edwards, A. (2009). *Engestrom's Developmental Work Research: Research as provoking change*. Retrieved August 21, 2011, from http://education.monash.edu.au/research/seminars/show.php?id=443&archive=tue

Effing, T., Monninkhof, E. M., van der Valk, P. D., van der Palen, J., van Herwaarden, C. L., & Partidge, M. R. et al. (2007). Self-management education for patients with chronic obstructive pulmonary disease. *Cochrane Database of Systematic Reviews*, 4. doi:10.1002/14651858.CD002990.pub2 PMID:17943778

Eichler, K., Wieser, S., & Brügger, U. (2009). The costs of limited health literacy: A systematic review. *International Journal of Public Health*, 54(5), 313–324. doi:10.1007/s00038-009-0058-2 PMID:19644651

Ellis, L., Showell, C., & Turner, P. (2013). Social Media and patient self management: Not all sites are created equal. In *Proceedings of Information Technology and Communications in Health (ITCH) Conference*. IOS Press.

EMBASE ®. (n.d.). Retrieved 6 November 2012, from http://www.embase.com/

Epic. (2013). *Epic Systems Corporation: Mobile Applications and Portals*. Retrieved October 8, 2013, from http://www.epic.com/software-phr.php

Epstein, M., & Howes, P. (2006, September-October). The Millennial Generation: Recruiting, Retaining and Managing. *Today's CPA*, 66-75.

European Environment Agency (EEA). (2011). *Air Pollution monitoring system*. Retrieved June 8, 2011, from http://www.eea.europa.eu/maps/ozone/map

Eurostat. (2011). Internet use in households and by individuals in 2011. *Statistics in Focus*, 66. Retrieved July 10, 2013, from http://epp.eurostat.ec.europa.eu/cache/ITY_OFFPUB/KS-SF-11-066/EN/KS-SF-11-066-EN.PDF

Eurostat. (2012). Internet use in households and by individuals in 2012. *Statistics in Focus*, 50. Retrieved July 10, 2013, from http://epp.eurostat.ec.europa.eu/cache/ITY_OFFPUB/KS-SF-12-050/EN/KS-SF-12-050-EN.PDF

Evans, R. S., Pestotnik, S. L., Classen, D. C., Clemmer, T. P., Weaver, L. K., Orme, J. F. Jr, & Burke, J. P. (1998). A computer-assisted management program for antibiotics and other antiinfective agents. *The New England Journal of Medicine*, *338*(4), 232–238. doi:10.1056/NEJM199801223380406 PMID:9435330

Evans, W. D., Wallace, J. L., & Snider, J. (2012). Pilot evaluation of the text4baby mobile health program. *BMC Public Health*, *12*(1), 1031. doi:10.1186/1471-2458-12-1031 PMID:23181985

Eysenbach, G., Yihune, G., Lampe, K., Cross, P., & Brickley, D. (2000). Quality management, certification and rating of health information on the net with medcertain: Using a medpics/rdf/xml metadata structure for implementing ehealth ethics and creating trust globally. *J Med Internet Res, 2*(2 Suppl), 2E1.

Eysenbach, G. (2005). The law of attrition. *Journal of Medical Internet Research*, *7*(1), e11. doi:10.2196/jmir.7.1.e11 PMID:15829473

Eysenbach, G. (2008). Medicine 2.0: Social networking, collaboration, participation, apomediation, and openness. *Journal of Medical Internet Research*, *10*(3), e22. doi:10.2196/jmir.1030 PMID:18725354

Eysenbach, G. (2008a). Credibility of Health Information and Digital Media: New Perspectives and Implications for Youth. In M. J. Metzger, & A. J. Flanagin (Eds.), *Digital Media, Youth, and Credibility* (pp. 123–154). Cambridge, MA: The MIT Press.

Eysenbach, G. (2011). Infodemiology and Infoveillance: Tracking Onlline Health Information and Cyberbehaviour for Public Health. *American Journal of Preventive Medicine*, *40*(5), 154–158. doi:10.1016/j.amepre.2011.02.006

Facebook. (2013). Retrieved May 7, 2013, from https://www.facebook.com/

Factbrowser.com. (2012a). Malaysia has 34MM mobile subscribers and 17.5MM internet users. *Factbrowser*. Retrieved May 6, 2013, from http://www.factbrowser.com/facts/6143/

Factbrowser.com. (2012b). 87.9% of Malaysians on the Internet access Facebook. *Factbrowser*. Retrieved May 6, 2013, from http://www.factbrowser.com/facts/3404/

Factbrowser.com. (2012c). Malaysia's mobile penetration is more than 100%, compared to 59% for internet and 41% for social media. *Factbrowser*. Retrieved May 6, 2013, from http://www.factbrowser.com/facts/4159/

Fang, Y. H., & Chiu, C. M. (2010). In justice we trust: Exploring knowledge-sharing continuance intentions in virtual communities of practice. *Computers in Human Behavior*, *26*(2), 235–246. doi:10.1016/j.chb.2009.09.005

Farin, E., Gramm, L., & Kosiol, D. (2011). Development of a questionnaire to assess communication preferences of patients with chronic illness. *Patient Education and Counseling*, *82*(1), 81–88. doi:10.1016/j.pec.2010.02.011 PMID:20219317

Farin, E., Gramm, L., & Schmidt, E. (2012). Taking into account patients' communication preferences: Instrument development and results in chronic back pain patients. *Patient Education and Counseling*, *86*(1), 41–48. doi:10.1016/j.pec.2011.04.012 PMID:21570795

Farvolden, P., Cunningham, J. A., van Mierlo, T., & Selby, P. (2009). Using E-health programs to overcome barriers to the effective treatment of mental health and addiction problems. *Journal of Technology in Human Services*, *27*(1), 5–22. doi:10.1080/15228830802458889

Fattori, G., & Pianelli, N. (2013). ASL e ospedali ai tempi di Twitter. *Il Sole24Ore Sanità, 16*(28), 8-9.

FDA. (2013). *Mobile Medical Applications - Food & Drug Administration (FDA): Draft Guidance for Industry and Food and Drug Administration Staff – Mobile Medical Applications*. Retrieved January 21, 2014 from http://www.fda.gov/medicaldevices/productsandmedicalprocedures/connectedhealth/mobilemedicalapplications/default.htm

Federal Drug Administration. (2011). *Draft Guidance for Industry and Food and Drug Administration Staff - Mobile Medical Applications*. Retrieved from http://x.co/1U9bc

Fernandez, I., Gonzalez, A., & Sabherwal, R. (2004). *Knowledge Management, solutions, technology*. Prentice-Hall, Inc.

Firefly. (2013). Social animals on the move in Asia: A social media & mobile perspective. *Firefly*. Retrieved May 5, 2013, from http://www.fireflymb.com/Libraries/Papers_and_Presentations/FireflyMillwardBrown_AMAP_Social_Animals.sflb.ashx

Fogg B. J. (2009). A behavior model for persuasive design. In Proceedings of the 4th International Conference on Persuasive Technology. ACM.

Fox, S. (2011). *Health Topics*. Pew Research Center's Internet & American Life Project. Retrieved from http://www.pewinternet.org/~/media//Files/Reports/2011/PIP_Health_Topics.pdf

Fox, S. (2011). *Health Topics: 80% of users look for health information online*. Washington, DC: Pew Internet & American Life Project. Retrieved from http://www.pewinternet.org/Reports/2011/HealthTopics.aspx

Fox, S. (2011). *The Social Life of Health Information*. Retrieved from http://www.pewinternet.org/Reports/2011/Social-Life-of-Health-Info.aspx

Fox, S., & Duggan, M. (2013). *Tracking for Health*. Pew Research Center's Internet & American Life Project. Retrieved from http://pewinternet.org/Reports/2013/Tracking-for-Health.aspx

Fox, S., & Duggan, M. (2013a). *Health Online 2013*. Washington, DC: Pew Internet & American Life Project. Retrieved July 20, 2013, from http://www.pewinternet.org/~/media//Files/Reports/PIP_HealthOnline.pdf

Fox, S., & Duggan, M. (2013b). *Tracking for Health*. Retrieved July 20, 2013, from http:pewinternet.org/Reports/2013/Tracking-for-Health.aspx

Fox, S., & Jones, S. (2009). *The social life of health information*. Washington, DC: Pew Internet & American Life Project. Retrieved from http://www.pewinternet.org/~/media//Files/Reports/009/PIP_Health_2009.pdf

Franco, O. H., de Laet, C., Peeters, A., Jonker, J., Mackenbach, J., & Nusselder, W. (2005). Effects of physical activity on life expectancy with cardiovascular disease. *Archives of Internal Medicine*, *165*(20), 2355–2360. doi:10.1001/archinte.165.20.2355 PMID:16287764

Free, C., Roberts, I., Knight, R., Robertson, S., Whittaker, R., Edwards, P., & Kenward, M. G. (2011). Smoking cessation support delivered via mobile phone text messaging (txt2stop), A single-blind, randomised trial. *Lancet*, *378*(9785), 49–55. doi:10.1016/S0140-6736(11)60701-0 PMID:21722952

Free, C., Whittaker, R., Knight, R., Abramsky, T., Rodgers, A., & Roberts, I. G. (2009). Txt2stop: A pilot randomised controlled trial of mobile phone-based smoking cessation support. *Tobacco Control*, *18*(2), 88–91. doi:10.1136/tc.2008.026146 PMID:19318534

Freedman, M. J., Lester, K. M., McNamara, C., Milby, J. B., & Schumacher, J. E. (2006). Cell phones for ecological momentary assessment with cocaine-addicted homeless patients in treatment. *Journal of Substance Abuse Treatment*, *30*(2), 105–111. doi:10.1016/j.jsat.2005.10.005 PMID:16490673

Freifeld, C., & Brownstein, J. (2007). *HealthMap*. Retrieved June 7, 2011, from http://www.healthmap.org/about/

Freyne, J., Berkovsky, S., Baghaei, N., Kimani, S., & Smith, G. (2011). Personalised Techniques For Lifestyle Change. In *Proceedings of the 13th International Conference on Artificial Intelligence in Medicine in Europe.* Bled, Slovenia: AIME.

Friedman, C. P. (2009). A fundamental theorem of biomedical informatics. *Journal of the American Medical Informatics Association, 16*(2), 169–170. doi:10.1197/jamia.M3092 PMID:19074294

Gao, G., McCullough, J. S., Agarwal, R., & Jha, J. K. (2012). *A Changing Landscape of Physician Quality Reporting: Analysis of Patients' Online Ratings of Their Physicians.* iPROCEEDINGS Medicine 2.0 Boston. Retrieved from http://www.medicine20congress.com/ocs/index.php/med/med2012/paper/view/954

Garg, A. X., Adhikari, N. K., McDonald, H., Rosas-Arellano, M. P., Devereaux, P. J., Beyene, J., & Haynes, R. B. (2005). Effects of computerized clinical decision support systems on practitioner performance and patient outcomes: A systematic review. *Journal of the American Medical Association, 293*(10), 1223–1238. doi:10.1001/jama.293.10.1223 PMID:15755945

Garrett, J. J. (2005). Ajax: A New Approach to Web Applications. *Adaptive Path.* Retrieved July 12, 2011, from http://www.adaptivepath.com/ideas/ajax-new-approach-web-applications

Geisler, B. P., Schuur, J. D., & Pallin, D. J. (2010). Estimates of electronic medical records in U.S. Emergency departments. *PLoS ONE, 5*(2), e9274. doi:10.1371/journal.pone.0009274 PMID:20174660

Geoffery, G. (2008). *A community-based model for the production of ideas.* (Master Thesis). Simon Fraser University.

Georgiev, T., Georgieva, E., & Smrikarov, A. (2004). *M-Learning - A New Stage of E- Learning.* Paper presented at the ComSysTech'2004. New York, NY.

Gerdes, A., & Øhrstrøm, P. (2011). The role of credibility in the design of mobile solutions to enhance the social skill-set of teenagers diagnosed with autism. *Journal of Information. Communication and Ethics in Society, 9*(4), 253–264. doi:10.1108/14779961111191057

Gerster Consulting. (2008). *ICT in Africa: Boosting Economic Growth and Poverty Reduction.* Paper presented at the 10th meeting of the Africa partnership forum. Tokyo, Japan.

Gilhooly, M. L., Gilhooly, K. J., & Jones, R. B. (2009). Quality of life: conceptual challenges in exploring the role of ICT in active ageing. In Information and Communication Technologies for Active Ageing – Opportunities and Challenges for the European Union. IOS Press.

G-I-N. (2010). *G-I-N Emergency Care Community of Interest Annual Report.* Guidelines International Network.

Glasgow, N. J., Jeon, Y.-H., Kraus, S. G., & Pearce-Brown, C. L. (2008). Chronic disease self-management support: The way forward for Australia. *Med J, 189*(10), 14.

Global HIV Prevention Working Group. (2008). *Behavior Change and HIV Prevention: Reconsiderations for the 21st Century.* Retrieved August 23, 2011, from http://www.globalhivprevention.org/pdfs/PWG_behavior%20report_FINAL.pdf

Google. (2012). Google Flu Trends. *Google.org.* Retrieved August 25, 2011, from http://www.google.org/flutrends/about/how.html

Google. (2014). *Android developer – Help: Upload applications.* Retrieved January 21, 2014 from https://support.google.com/googleplay/android-developer/answer/113469?hl=en

Gross, A. M., Levin, R. B., Mulvihill, M., Richardson, P., & Davidson, P. C. (1984). Blood glucose discrimination training with insulin-dependent diabetics: A clinical note. *Biofeedback and Self-Regulation, 9*(1), 49–54. doi:10.1007/BF00998845 PMID:6487674

Gustafson, D., Boyle, M., Shaw, B., Isham, A., McTavish, F., & Richards, S. et al. (2011). An E-Health Solution for People with Alcohol Problems. *Alcohol Research & Health, 33*(4), 327–337. PMID:23293549

H. R. 2157. (2001). *Rural Health Care Improvement Act of 2001.* 107th Congress. 1st, Session.

Haggstrom, D. A., Saleem, J. J., Russ, A. L., Jones, J., Russell, S. A., & Chumbler, N. R. (2011). Lessons learned from usability testing of the VA's personal health record. *Journal of the American Medical Informatics Association, 18*(Suppl 1), i13–i17. doi:10.1136/amiajnl-2010-000082 PMID:21984604

Halamka, J., Mandl, K., & Tang, P. (2007). Early experiences with personal health records. *Journal of the American Medical Informatics Association, 15*(1), 1–7. doi:10.1197/jamia.M2562 PMID:17947615

Hannawa, A. F., Kreps, G. L., Paek, H.-J., Schulz, P. J., Smith, S., & Street, R. L. (2014). Emerging Issues and Future Directions of the Field of Health Communication. *Health Communication.* doi: doi:10.1080/10410236.2013.814959 PMID:24345246

Hanson, C. L., Cannon, B., Burton, S., & Giraud-Carrier, C. (2013). An Exploration of Social Circles and Prescription Drug Abuse Through Twitter. *Journal of Medical Internet Research, 15*(9), e189. doi:10.2196/jmir.2741 PMID:24014109

Happtique. (2014). *App. certification: Draft standards.* Retrieved January 21, 2014 from http://www.happtique.com/app-certification/

Harris, J.K., Snider, D., & Mueller, N. (2013). Social Media Adoption in Health Departments Nationwide: The State of the States. *Frontiers in Public Services and System Research, 2*(1), art.5.

Harris, J., Felix, L., Miners, A., Murray, E., Michie, S., & Ferguson, E. et al. (2011). Adaptive e-learning to improve dietary behavior: A systematic review and cost-effectiveness analysis. *Health Technology Assessment, 15*(37), 1–160. PMID:22030014

Hawkins, A. O., Kantayya, V. S., & Sharkey-Asner, C. (2010). Health literacy: A potential barrier in caring for underserved populations. *Disease-a-Month, 56*(12), 734–740. doi:10.1016/j.disamonth.2010.10.006 PMID:21168579

Health and Social Care Information Centre. 1 Trevelyan Square. (2013, September 26). *Care.data. standard.* Retrieved April 10, 2014, from http://www.hscic.gov.uk/article/3525/Caredata

Health Council of Canada. (2010). *Helping patients help themselves: Are Canadians with chronic conditions getting the support they need to manage their health?* Toronto, Canada: Health Council of Canada.

Health Literacy. (n.d.). Retrieved from http://healthliteracy.ca/en/professionals-and-service-providers.html

Health on the Net Foundation. (2010). *Operational definition of the HONcode principles.* Retrieved January 21, 2014 from http://www.hon.ch/HONcode/Webmasters/Guidelines/guidelines.html

Health Protection Agency. (2010). Introduction to environmental public health tracking. *Health Protection Agency.* Retrieved May 8, 2013, from http://www.hpa.org.uk/webc/HPAwebFile/HPAweb_C/1287143109858

Healthmap. (2012). Healthmap. *Boston Children Hospital.* Retrieved June 4, 2012, from http://healthmap.org/en/

HealthOn. (2014). *App-Testberichte – HealthOn-Apps.* Retrieved January 21, 2014 from http://tests.healthon.de/app-testberichte.html

Henkleman, D. (2003). The Evolution of a Health Information Brokering Service in the Province of British Columbia. *Electronic Healthcare, 2*(2), 16–21.

Hesse, B. W., O'Connell, M., Auguston, E. M., Chou, W. S., Shaikh, A. R., & Finney Rutten, L. J. (2011). Realizing the Promise of Web 2.0: Engaging Community Intelligence. *Journal of Health Communication: International Perspectives, 16*(1), 10–31. PMID:21843093

Hibbard, J. H., & Greene, J. (2013). What the evidence shows about patient activation: Better health outcomes and care experiences, fewer data on costs. *Health Affairs (Project Hope)*, *32*(2), 207–214. doi:10.1377/hlthaff.2012.1061 PMID:23381511

Hibbard, J., & Cunningham, P. J. (2008). How engaged are consumers in their health and health care, and why does it matter? *Research Briefs*, *8*, 1–9. PMID:18946947

Hibbard, J., Mahoney, E., Stock, R., & Tusler, M. (2007). Self-management and health care utilization: Do increases in patient activation result in improved self-management behaviors? *Health Services Research*, *42*(4), 1443–1463. doi:10.1111/j.1475-6773.2006.00669.x PMID:17610432

HIMSS. (2012). *Selecting a Mobile App: Evaluating the Useability of Medical Applications.* Retrieved 17 December, 2012, from http://www.yumpu.com/en/document/view/10378687/himssguidetoappusabilityv1mhimss

Ho, W. H., Weinstein, P., De Sousa, D., Husain, J. T., Wu, R. A., Cafazzo, J. A., & Armour, K. (2012). *A Mobile Clinical Collaboration System for Inter-Professional Team Based Care in an Outpatient Setting.* iPROCEEDINGS Medicine 2.0 Boston. Retrieved from http://www.medicine20congress.com/ocs/index.php/med/med2012/paper/view/1243

Ho, K., Jarvis Selinger, S., Norman, C. D., Li, L. C., Olatunbosun, T., Cressman, C., & Nguyen, A. (2010). Electronic communities of practice: Guidelines from a project. *The Journal of Continuing Education in the Health Professions*, *30*(2), 139–143. doi:10.1002/chp.20071 PMID:20564704

Holbrook, A., Pullenayegum, E., Thabane, L., Troyan, S., Foster, G., & Keshavjee, K. et al. (2011). Shared electronic vascular risk decision support in primary care: Computerization of Medical Practices for the Enhancement of Therapeutic Effectiveness (COMPETE III) randomized trial. *Archives of Internal Medicine*, *171*(19), 1736–1744. doi:10.1001/archinternmed.2011.471 PMID:22025430

Holtz, B., & Lauckner, C. (2012). Diabetes management via mobile phones: A systematic review. *Telemedicine Journal and e-Health*, *18*(3), 175–184. doi:10.1089/tmj.2011.0119 PMID:22356525

Hopgood, A. A. (2005). The State of Aritificial Intelligence. *Advanced in Computers*, *65*, 1–75. doi:10.1016/S0065-2458(05)65001-2

Househ, M. (2013). The Use of Social Media in Health-Care: Organisational, Clinical and Patient Perspectives. In *Proceedings of Information Technology and Communications in Health (ITCH) Conference.* IOS Press.

Househ, M., Borycki, E., Kushniruk, A., & Alofaysan, S. (2012). mHealth: A passing fad or here to stay? In Telemedicine and E-health Services, Policies, and Applications: Advancements and Developments. Hershey, PA: IGI Global.

Househ, M. (2013). The Use of Social Media in Healthcare: Organizational, Clinical, and Patient Perspectives. In K. L. Courtney et al. (Eds.), *Enabling Health and Healthcare through ICT* (pp. 244–248). IOS Press.

Houston, T., & Ehrenberger, H. (2001). The Potential of Consumer Health Informatics. *Seminars in Oncology Nursing*, *17*(1), 41–47. doi:10.1053/sonu.2001.20418 PMID:11236364

Hsu, M. H., Ju, T. L., Yen, C. H., & Chang, C. M. (2007). Knowledge sharing behavior in virtual communities: The relationship between trust, self-efficacy, and outcome expectations. *International Journal of Human-Computer Studies*, *65*(2), 153–169. doi:10.1016/j.ijhcs.2006.09.003

Huber, J., Ihrig, A., & Peters, T. et al. (2011). Decision-making in localized prostate cancer: Lessons learned from an online support group. *BJU International*, *107*(10), 1570–1575. doi:10.1111/j.1464-410X.2010.09859.x PMID:21105988

Huber, M., Knottnerus, J. A., Green, L., Horst, H. V. D., Jadad, A. R., Kromhout, D., & Smid, H. (2011). How should we define health? *British Medical Journal*, *343*(6). doi: doi:10.1136/bmj.d4163 PMID:21791490

Hu, P. J., Chau, P. K., Liu Sheng, O. R., & Kar Yan, T. (1999). Examining the Technology Acceptance Model Using Physician Acceptance of Telemedicine Technology. *Journal of Management Information Systems*, *16*(2), 91–112.

Hurling, R., Catt, M., Boni, M. D., Fairley, B. W., Hurst, T., Murray, P., & Sodhi, J. S. (2007). Using internet and mobile phone technology to deliver an automated physical activity program: Randomized controlled trial. *Journal of Medical Internet Research*, *9*(2), e7. doi:10.2196/jmir.9.2.e7 PMID:17478409

HWA. (2013a). Nurses in focus. *Australia's Health Workforce Series*. Retrieved 23 July 2013, from https://www.hwa.gov.au/sites/uploads/Nurses-in-Focus-FINAL.pdf

HWA. (2013b). NHETsim. *Training the Healthcare simulation community*. Retrieved 23 July, from http://www.nhet-sim.edu.au/

IAPP. (2011). *US Privacy Enforcement Case Studies Guide*. Retrieved 17 December, 2012, from https://www.privacyassociation.org/media/pdf/certification/CIPP_Case_Studies_0211.pdf

iHealthBeat. (2011). Mayo Clinic launches social networking site on health care issues. *iHealthBeat, 15*. Retrieved 17 August 2011, from http://www.ihealthbeat.org/articles/2011/7/15/mayo-clinic-launches-social-networking-site-on-health-care-issues.aspx

Ingrosso, M. (Ed.). (2008). *La salute comunicata: Ricerche e valutazioni nei media e nei servizi sanitari*. Milano: Franco Angeli.

Institute of Medicine (IoM). (2012). *Living well with chronic illness: A call for public health action*. Washington, DC: The National Academies Press.

International Organization for Standardization. (2006). *ISO 9241-110:2006 Ergonomics of human-system interaction -- Part 110: Dialogue principles*. Geneva, Switzerland: ISO.

International Organization for Standardization. (2007). [*Medical devices -- Application of usability engineering to medical devices*. Arlington, VA: AAMI.]. *IEC*, *62366*, 2007.

International Organization for Standardization. (2010). *ISO 9241-210:2010 Ergonomics of human-system interaction -- Part 210: Human-centred design for interactive systems*. Geneva, Switzerland: ISO.

International Telecommunications Union (ITU). (n.d.). *ICT data and statistics*. Retrieved from http://www.itu.int/ITU-D/ict/statistics/

ISI Web of Knowledge. (n.d.). Retrieved 1 August 2012, from http://apps.webofknowledge.com/UA_GeneralSearch_input.do?product=UA&search_mode=GeneralSearch&SID=2DPDdNGBCKHI7NPmmI5&preferencesSaved=

Istat. (2013a). *Cittadini e nuove tecnologie*. Retrieved December 20, 2013, from http://www.istat.it/it/archivio/108009

Istat. (2013b). *Popolazione residente al 1° gennaio 2013*. Retrieved December 20, 2013, from http://demo.istat.it/pop2013/index.html

Istepanian, R. S. H., Jovanov, E., & Zhang, Y. T. (2004). Guest editorial introduction to the special section on M-health: Beyond seamless mobility and global wireless health-care connectivity. *IEEE Transactions on Information Technology in Biomedicine*, *8*(4), 405–414. doi:10.1109/TITB.2004.840019 PMID:15615031

Jain, N., Dahlin, M., & Tewari, R. (2005). TAPER: Tiered approach for eliminating redundancy in replica synchronization. In *Proceedings of the 4th conference FAST 2005 on USEUNIX Conference on File and Storage Technologies*. USEUNIX.

James, J. (2013). *Apple's app. store marks historic 50 billionth download*. Retrieved January 21, 2014 from http://www.apple.com/au/pr/library/2013/05/16Apples-App-Store-Marks-Historic-50-Bill

Jamoom, E., Beatty, P., Bercovitz, A., Woodwell, D., Palso, K., & Rechtsteiner, E. (2012). Physician adoption of electronic health record systems: United States, 2011. *NCHS Data Brief*, (98), 1-8.

Jaspers, M. W. M. (2009). A comparison of usability methods for testing interactive health technologies: Methodological aspects and empirical evidence. *International Journal of Medical Informatics*, *78*(5), 340–353. doi:10.1016/j.ijmedinf.2008.10.002 PMID:19046928

Jennex, M. E., Smolnik, S., & Croasdell, D. (2008). Towards measuring knowledge management success. In *Proceedings of Hawaii International Conference on System Sciences*. IEEE.

Jennex, M. E. (2008). Knowledge Management Success Models. In *Knowledge Management: Concepts, Methodologies,Tools, and Applications* (pp. 32–40). Hershey, PA: IGI Global.

Jessup, M., Courtney-Pratt, H., Robinson, A., Cameron-Tucker, H., Walters, H., & Wood-Baker, R. et al. (2006). Cementing Pathways Home: Enhancing quality of life for people with chronic obstructive pulmonary disease (COPD). *Ageing International, 31*, 232–240. doi:10.1007/BF02915231

Jin, X. L., Cheung, C. M. K., Lee, M. K. O., & Chen, H. P. (2009). How to keep members using the information in a computer-supported social network. *Computers in Human Behavior, 25*(5), 1172–1181. doi:10.1016/j.chb.2009.04.008

Jones, J., Hook, S., Park, S., & Scott, L. (2011). *Privacy, security and interoperability of mobile health applications*. Paper presented at the 6th International Conference on Universal Access in Human-Computer Interaction. New York, NY.

Jones, D. A., Shipman, J. P., Plaut, D. A., & Selden, C. R. (2010). Characteristics of personal health records: Findings of the medical library association/national library of medicine joint electronic personal health record task force. *Journal of the Medical Library Association: JMLA, 98*(3), 243–249. doi:10.3163/1536-5050.98.3.013 PMID:20648259

Jordan, J. E., Briggs, A., Brand, C., & Osborne, R. H. (2008). Enhancing patient engagement in chronic disease self management support initiatives in Australia: The need for an integrated approach. *The Medical Journal of Australia, 189*(10). PMID:19143585

Jordan, J. E., Buchbinderb, R., & Osbourne, R. H. (2010). Conceptualising health literacy from the patient perspective. *Patient Education and Counseling, 79*(1), 36–42. doi:10.1016/j.pec.2009.10.001 PMID:19896320

Kaelber, D., & Pan, E. C. (2008). The value of personal health record (PHR) systems. In *Proceedings of AMIA Annual Symposium*. American Medical Informatics Association.

Kankanhalli, A., & Tan, B. C. Y. (2005). Knowledge Management Metrics: A Review and Directions for Future Research. *International Journal of Knowledge Management, 1*(2), 20–32. doi:10.4018/jkm.2005040103

Kankanhalli, A., Tan, B. C. Y., & Wei, K. K. (2005a). Contributing knowledge to electronic knowledge repositories: An empirical investigation. *Management Information Systems Quarterly, 29*(1), 113–143.

Kankanhalli, A., Tan, B. C. Y., & Wei, K. K. (2005b). Understanding seeking from electronic knowledge repositories: An empirical study. *Journal of the American Society for Information Science and Technology, 56*(11), 1156–1166. doi:10.1002/asi.20219

Kaplan, A. M., & Haenlein, M. (2010). Users of the world, unite! The challenges and opportunities of social media. *Business Horizons, 53*(1), 59–68. doi:10.1016/j.bushor.2009.09.003

Katz, R., Mesfin, T., & Barr, K. (2012). Lessons from a community-based mHealth diabetes self-management program: It's not just about the cell phone. *Journal of Health Communication, 17*(1), 67–72. doi:10.1080/108 10730.2012.650613 PMID:22548601

Kawamoto, K., Houlihan, C. A., Balas, E. A., & Lobach, D. F. (2005). Improving clinical practice using clinical decision support systems: A systematic review of trials to identify features critical to success. *British Medical Journal, 330*(7494), 765. doi:10.1136/bmj.38398.500764.8F PMID:15767266

Kay, M., Santos, J., & Takane, M. (2011). mHealth: New horizons for health through mobile technologies. Geneva, Switerland: World Health Organization.

Keckley, P. H., & Hoffman, M. (2010). *2010 Survey of Health Care Consumers: Key Findings, Strategic Implications*. Deloitte Center for Health Solutions. Retrieved October 10, 2013, from http://www.deloitte.com/assets/Dcom-UnitedStates/Local%20Assets/Documents/US_CHS_2010SurveyofHealthCareConsumers_050310.pdf

Keehan, S., Sisko, A., Truffer, C., Smith, S., Cowan, C., Poisal, J., & Clemens, M. (2008). Health spending projections through 2017: The baby-boom generation is coming to medicare. *Health Affairs*, *27*(2), 145–155. doi:10.1377/hlthaff.27.2.w145 PMID:18303038

Kelly, N. (2013, June 6). 7 Trends in Global Internet Growth You Can't Afford to Ignore. *Huffington Post*. Retrieved from http://www.huffingtonpost.com/nataly-kelly/seven-trends-in-global-in_b_3382907.html

Kenny, R., Neste-Kenny, J., Park, C., Burton, P., & Meiers, J. (2009). Mobile learning in Nursing practice education: Applying Koole's FRAME model. *Journal of Distance Education*, *23*(3), 75–96.

KeshavjeeK.BosomworthJ.CopenJ.LaiJ.KucukyaziciB. LilaniR.HolbrookA. M. (2006). Best Practices in EMR Implementation: A Systematic Review. In Proceedings of AMIA Annual Symposium. AMIA.

Khairat, S., & Garcia, C. (2012). *Introducing a Wireless Mobile Technology to Improve Diabetes Care Outcomes among Specific Minority Groups*. iPROCEEDINGS Medicine 2.0 Boston. Retrieved from http://www.medicine20congress.com/ocs/index.php/med/med2012/paper/view/900

Kharrazi, H., Chisholm, R., VanNasdale, D., & Thompson, B. (2012). Mobile personal health records: An evaluation of features and functionality. *International Journal of Medical Informatics*, *81*(9), 579–593. doi:10.1016/j.ijmedinf.2012.04.007 PMID:22809779

Khdour, M. R., Agus, A. M., Kidney, J. C., Smyth, B. M., Elnay, J. C., & Crealey, G. E. (2011). Cost-utility analysis of a pharmacy-led self-management programme for patients with COPD. *International Journal of Clinical Pharmacology, Therapy and Toxicology*, *33*(4), 665–673. PMID:21643784

Kiecolt-Glaser, J., & Glaser, R. (2001). Stress and immunity: age enhances the risks. *Current Directions in Psychological Science*, *10*(1), 18–21. doi:10.1111/1467-8721.00105

Kietzmann, J. H., Hermkens, K., McCarthy, I. P., & Silvestre, B. S. (2011). Social media? Get serious! Understanding the functional building blocks of social media. *Business Horizons*, *54*(3), 241–251. doi:10.1016/j.bushor.2011.01.005

Kim, J. N., Park, S. C., Yoo, S. W., & Shen, H. (2010). Mapping Health Communication Scholarship: Breadth, depth, and agenda of published research in Health Communication. *Health Communication*, *25*(6-7), 487–503. doi:10.1080/10410236.2010.507160 PMID:20845126

King, G., Tomz, M., & Wittenberg, J. (2000). Making the most of statistical analysis: Improving interpretation and presentation. *American Journal of Political Science*, *44*(2), 347–361. doi:10.2307/2669316

Klersy, C., De Silvestri, A., Gabutti, G., Regoli, F., & Auricchio, A. (2009). A meta-analysis of remote monitoring of heart failure patients. *Journal of the American College of Cardiology*, *54*(18), 1683–1694. doi:10.1016/j.jacc.2009.08.017 PMID:19850208

Kocoglu, Z. (2008). Turkish EFL student teachers' perceptions on the role of Electronic portfolios in their professional development. *The Turkish Online Journal of Educational Technology, 7*, Article 8,

Koff, P. B., Jones, R. H., Cashman, J. M., Voelkel, N. F., & Vandivier, R. W. (2009). Proactive integrated care improves quality of life in patients with COPD. *The European Respiratory Journal*, *33*(5), 1031–1038. doi:10.1183/09031936.00063108 PMID:19129289

Kontos, E. Z., Emmons, K. M., Puleo, E., & Viswanath, K. (2010). Communication inequalities and public health implications of adult social networking site use in the United States. *Journal of Health Communication*, *15*(Suppl 3), 216–235. doi:10.1080/10810730.2010.522689 PMID:21154095

Korda, H., & Itani, Z. (2013). Harnessing Social Media for Health Promotion and Behavior Change. *Health Promotion Practice*, *14*(1), 15–23. doi:10.1177/1524839911405850 PMID:21558472

Kortum, P., & Safari Technical Books. (2008). *HCI beyond the GUI design for haptic, speech, olfactory and other nontraditional interfaces.* San Francisco: Morgan Kaufmann.

Kout, A. (2012). *Social Networking Popular Across Globe.* Washington, DC: Pew Internet & American Life Project. Retrieved July 15, 2013, from http://www.pewglobal.org/files/2012/12/Pew-Global-Attitudes-Project-Technology-Report-FINAL-December-12-2012.pdf

Kovachev, D., Aksakali, G., & Klamma, R. (2012). *A real-time collaboration-enabled Mobile Augmented Reality system with semantic multimedia.* Paper presented at the Collaborative Computing: Networking, Applications and Worksharing (CollaborateCom), 8th International Conference. Pittsburgh, PA. doi:10.4108/icst.collaboratecom.2012.25043610.4108/icst.collaboratecom.2012.250436

Kovatchev, B. P., Cox, D. J., Gonder-Frederick, L., & Clarke, W. L. (2002). Methods for quantifying self-monitoring blood glucose profiles exemplified by an examination of blood glucose patterns in patients with type 1 and type 2 diabetes. *Diabetes Technology & Therapeutics, 4*(3), 295–303. doi:10.1089/152091502760098438 PMID:12165168

Kubota, A., Fujita, M., & Hatano, Y. (2004). Development and effects of a health promotion program utilizing the mail function of mobile phones. *Japanese Journal of Public Health, 51*(10), 862. PMID:15565995

Kuijpers, W., Groen, W. G., Aaronson, N. K., & Van Harten, W. (2013). A Systematic Review of Web-Based Interventions for Patient Empowerment and Physical Activity in Chronic Diseases: Relevance for Cancer Survivors. *Journal of Medical Internet Research, 15*(2), e37. doi:10.2196/jmir.2281 PMID:23425685

Kuo, B., Young, M. L., Hsu, M. H., Lin, C., & Chiang, P. C. (2003). *A study of the cognition-action gap in knowledge management.* Paper presented at the International Conference on Information Systems (ICIS) 2003. New York, NY.

Kurniawan, S., Mahmud, M., & Nugroho, Y. (2006). *A study of the use of mobile phones by older persons.* doi:10.1145/1125451.1125641

Kurzweil, R. (2001). Law of Accelerating returns. *KurzweilAI.net.* Retrieved 23 July 2013, from http://www.kurzweilai.net/articles/art0134.html?printable=1

Kushniruk, A. W., Patel, V. L., & Cimino, J. J. (1997). Usability testing in medical informatics: Cognitive approaches to evaluation of information systems and user interfaces. In *Proceedings of the AMIA Annual Fall Symposium* (pp. 218). American Medical Informatics Association.

Kushniruk, A. (2002). Evaluation in the design of health information systems: Application of approaches emerging from usability engineering. *Computers in Biology and Medicine, 32*(3), 141–149. doi:10.1016/S0010-4825(02)00011-2 PMID:11922931

Kushniruk, A. W., Borycki, E. M., Kuwata, S., & Kannry, J. (2011). Emerging approaches to usability evaluation of health information systems: Towards in-situ analysis of complex healthcare systems and environments. *Studies in Health Technology and Informatics, 169*, 915. PMID:21893879

Kushniruk, A. W., & Patel, V. L. (2004). Cognitive and usability engineering methods for the evaluation of clinical information systems. *Journal of Biomedical Informatics, 37*(1), 56–76. doi:10.1016/j.jbi.2004.01.003 PMID:15016386

Kushniruk, A., Borycki, E., Kuwata, S., & Kannry, J. (2006). Predicting changes in workflow resulting from healthcare information systems: Ensuring the safety of healthcare. *Healthcare Quarterly, 9*, 114–118. doi:10.12927/hcq..18469 PMID:17087179

Kushniruk, A., Triola, B., Borycki, E., Stein, B., & Kannry, J. (2005). Technology Induced Error and Usability: The Relationship Between Usability Problems and Prescription Errors When Using a Handheld Application. *International Journal of Medical Informatics, 74*(7-8), 519–526. doi:10.1016/j.ijmedinf.2005.01.003 PMID:16043081

Kwankam, Y. S., & Ntomambang, N. N. (n.d.). *Information Technology in Africa: A proactive approach and the prospects of leapfrogging decades in the development process.* Retrieved August 21, 2011, from http://www.isoc.org/inet97/proceedings/B7/B7_1.HTM

Laakko, T., Leppanen, J., Lahteenmaki, J., & Nummiaho, A. (2008). Mobile Health and Wellness Application Framework. *Methods of Information in Medicine, 47*(3), 217–222. PMID:18473087

Laird, S. (2012). How social media is taking over the news industry. *Mashable.* Retrieved May 20, 2013, from http://mashable.com/2012/04/18/social-media-and-the-news/

Lam, R., Lin, V. S., Senelick, W. S., Tran, H. P., Moore, A. A., & Koretz, B. (2013). Older adult consumers' attitudes and preferences on electronic patient-physician messaging. *The American Journal of Managed Care, 19*(10), eSP7–eSP11. PMID:24511886

Landa, A. H., Szabo, I., Le Brun, L., Owen, I., Fletcher, G., & Hill, M. (2011). An Evidence-Based Approach to Scoping Reviews. *Electronic Journal of Information Systems Evaluation, 14*(1), 46–52.

Lapointe, L., & Rivard, S. (2005). A multilevel model of resistance to information technology implementation. *MIS Quart, 29*(3), 461–491.

Lau, A. Y., Siek, K. A., Fernandez-Luque, L., Tange, H., Chhanabhai, P., & Li, S. Y. et al. (2011). The Role of Social Media for Patients and Consumer Health: Contribution of the IMIA Consumer Health Informatics Working Group. *Yearbook of Medical Informatics, 6*(1), 131–138. PMID:21938338

Lau, J. K., Lowres, N., Neubeck, L., Brieger, D. B., Sy, R. W., Galloway, C. D., & Freedman, S. B. (2013). iPhone ECG application for community screening to detect silent atrial fibrillation: A novel technology to prevent stroke. *International Journal of Cardiology, 165*(1), 193–194. doi:10.1016/j.ijcard.2013.01.220 PMID:23465249

Lazev, A., Vidrine, D., Arduino, R., & Gritz, E. (2004). Increasing access to smoking cessation treatment in a low-income, HIV-positive population: The feasibility of using cellular telephones. *Nicotine & Tobacco Research: Official Journal of the Society for Research on Nicotine and Tobacco, 6*(2), 281–286. doi:10.1080/14622200410 001676314 PMID:15203801

Lee, R. Y. W., & Carlisle, A. J. (2011). Detection of falls using accelerometers and mobile phone technology. *Age and Ageing, 40*(6), 690–696. doi:10.1093/ageing/afr050 PMID:21596711

Lemon, S. M., Hamburg, M. A., Sparling, P. F., Choffnes, E. R., & Mack, A. (2007). Global infectious disease surveillance and detection: Assessing the challenges – Finding solutions. *Forum on Microbial Threats.* Retrieved May 8, 2013, from http://www.ncbi.nlm.nih.gov/books/NBK52867/pdf/TOC.pdf

Leung, R., McGrenere, J., & Graf, P. (2011). Age-related differences in the initial usability of mobile device icons. *Behaviour & Information Technology, 30*(5), 629–642. doi:10.1080/01449290903171308

Leung, R., Tang, C., Haddad, S., Mcgrenere, J., Graf, P., & Ingriany, V. (2012). How older adults learn to use mobile devices: Survey and field investigations. *ACM Transactions on Accessible Computing, 4*(3), 1–33. doi:10.1145/2399193.2399195

Levine, D., Madsen, A., Wright, E., Barar, R. E., Santelli, J., & Bull, S. (2011). Formative research on MySpace: online methods to engage hard-to-reach populations. *Journal of Health Communication, 16*(4), 448–454. doi:10.1080/10810730.2010.546486 PMID:21391040

Lewis, T. L. (2013). A systematic self-certification model for mobile medical apps. *Journal of Medical Internet Research, 15*(4), e89. doi:10.2196/jmir.2446 PMID:23615332

Lin, H., Fan, W., Wallace, L., & Zhang, Z. (2007). An empirical study of web-based knowledge community success. In *Proceedings of the 40th Hawaii International Conference on System Sciences.* IEEE.

Lin, H. F. (2007). Effects of extrinsic and intrinsic motivation on employee knowledge sharing intentions. *Journal of Information Science, 33*(2), 135–149. doi:10.1177/0165551506068174

Lin, H. F. (2008a). Antecedents of virtual community satisfaction and loyalty: An empirical test of competing theories. *Cyberpsychology & Behavior, 11*(2), 138–144. doi:10.1089/cpb.2007.0003 PMID:18422404

Lin, H. F. (2008b). Determinants of successful virtual communities: Contributions from system characteristics and social factors. *Information & Management, 45*(8), 522–527. doi:10.1016/j.im.2008.08.002

Lin, H. F., & Lee, G. G. (2006). Determinants of success for online communities: An empirical study. *Behaviour & Information Technology, 25*(6), 479–488. doi:10.1080/01449290500330422

Lin, M. J. J., Hung, S. W., & Chen, C. J. (2009). Fostering the determinants of knowledge sharing in professional virtual communities. *Computers in Human Behavior, 25*(4), 929–939. doi:10.1016/j.chb.2009.03.008

Lin, T. C., & Huang, C. C. (2008). Understanding the determinants of EKR usage from social, technological and personal perspectives. *Journal of Information Science, 35*(2), 165–179. doi:10.1177/0165551508095780

Li, T., Wu, H. M., Wang, F., Huang, C. Q., Yang, M., Dong, B. R., & Liu, G. J. (2011). Education programmes for people with diabetic kidney disease. *Cochrane Database of Systematic Reviews, 6.* doi:10.1002/14651858. CD007374.pub2 PMID:21678365

Little, M. A., McSharry, P. E., Hunter, E. J., Spielman, J., & Ramig, L. O. (2009). Suitability of dysphonia measurements for telemonitoring of Parkinson's disease. *IEEE Transactions on Bio-Medical Engineering, 56*(4), 1015–1022. doi:10.1109/TBME.2008.2005954 PMID:21399744

Lober, W. B., & Flowers, J. L. (2011). Consumer Empowerment in Health Amid the Internet and Social Media. *Seminars in Oncology Nursing, 27*(3), 169–182. doi:10.1016/j.soncn.2011.04.002 PMID:21783008

Lorenzo, G., & Ittelson, G. (2005). An overview of e-portfolios. *Educause Learning Initiative.* Retrieved 14 February 2010, from www.educause.edu

Lorig, K., Ritter, P., Laurent, D., & Plant, K. (2006). Internet-Based Chronic Disease Self-Management: A Randomized Trial. *Medical Care, 44,* 964–971. doi:10.1097/01. mlr.0000233678.80203.c1 PMID:17063127

Lovari, A., & Giglietto, F. (2012). *Social Media and Italian Universities: An Empirical Study on the Adoption and Use of Facebook, Twitter and YouTube.* Retrieved July 20, 2013, from http://papers.ssrn.com/sol3/papers.cfm?abstract_id=1978393

Lovari, A., Kim, S., Vibber, K., & Kim, J.-N. (2011). Digitisation's impacts on publics: Public knowledge and civic conversation. *PRism, 8* (2).

Lovari, A. (2013). *Networked citizens: Comunicazione pubblica e amministrazioni digitali.* Milano: Franco Angeli.

Lovari, A., & Parisi, L. (2012). Public Administrations and Citizens 2.0: Exploring Digital Public Communication Strategies and Civic Interaction within Italian Municipality Pages on Facebook. In F. Comunello (Ed.), *Networked Sociability and Individualism: Technology for Personal and Professional Rellationships* (pp. 239–264). Hershey, PA: IGI Global.

Lowensohn, J. (2008). Google now tracking flu trends via search. *CNET.* Retrieved August 18, 2011, from http://news.cnet.com/google-now-tracking-flu-trends-via-search/

Lubon, L. (2005). *Information by country.* UNICEF. Retrieved June 1, 2010, from http://www.unicef.org/infobycountry/malaysia_34164.html

Lupiañez-Villanueva, F., Maghiros, I., & Abadie, F. (2012). *Citizens and ICT for Health in 14 EU Countries: Results from an Online Panel.* Luxembourg: Publications Office of the European Union. Retrieved March 20, 2013, from http://is.jrc.ec.europa.eu/pages/TFS/documents/SIMPHS2_D3.2CitizenPanelfinal.pdf

Lupiáñez-Villanueva, F., Mayer, M. A., & Torrent, J. (2009). Opportunities and challenges of Web 2.0 within the health care systems: An empirical exploration. *Informatics for Health & Social Care, 34*(3), 117–126. doi:10.1080/17538150903102265 PMID:19670002

Lupton, D. (2012). M-health and health promotion: The digital cyborg and surveillance society. *Social Theory & Health, 10*(3), 229–244. doi:10.1057/sth.2012.6

Luxton, D., McCann, R., Bush, N., Mishkind, M., & Reger, G. (2011). mHealth for mental health: Integrating smartphone technology in behavioral healthcare. *Professional Psychology, Research and Practice, 42*(6), 505–512. doi:10.1037/a0024485

Lyytinen, K., & Rose, G. M. (2003). Disruptive information system innovation: The case of internet computing. *Information Systems Journal, 13*(4), 301–330. doi:10.1046/j.1365-2575.2003.00155.x

Mack, K., & Thompson, L. (2001). *Data: Profiles, family caregivers of older persons: Adult children.* Georgetown University, The Center on an Aging Society.

MacKay, B., & Harding, T. (2009). M-support: Keeping in touch on placement in primary health care settings. *Nursing Praxis in New Zealand Inc, 25*(2), 30–40. PMID:19928649

Madden, T. (2007). *Supporting student e-Portfolios: A physical sciences practice guide.* Hull, UK: Higher Education Academy Physical Sciences Centre.

Maier, R. (2007). *Knowledge Management Systems Information and Communication Technologies for Knowledge Management.* New York: Springer.

Manary, M. P., Boulding, W., Staelin, R., & Glickman, S. W. (2013). The patient experience and health outcomes. *The New England Journal of Medicine, 368*(3), 201–203. doi:10.1056/NEJMp1211775 PMID:23268647

Manson, J. E., Stampfer, M. J., Colditz, G. A., Willett, W. C., Rosner, B., & Hennekens, C. H. et al. (1991). Physical activity and incidence of non-insulin-dependent diabetes mellitus in women. *Lancet, 338*(8770), 774–778. doi:10.1016/0140-6736(91)90664-B PMID:1681160

Martin, R. (2011). *Onsite: The iPad Revolution at the Ottawa Hospital Deploying Mobile Technology in a Large Hospital.* Retrieved from http://www.mobilehealthcaretoday.com/onsites/2011/01/the-ottawa-hospitals-ipad-revolution.aspx

Mason, R., Pegler, C., & Weller, M. (2004). E-portfolios: An assessment tool for online courses. *British Journal of Educational Technology, 35*(6), 717–727. doi:10.1111/j.1467-8535.2004.00429.x

Mather, C. A. (2010). *Human interface technology: Enhancing tertiary nursing education to ensure workplace readiness.* Paper presented at the International Technology, Education and Development Conference. New York, NY.

Mather, C. A. (2011). *E-portfolios: Lessons from an interdisciplinary collaboration: The School of nursing and Midwifery experience abstract.* Paper presented at the EDULEARN11 (3rd International Conference on Education and New Learning Technologies). Barcelona, Spain.

Mather, C. A. (2012b). *Embedding an e-portfolio into a work Integrated learning environment: The School of Nursing and Midwifery experience.* Paper presented at the EDULEARN12 (4th International Conference on Education and New Learning Technologies). Barcelona, Spain.

Mather, C. A., Marlow, A., & Cummings, E. (2013b). *Web 2.0 strategies to enhance support of clinical supervisors of undergraduate nursing students: An Australian experience.* Paper presented at the EDULEARN13 (5th International Conference on Education and New Learning Technologies). New York, NY.

Mather, C. A. (2012a). An Interdisciplinary evaluation of an e-portfolio: WIL at the University of Tasmania. In C. Simmons, W. Sher, A. Williams, & T. Levett-Jones (Eds.), *Workready. E-portfolios to support professional placements in nursing and construction management degrees in Australia* (pp. 73–88). Sydney: Office for Learning and Teaching.

Mather, C. A., & Marlow, A. (2012). Audio teleconferencing: Creative use of a forgotten innovation. *Contemporary Nurse, 41*(2), 177–183. doi:10.5172/conu.2012.41.2.177 PMID:22800383

Mather, C. A., Marlow, A., & Cummings, E. (2013a). Digital communication to support clinical supervision: Considering the human factors. *Studies in Health Technology and Informatics, 194*, 160–165. PMID:23941949

Maxis. (2012). Maxis and IJN establish partnership to bring healthcare content and awareness to maxis customers. *Maxis.* Retrieved 15 May, 2013, from http://www.maxis.com.my/mmc/index.asp?fuseaction=home.article&aid=618&status=1

Mayer, R. C., Davis, J. H., & Schoorman, F. D. (1995). An integrative model of organizational trust. *Academy of Management Review, 20*(3), 709–734.

Mayhew, D. J. (1999). *The usability engineering lifecycle: A practitioner's handbook for user interface design*. San Francisco: Morgan Kaufmann Publishers. doi:10.1145/632780.632805

Mayo Clinic Center. (2012). *Bringing the Social Media #Revolution to Health Care*. Mayo Foundation for Medical Education and Research.

McCallum, S. (2012). Gamification and serious games for personalized health. *Studies in Health Technology and Informatics*, 85–96. doi: doi:10.3233/978-1-61499-069-7-85 PMID:22942036

McCarthy, R. L., Kenneth, W., Schafermeyer, K., & Plake, S. (2012). *Introduction to Health Care Delivery: A Primer for Pharmacists*. Sudbury, MA: Jones & Bartlett Learning.

McCurdie, T., Taneva, S., Casselman, M., Yeung, M., McDaniel, C., Ho, W., & Cafazzo, J. (2012). mHealth consumer apps: The case for user-centered design. *Biomedical Instrumentation & Technology*, 49–56. doi:10.2345/0899-8205-46.s2.49 PMID:23039777

McDonough, R. P., & Doucette, W. R. (2001). Developing CWRs between pharmacists and physicians. *Journal of the American Pharmaceutical Association*, (41): 682–692.

McGillicuddy, J. W., Weiland, A. K., Frenzel, R. M., Mueller, M., Brunner-Jackson, B. M., Taber, D. J., & Treiber, F. A. (2013). Patient attitudes toward mobile phone-based health monitoring: Questionnaire study among kidney transplant recipients. *Journal of Medical Internet Research, 15*(1), e6. doi:10.2196/jmir.2284 PMID:23305649

McGowan, B. S., Wasko, M., Vartabedian, B. S., Miller, R. S., Freiherr, D. D., & Abdolrasulnia, M. (2012). Understanding the factors that influence the adoption and meaningful use of social media by physicians to share medical information. *Journal of Medical Internet Research, 14*(5), e117. doi:10.2196/jmir.2138 PMID:23006336

McLaughlin, K., Osborne, S. P., & Ferlie, E. (Eds.). (2002). *New public management: Current trends and future prospects*. London: Routledge.

MedLinePlus Health. (n.d.). Environmental Health Ontology. *BioPortal*. Retrieved June 10, 2011, from http://bioportal.bioontology.org/search

Meneghetti, A. (2013). Challenges and benefits in a mobile medical world: Institutions should create a set of byod guidelines that foster mobile device usage. *Health Management Technology, 34*(2), 6–7. PMID:23469466

Mergel, I. (2010). Gov 2.0 revisited: Social media strategies in the public sector. *PA Times, 33*(3).

Mergel, I. (2013). *Social media in the public sector: A guide to participation, collaboration and transparency in the networked world*. San Francisco, CA: Jossey-Bass.

Mergel, I., & Bretschneider, I. (2013). A Three-Stage Adoption Process for Social Media Use in Government. *Public Administration Review, 73*(3), 390–400. doi:10.1111/puar.12021

Merolli, M., Gray, K., & Martin-Sanchez, F. (2013). Health Outcomes And Related Effects Of Using Social Media In Chronic Disease Management: A Literature Review And Analysis Of Affordances. *Journal of Biomedical Informatics, 46*(6), 957–969. doi:10.1016/j.jbi.2013.04.010 PMID:23702104

Merriam-Webster. (2014). *Definition of medicine*. Retrieved January 21, 2014 from http://www.merriam-webster.com/dictionary/medicine

Merrill, J., & Hripcsak, G. (2008). Using social network analysis within a department of biomedical informatics to induce a discussion of academic communities of practice. *Journal of the American Medical Informatics Association, 15*(6), 780–782. doi:10.1197/jamia.M2717 PMID:18756000

Meskó, B. (2013). *Social Media in Clinical Practice*. London: Springer-Verlag. doi:10.1007/978-1-4471-4306-2

Microsoft. (2013). *Microsoft HealthVault Personal Health Record Goes Mobile in 2012 with iTriage.* Retrieved October 8, 2013, from http://www.prweb.com/releases/2011/12/prweb9064141.htm

Miller, R. A., Waitman, L. R., Chen, S., & Rosenbloom, S. T. (2005). The anatomy of decision support during inpatient care provider order entry (CPOE), empirical observations from a decade of CPOE experience at Vanderbilt. *Journal of Biomedical Informatics*, *38*(6), 469–485. doi:10.1016/j.jbi.2005.08.009 PMID:16290243

Miluzzo, E., Wang, T., & Campbell, A. (2010). *Eye-Phone: Activating mobile phones with your eyes.* doi:10.1145/1851322.1851328

Ministero della Salute. Direzione Generale del Sistema Informativo e Statistico Sanitario. (2012). *Relazione sullo Stato Sanitario del Paese 2011.* Centro stampa del Ministero della salute. Retrieved March 20, 2013 from hhtp://rssp.salute.gov.it

Ministry of Health. (2007). Communicable Disease Control Information System. *Ministry of Health.* Retrieved July 15, 2011, http://www.unescap.org/idd/events/2007_REM-avian-influenza/Surveillance-of-infectious-diseases-in-Malaysia.pdf

Ministry of Health. (2013). MyHealth. *Ministry of Health.* Retrieved 8 May, 2013, from http://www.myhealth.gov.my/v2/

Miskelly, F. (2005). Electronic tracking of patients with dementia and wandering using mobile phone technology. *Age and Ageing*, *34*(5), 497–499. doi:10.1093/ageing/afi145 PMID:16107453

Moen, A., Smørdal, O., & Sem, I. (2009). Web-based resources for peer support-opportunities and challenges. *Studies in Health Technology and Informatics*, *150*, 302–306. PMID:19745318

Moher, D., Liberati, A., Tetzlaff, J., & Altman, D. G. The PRISMA Group. (2009). Preferred reporting items for systematic reviews and meta-analyses: The PRISMA statement. *PLoS Medicine*, *6*(7), e1000097. doi:10.1371/journal.pmed.1000097 PMID:19621072

Mokhtar, M. B., & Murad, M. D. W. (2010). Issues and framework of environmental health in Malaysia. *The Free Library by Farlex.* Retrieved June 1, 2011, http://www.thefreelibrary.com/Issues+and+framework+of+environmental+health+in+Malaysia.-a0222252556

Monkman, H., & Kushniruk, A. W. (2013a). A Health Literacy and Usability Heuristic Evaluation of a Mobile Consumer Health Application. *Studies in Health Technology and Informatics*, *192*, 724. PMID:23920652

Monkman, H., & Kushniruk, A. W. (2013b). Applying Usability Methods to Identify Health Literacy Issues: An Example Using a Personal Health Record. *Studies in Health Technology and Informatics*, *183*, 179–185. PMID:23388278

Moore, G. (1965). Cramming more components into integrated circuits. *Electronics*, *38*(8), 114.

Moorhead, S. A., Hzlett, D. E., Harrison, L., Carroll, J. K., Irwin, A., & Hoving, C. (2013). New Dimension of Health Care: Systematic Review of the Uses, Benefits, and Limitations of Social Media for Health Communication. *Journal of Medical Internet Research*, *15*(4), e85. doi:10.2196/jmir.1933 PMID:23615206

Morgan, M. (2003). The Doctor-Patient Relationship. In *Sociology as Applied to Medicine* (5th ed., pp. 49–65). London: Saunders.

Mosa, A. S. M., Yoo, I., & Sheets, L. (2012). A Systematic Review of Healthcare Applications for Smartphones. *BMC Medical Informatics and Decision Making*, *12*(67). PMID:22781312

Mosen, D. M., Schmittdiel, J., Hibbard, J., Sobel, D., Remmers, C., & Bellows, J. (2007). Is patient activation associated with outcomes of care for adults with chronic conditions? *The Journal of Ambulatory Care Management*, *30*(1), 21–29. doi:10.1097/00004479-200701000-00005 PMID:17170635

Mossberger, K., Tolbert, C., & Gilbert, M. (2006). Race, concentrated poverty and information technology. *Urban Affairs Review*, *41*(5), 583–620. doi:10.1177/1078087405283511

Mossberger, K., Tolbert, C., & McNeal, R. (2007). *Digital citizenship: The internet, society and participation.* Cambridge, MA: MIT Press.

Mossberger, K., Tolbert, C., & Stansbury, M. (2003). *Virtual inequality: Beyond the digital divide.* Washington, DC: Georgetown Press.

Mulvaney, S. A., Anders, S., Smith, A. K., Pittel, E. J., & Johnson, K. B. (2012). A pilot test of a tailored mobile and web-based diabetes messaging system for adolescents. *Journal of Telemedicine and Telecare, 18*(2), 115–118. doi:10.1258/jtt.2011.111006 PMID:22383802

Murphy, K. (2005, June 30). *Aging surge poses challenge for states.* Retrieved June 3, 2013, from http://www.pewstates.org/projects/stateline/headlines/aging-surge-poses-challenge-for-states-85899389790

Murphy, K. (2007). *Evaluating the Use of Tablet PCs in an Ambulatory Clinic Setting.* Retrieved from http://www.medicalcomputing.org/mcr/openaccess.php

Musen, M. A., Shakar, Y., & Shortliffe, E. H. (2006). Clinical Decision-Support Systems. In E. H. Shortliffe, & J. J. Cimino (Eds.), *Biomedical informatics: Computer applications in health care and biomedicine* (3rd ed., pp. 698–736). New York: Springer. doi:10.1007/0-387-36278-9_20

Nabatchi, T., & Mergel, I. (2010). Participation 2.0: Using Internet and social media: Technologies to promote distributed democracy and create digital neighborhoods. In J. H. Svara & J. Denhardt (Eds.), *Connected communities, local government as partners in citizens engagement and community building* (pp. 80-87). Retrieved March 10, 2011, from http://www.tlgconference.org/communityconnectionswhitepaper.pdf

Nahapiet, J., & Ghoshal, S. (1998). Social capital, intellectual capital, and the organizational advantage. *Academy of Management Review, 23*(2), 242–266.

Nakamura, M. M., Ferris, T. G., DesRoches, C. M., & Jha, A. K. (2010). Electronic health record adoption by children's hospitals in the United States. *Archives of Pediatrics & Adolescent Medicine, 164*(12), 1145–1151. doi:10.1001/archpediatrics.2010.234 PMID:21135344

National AIDS Coordinating Agency (NACA). (2005). *Botswana AIDS impact survey II.* Retrieved August 10, 2011, from http://unbotswana.org.bw/undp/documents/final_popular_report_feb06.pdf

National Alliance for Caregiving. (2009). *Caregiving in the U.S. 2009.* Retrieved June 8, 2013, from http://www.caregiving.org/data/Caregiving_in_the_US_2009_full_report.pdf

National Library of Medicine. (2014). *Greek medicine – The Hippocratic Oath.* Retrieved January 21, 2014 from http://www.nlm.nih.gov/hmd/greek/greek_oath.html

National Telecommunications and Information Administration. (2011). *Digital nation: Expanding internet usage.* Retrieved March 15, 2012, from http://www.ntia.doc.gov/files/ntia/publications/ntia_internet_use_report_february_2011.pdf

Nations, D. (2011). *What is social networking? Social networking explained.* Academic Press.

Nehring, W., & Lashley, F. (2009). Nursing Simulation: A Review of the Past 40 Years. *Simulation & Gaming, 40*(4), 528–552. doi:10.1177/1046878109332282

Neiger, B. L., Thackeray, R., Van Wagenen, S. A., Hanson, C. L., West, J. H., Barnes, M. D., & Fagen, M. C. (2012). Use of Social Media in Health Promotion Purposes, Key Performance Indicators, and Evaluation Metrics. *Health Promotion Practice, 13*(2), 159–164. doi:10.1177/1524839911433467 PMID:22382491

Nelsey, L., & Brownie, S. (2012). Effective leadership, teamwork and mentoring – Essential elements in promoting generational cohesion in the nursing workforce and retaining nurses. *Collegian (Royal College of Nursing, Australia), 19*(4), 197–202. doi:10.1016/j.colegn.2012.03.002 PMID:23362605

New York Department of Health. (2009). Glossary. *Environmental Health Tracking.* Retrieved May 20, 2013, from http://www.health.ny.gov/environmental/public_health_tracking/about/glossary.htm

Ng, H. S., Sim, M. L., & Tan, C. M. (2006). Security issues of wireless sensor networks in healthcare applications. *BT Technology Journal, 24*(2), 138–144. doi:10.1007/s10550-006-0051-8

Niehaves, B., & Plattfaut, R. (2010). *T-Government for the Citizens: Digital Divide and Internet Technology Acceptance among the Elderly*. Paper presented at the T-Gov Workshop. London, UK.

Nielsen. (2011). *State of the media: The social media report*. Retrieved June 30, 2013, from http://blog.nielsen.com/nielsenwire/social/

Nielsen, J. (1993). *Usability engineering*. Boston: Academic Press.

Nielsen, J., & Budiu, R. (2012). *Mobile usability*. Pearson Education.

Nielson Company. (2013). *The Mobile Consumer: A Global Snapshot*. Retrieved from http://www.nielsen.com/content/dam/corporate/us/en/reports-downloads/2013 Reports/Mobile-Consumer-Report-2013.pdf

Nistor, N., Schworm, S., & Werner, M. (2012). Online help-seeking in communities of practice: Modeling the acceptance of conceptual artifacts. *Computers & Education, 59*(2), 774–784. doi:10.1016/j.compedu.2012.03.017

Nmawston. (2012, October 17). Worldwide smartphone population tops 1 billion in Q3 2012. *Strategy Analytics*.

NMBA. (2013). *Nursing and Midwifery Continuing Professional Development Registration Standard*. Retrieved 23 July 2013, from http://www.nursingmidwiferyboard.gov.au/Registration-Standards.aspx

Nonaka, I., & Takeuchi, H. (1995). *The knowledge-creating company: How Japanese companies create the dynamics of innovation*. Oxford University Press.

Noveck, B. S. (2009). *Wiki government: How technology can make government better, democracy stronger, and citizens more powerful*. Washington, DC: Brookings Institution Press.

Nsubuga, P., White, M. E., Thacker, S. B., Anderson, M. A., Blount, S. B., & Broome, C. V. ... Trostle, M. (2006). *Public Health Surveillance: A tool for targeting and monitoring interventions disease control priorities in developing countries* (2nd ed.). Retrieved May 20, 2013, from http://www.ncbi.nlm.nih.gov/books/NBK11770/

Nutbeam, D. (1998). Health promotion glossary. *Health Promotion International, 13*(4), 349–364. doi:10.1093/heapro/13.4.349

O'Mally, G. (2010, April 8). Study: Social Media Vital To Consumers Seeking Healthcare Information. *OnlineMediaDaily*. Retrieved July 25th 2013 from www.mediapost.com/publications/article/125801/?print

O'Reilly, T. (2005). What is Web 2.0: Design patterns and business models for the next generation of software. *O'Reilly*. Retrieved July 16, 2011, from http://oreilly.com/web2/archive/what-is-web-20.html

Obermayer, J. L., Riley, W. T., Asif, O., & Jean-Mary, J. (2004). College smoking-cessation using cell phone text messaging. *Journal of American College Health, 53*(2), 71–78. doi:10.3200/JACH.53.2.71-78 PMID:15495883

Oblinger, D. (2003). Boomers, Gen-Xers and Millenials: Understanding the New Students. *Educause Review*. Retrieved 14 February 2010, from www.educause.edu/educatingthenetgen

Oblinger, D., & Oblinger, J. (2005). *Educating the Net Generation*. Retrieved 23 December 2009, from http://www.educause.edu/educatingthenetgen

Ogungbure, A. A. (2011). The possibilities of technological development in Africa: An evaluation of the role of culture. *The Journal of Pan African Studies, 14*(3).

Olphert, C. W., Damodaran, L., & May, A. J. (2005). *Towards digital inclusion – Engaging older people in the 'digital world'*. Paper presented at the Accessible Design in the Digital World Conference. Dundee, UK.

Organisation for Economic Co-operation and Development (OECD). (2009). *The long-term care workforce: Overview and strategies to adapt supply to a growing demand*. Paris: OCED.

Osborne, S. P. (Ed.). (2010). *The New Public Governance? Emerging Perspectives on the Theory and Practice of Public Governance*. London: Routledge.

Østbye, T., Yarnall, K. S. H., Krause, K. M., Pollak, K., Gradison, M., & Lloyd Michener, J. (2005). Is There Time for Management of Patients With Chronic Diseases in Primary Care? *Annals of Family Medicine, 3*(3), 209–214. doi:10.1370/afm.310 PMID:15928223

Ottenhoff, M. (2012). Infographic: Rising Use of Social and Mobile in Healthcare. *The Spark Report*. Retrieved from http://x.co/1U9fJ

Ozdalga, E., Ozdalga, A., & Ahuja, N. (2012). The Smartphone in Medicine: A Review of Current and Potential Use Among Physicians and Students. *Journal of Medical Internet Research*, *14*(5), e128. doi:10.2196/jmir.1994 PMID:23017375

Pagan, J., Higgs, P., & Cunningham, S. (2008). *Getting Creative in Healthcare: The contribution of creative activities to Australian Healthcare*. Retrieved 23 july 2013, from http://eprints.qut.edu.au/14757/

Pagliari, C., Detmer, D., & Singleton, P. (2007). Potential of electronic personal health records. *BMJ (Clinical Research Ed.)*, *335*(7615), 330–333. doi:10.1136/bmj.39279.482963.AD PMID:17703042

Paiva, A. L., Lipschitz, J. M., Fernandez, A. C., Redding, C. A., & Prochaska, J. O. (2014). Evaluation of the acceptability and feasibility of a computer-tailored intervention to increase human papillomavirus vaccination among young adult women. *Journal of American College Health*, *62*(1), 32–38. doi:10.1080/07448481.2013.843534 PMID:24313694

Pal, K., Eastwood, S. V., Michie, S., Farmer, A. J., Barnard, M. L., & Peacock, R. et al. (2013). Computer-based diabetes self-management interventions for adults with type 2 diabetes mellitus. *Cochrane Database of Systematic Reviews*, *3*. doi:10.1002/14651858.CD008776.pub2 PMID:23543567

Palmier-Claus, J., Ainsworth, J., Machin, M., Barrowclough, C., Dunn, G., & Barkus, E. et al. (2012). The feasibility and validity of ambulatory self-report of psychotic symptoms using a smartphone software application. *BMC Psychiatry*, *12*, 72. doi:10.1186/1471-244X-12-172 PMID:22759565

Pan-Canadian Change Management Network - Communications Working Group. (2012). *Why Change Matters - Investing in Change Management*. Retrieved from https://www.infoway-inforoute.ca/index.php/resources/toolkits/change-management/national-framework/governance-and-leadership/resources-and-tools/doc_download/1330-why-change-matters-investing-in-change-management-healthcare-information-management-communications-hcim-c-2012-26-3-44-46

Parcell, G. (2005). *The Bulletin interview with Geoff Parcell*. World Health Organization. Retrieved June 13, 2012, from http://www.who.int/bulletin/volumes/83/10/interview1005/en/index.html

Paré, G., Moqadem, K., Pineau, G., & St-Hilaire, C. (2010). Clinical effects of home telemonitoring in the context of diabetes, asthma, heart failure and hypertension: A systematic review. *Journal of Medical Internet Research*, *12*(2), e21. doi:10.2196/jmir.1357 PMID:20554500

Parsons, T. (1951). *The social system*. Glencoe, IL: Free Press.

Pathuru Raj, D., Ravichandiran, C. C., & Vaithiyanathan, D. R. (2010). A Comparison and SWOT Analysis of Towards 4G Technologies: 802.16e and 3GPP-LTE. *International Journal on Computer Science & Engineering*, *2*(2), 109–114.

Patrick, K., Raab, F., Adams, M. A., Dillon, L., Zabinski, M., Rock, C. L., & Norman, G. J. (2009). A text message-based intervention for weight loss: Randomized controlled trial. *Journal of Medical Internet Research*, *11*(1), e1. doi:10.2196/jmir.1100 PMID:19141433

Patterson, E. S., Cook, R. I., & Render, M. L. (2002). Improving patient safety by identifying side effects from introducing bar coding in medication administration. *Journal of the American Medical Informatics Association*, *9*(5), 540–553. doi:10.1197/jamia.M1061 PMID:12223506

Patterson, E. S., Doebbeling, B. N., Fung, C. H., Militello, L., Anders, S., & Asch, S. M. (2005). Identifying barriers to the effective use of clinical reminders: Bootstrapping multiple methods. *Journal of Biomedical Informatics*, *38*(3), 189–199. doi:10.1016/j.jbi.2004.11.015 PMID:15896692

Pavlou, P. A. (2003). Consumer Acceptance of Electronic Commerce: Integrating Trust and Risk with the Technology Acceptance Model. *International Journal of Electronic Commerce*, *7*(3), 101.

Pearce-Brown, C., Glasgow, N., Jeon, H., Jenkins, S., & Douglas, K. (2009). *Health literacy and self management in COPD: The same, different or misunderstood?* Paper presented at the PHC Research Conference. New York, NY.

Perficient. (2013). *The Driving Force of Social Media in Healthcare*. Retrieved July 25th 2013 from http://www.perficient.com/Thought-Leadership/Perficient-Perspectives/2013/Social-Media-in-Healthcare

Perrig, A., Stankovic, J., & Wagner, D. (2004). Security in wireless sensor networks. *Communications of the ACM*, *47*(6), 53–57. doi:10.1145/990680.990707

Pew Internet & American Life Project, & Zickuhr, K. (2013, June). *Tablet Ownership 2013*. Retrieved September 30, 2013, from http://pewinternet.org/Reports/2013/Tablet-Ownership-2013.aspx

Pew Internet and American Life Project. (2012). *CHCF Health Survey Aug 7-Sep 6, 2012*. Retrieved from http://www.pewinternet.org/Reports/2013/Tracking-for-Health/Summary-of-Findings.aspx

Pew Research Center's Internet & American Life Project. (2011, May 12). *The social life of health information, 2011*. Retrieved April 8, 2012, from http://www.pewinternet.org/Reports/2011/Social-Life-of-Health-Info.aspx

Pew Research Center's Internet & American Life Project. (2012a). *Mobile health 2012*. Retrieved March 9, 2013, from http://www.pewinternet.org/Reports/2012/Mobile-Health.aspx

Pew Research Center's Internet & American Life Project. (2012b). *Family caregivers online*. Retrieved February 10, 2013, from http://www.pewinternet.org/Reports/2012/Caregivers-online.aspx

Phillips, R., Kennedy, G., & McNaught, C. (2012). The role of theory in learning technology evaluation research. *Australasian Journal of Educational Technology*, *28*(7), 1103–1118.

Picot, J. (1998). Telemedicine and Telehealth in Canada: Forty Years of Change in the Use of Information and Communications Technologies in a Publicly Administered Health Care System. *Telemedicine Journal*, *4*(3), 199–205. doi:10.1089/tmj.1.1998.4.199 PMID:9831745

Pino, C., & Kavasidis, I. (2012). Improving mobile device interaction by eye tracking analysis. In *Proceedings of Computer Science and Information Systems (FedCSIS), 2012 Federated Conference on* (pp. 1199-1202). IEEE.

Pitts, S. R., Niska, R. W., Xu, J., & Burt, C. W. (2008). National Hospital Ambulatory Medical Care Survey: 2006 emergency department summary. *National Health Statistics Reports*, (7), 1-38.

Plint, A. C., Moher, D., Morrison, A., Schulz, K., Altman, D. G., Hill, C., & Gaboury, I. (2006). Does the CONSORT checklist improve the quality of reports of randomized controlled trials? A systematic review. *The Medical Journal of Australia*, *185*(5), 263–267. PMID:16948622

Pope, L., Silva, P., & Almeyda, R. (2010). i-Phone applications for the modern day otolaryngologist. *Clinical Otolaryngology: Official Journal of ENT-UK. Official Journal of Netherlands Society for Oto-Rhino-Laryngology & Cervico-Facial Surgery*, *35*(4), 350. doi:10.1111/j.1749-4486.2010.02170.x

Popoiu, M. C., Grosseck, G., & Holetescu, C. (2012). What do we know about the use of social media in medical education? *Procedia: Social and Behavioral Sciences*, *46*, 2262–2266. doi:10.1016/j.sbspro.2012.05.466

Porter, M. E. (2009). A Strategy for Health Care Reform - Toward a Value-Based System. *The New England Journal of Medicine*, *361*(2), 109–112. doi:10.1056/NEJMp0904131 PMID:19494209

Portnoy, D. B., Scott-Sheldon, L. A., Johnson, B. T., & Carey, M. P. (2008). Computer-delivered interventions for health promotion and behavioural risk reduction: A meta-analysis of 75 randomized controlled trials, 1988 – 2007. *Preventive Medicine*, *47*, 3–16. doi:10.1016/j.ypmed.2008.02.014 PMID:18403003

Preece, J. (1995). *Human-computer interaction*. Wokingham, UK: Addison-Wesley Pub. Co.

Preece, J. (2001). Sociability and usability in online communities: Determining and measuring success. *Behaviour & Information Technology*, *20*(5), 347–356. doi:10.1080/01449290110084683

Prensky, M. (2001). Digital Natives, Digital Immigrants On the Horizon. MCB University Press, 9(5).

Price Waterhouse Coopers. (2010). *Healthcare unwired: New business models delivering care anywhere*. Retrieved from http://www.pwc.com/us/en/health-industries/publications/healthcare-unwired.jhtml

Price WaterHouse Coopers. (2012). *Emerging mHealth: Paths for growth*. Retrieved July 15, 2013, from http://www.pwc.com/en_GX/gx/healthcare/mhealth/assets/pwc-emerging-mhealth-full.pdf

Primack, B. A., Carroll, M. V., McNamara, M., Klem, M. L., King, B., & Rich, M. et al. (2012). Role of video games in improving health-related outcomes: A systematic review. *American Journal of Preventive Medicine*, *42*(6), 630–638. doi:10.1016/j.amepre.2012.02.023 PMID:22608382

Prochaska, J. O., Butterworth, S., Redding, C. A., Burden, V., Perrin, N., & Leo, M. et al. (2008). Initial efficacy of MI, TTM tailoring and HRI's with multiple behaviors for employee health promotion. *Preventive Medicine*, *46*(3), 226–231. doi:10.1016/j.ypmed.2007.11.007 PMID:18155287

Prochaska, J. O., DiClemente, C. C., & Norcross, J. C. (1992). In search of how people change: Applications to addictive behaviors. *The American Psychologist*, *47*(9), 1102–1114. doi:10.1037/0003-066X.47.9.1102 PMID:1329589

Proper, K. I., Van den Heuvel, S. G., De Vroome, E. M., Hildebrandt, V. H., & Van der Beek, A. J. (2006). Dose–response relation between physical activity and sick leave. *British Journal of Sports Medicine*, *40*(2), 173–178. doi:10.1136/bjsm.2005.022327 PMID:16432007

Protti, D. (2008). A comparison of how Canada, England and Demark are managing their electronic health record journeys. In *Human, Social and Organizational Aspects of Healthcare Information Systems*. Hershey, PA: IGI Global. doi:10.4018/978-1-59904-792-8.ch012

Proudfoot, J., Parker, G., Hadzi Pavlovic, D., Manicavasagar, V., Adler, E., & Whitton, A. (2010). Community attitudes to the appropriation of mobile phones for monitoring and managing depression, anxiety, and stress. *Journal of Medical Internet Research*, *12*(5), e64. doi:10.2196/jmir.1475 PMID:21169174

Public Health Agency of Canada. (n.d.). Retrieved from http://www.phac-aspc.gc.ca/cd-mc/hl-ls/index-eng.php

Public Law (111-148). (2010). *Patient Protection and Affordable Care Act.*

Public Law 103-3. (1993). *Family and Medical Leave Act.*

Public Law 109-442. (2006). *Lifespan Respite Care Act.*

Public Law 110-246. (2008). *The Older Americans Act.*

Public Law 78-410. (1991). *Public Health Service Act.*

Public Law 89-73. (1965). *Older Americans Act.*

PUBMED. (n.d.). Retrieved 1 August 2012, from http://www.ncbi.nlm.nih.gov/pubmed/

PwC Health Research Institute. (2013). *Top health industry issues of 2013: Picking up the pace on health reform*. Retrieved July 15, 2013, from http://pwchealth.com/cgi-local/hregister.cgi/reg/pwc-hri-top-health-industry-issues-2013.pdf

Qiang, C. Z., Yamamichi, M., Hausman, V., & Altman, D. (2011). *Mobile Applications for the Health Sector*. Washington, DC: ICT Sector Unit, World Bank.

Qualman, E. (2009). *Socialnomics: How social media transforms the way we live and do business*. Hoboken, NJ: John Wiley & Sons.

Qualman, E. (2013). *Socialnomics: How Social Media Transforms the way we live and do business* (2nd ed.). John Wiley & Sons.

Ramsay Health Care. (2012). *Ramsay Health Care's Social Media Policy*. Retrieved 6 May 2013, from http://www.youtube.com/watch?v=f-xo0237n6U

Raschke, R. A., Gollihare, B., Wunderlich, T. A., Guidry, J. R., Leibowitz, A. I., Peirce, J. C., & Susong, C. (1998). A computer alert system to prevent injury from adverse drug events: Development and evaluation in a community teaching hospital. *Journal of the American Medical Association*, *280*(15), 1317–1320. doi:10.1001/jama.280.15.1317 PMID:9794309

Rask, K. J., Ziemer, D. C., Kohler, S. A., Hawley, J. N., Arinde, F. J., & Barnes, C. S. (2009). Patient activation is associated with healthy behaviors and ease in managing diabetes in an indigent population. *The Diabetes Educator*, *35*(4), 622–630. doi:10.1177/0145721709335004 PMID:19419972

RCNA. (2011). *RCNA Social Media Guidelines for Nurses*. Canberra, Australia: Royal College of Nursing Australia.

Reason, J. (1995). Understanding adverse events: human factors. *Quality in Health Care*, *4*(2), 80–89. doi:10.1136/qshc.4.2.80 PMID:10151618

Report, W. H. (2013). *Research for Universal Health Coverage*. World Health Organization.

Research2Guidance. (2013). *Mobile Health market Report 2013-2017*. Retrieved January 21, 2014 from http://www.research2guidance.com/shop/index.php/mhealth-report-2

Rhodes, P., & Shaw, S. (1999). Informal care and terminal illness. *Health & Social Care in the Community*, *7*(1), 39–50. doi:10.1046/j.1365-2524.1999.00147.x PMID:11560621

Richards, T. B., Croner, C. M., Rushton, G., Brown, C. K., & Fowler, L. (1999). Geographical Information Systems and Public Health. *The Long Island Breast Cancer Study Project*. Retrieved March 10, 2011, from http://healthcybermap.org/HGeo/res/phr.pdf

Riddle, D. I. (2008). *Managing service innovation*. CMC Service-Growth Consultants Inc.

Robertson, C., Sawford, K., Daniel, S. L. A., Nelson, T. A., & Stephen, C. (2010). *Mobile phone-based infectious disease surveillance system, Sri Lanka*. Retrieved May 13, 2013, from http://wwwnc.cdc.gov/eid/article/16/10/pdfs/10-0249.pdf

Rock, D. (2009). Managing with the Brain in Mind. *Strategy+ Business, 56*, 1-11.

Rodgers, A., Corbett, T., Bramley, D., Riddell, T., Wills, M., Lin, R., & Jones, M. (2005). Do u smoke after txt? Results of a randomised trial of smoking cessation using mobile phone text messaging. *Tobacco Control*, *14*(4), 255–261. doi:10.1136/tc.2005.011577 PMID:16046689

Roehrer, E., Cummings, E., Beggs, S., Turner, P., Hauser, J., & Micallef, N. et al. (2013). Pilot evaluation of web enabled symptom monitoring in cystic fibrosis. *Informatics for Health & Social Care*. doi:10.3109/17538157.2013.812646 PMID:23957685

Roehrer, E., Cummings, E., Ellis, L., & Turner, P. (2011). The role of user-centred design within online community development. *Studies in Health Technology and Informatics*, *164*, 256–260. PMID:21335720

Roehrer, E., Cummings, E., Turner, P., Hauser, J., Cameron-Tucker, H., & Beggs, S. et al. (2013). Supporting cystic fibrosis with ICT. *Studies in Health Technology and Informatics*, *183*, 137–141. PMID:23388270

Rogers, E. (1995). *Diffusion of Innovations* (5th ed.). New York: Free Press.

Roher, D., & Hall, J. A. (2006). *Doctors talking with patients/patients talking with doctors: Improving communication in medical visits* (2nd ed.). Westport, CT: Praeger.

Rolland, J., Wright, D., & Kancherla, A. (1996). Towards a Novel Augmented-Reality Tool to Visualise Dynamic 3-D Anatomy. In J. Westwood, S. Westwood, L. Felländer-Tsai, R. Haluck, R. Robb, S. Senger, & K. Vosburgh (Eds.), *Medicine Meets Virtual Reality: Global healthcare grid* (pp. 337–348). Washington, DC: IOS Press.

Rosenbaum, H., & Shachaf, P. (2010). A structuration approach to online communities of practice: The case of Q&A communities. *Journal of the American Society for Information Science and Technology*, *61*(9), 1933–1944. doi:10.1002/asi.21340

Rosser, B. A., Vowles, K. E., Keogh, E., Eccleston, C., & Mountain, G. A. (2009). Technologically assisted behavior change: A systematic review of studies of novel technologies for the management of chronic illness. *Journal of Telemedicine and Telecare*, *15*(7), 327–338. doi:10.1258/jtt.2009.090116 PMID:19815901

Rubinelli, S., Camerini, L., & Schulz, P. J. (2010). *Comunicazione e salute*. Milano: Apogeo.

Rubin, J. (1994). *Handbook of usability testing: How to plan, design, and conduct effective tests*. New York: Wiley.

Rudansky, A. K. (2013, June 23). PayPal Founder's Fellowship Hatches Medication Reminder App. *Information Week Health Care*. Retrieved from http://x.co/1U6Xp

Ruiz, J., Mintzer, M., & Leipzig, R. (2006). The impact of E-learning in medical education. *Academic Medicine*, *81*(3), 207–212. doi:10.1097/00001888-200603000-00002 PMID:16501260

Russ, A. L., Weiner, M., Russell, S. A., Baker, D. A., Fahner, W. J., & Saleem, J. J. (2012). Design and implementation of a hospital-based usability laboratory: Insights from a Department of Veterans Affairs laboratory for health information technology. *Joint Commission Journal on Quality and Patient Safety, 38*(12), 531–540. PMID:23240261

Russell, J., Greenhalgh, T., Boynton, P., & Rigby, M. (2004). Soft networks for bridging the gap between research and practice: Illuminative evaluation of CHAIN. *BMJ (Clinical Research Ed.), 328*(7449), 1174. doi:10.1136/bmj.328.7449.1174 PMID:15142924

Russin, M., & Davis, J. (1990). Continuing education electronic bulletin board system: Provider readiness and interest. *Journal of Continuing Education in Nursing, 21*(1), 23–27. PMID:2106537

Salvendy, G. (2006). *Handbook of human factors and ergonomics* (3rd ed.). Hoboken, NJ: John Wiley. doi:10.1002/0470048204

Samie, N. (2011, October 19). *Social media popular with South African youth*. Voice of America.

Samsung. (2013). How do I use Air Gestures to control my Samsung Galaxy S® 4? In *How to Guides*. Retrieved, November 1, 2013, from http://www.samsung.com/us/support/howtoguide/N0000003/10141/120552

Sánchez, J., & Olivares, R. (2011). Problem solving and collaboration using mobile serious games. *Computers & Education, 57*(3), 1943–1952. doi:10.1016/j.compedu.2011.04.012

Sanson-Fisher, R. (2004). Diffusion of innovation theory for clinical change. *The Medical Journal of Australia, 180*, S55–S56. PMID:15012582

Santoro, E. (2011). *Web 2.0 e Social Media in medicina*. Milano: Il Pensiero Scientifico Editore.

Savage, E., Beirne, P. V., Ni Chroinin, M., Duff, A., Fitzgerald, T., & Farrell, D. (2011). Self-management education for cystic fibrosis. *Cochrane Database of Systematic Reviews, 7*. doi:10.1002/14651858.CD007641.pub2 PMID:21735415

Savitz, E. (2012). 5 Ways Mobile Apps Will Transform Healthcare. *CIO Network: Insights and Ideas for Technology Leaders*. Retrieved 10 Jan 2013, from http://www.forbes.com/sites/ciocentral/2012/06/04/5-ways-mobile-apps-will-transform-healthcare/

Schaefer, J., Miller, D., Goldstein, M., & Simmons, L. (2009). *Partnering in Self-Management Support: A Toolkit for Clinicians*. Institute for Healthcare Improvement. Retrieved from http://www.ihi.org/resources/Pages/Tools/SelfManagementToolkitforClinicians.aspx

Schein, R., Wilson, K., & Keelan, J. (2011). *Literature review on effectiveness of the use of social media: A report for Peel Public Health*. Retrieved June 25, 2013, from http://www.innonet.org/resources/files/socialmediaLitReview.pdf

Schmeida, M. (2005). *Telehealth innovation in the American states*. Ann Arbor, MI: ProQuest.

Schmeida, M., & McNeal, R. (2007). The telehealth divide: disparities to searching public health information online. *Journal of Health Care for the Poor and Underserved, 18*(3), 637–647. doi:10.1353/hpu.2007.0068 PMID:17675719

Schmeida, M., & McNeal, R. (2013). Bridging the inequality gap to searching Medicare and Medicaid information online: An empirical analysis of e-government success 2002 through 2010. In J. Ramon Gil-Garcia (Ed.), *E-government success around the world: Cases, empirical studies, and practical recommendations*. Hershey, PA: IGI Global. doi:10.4018/978-1-4666-4173-0.ch004

Schmidt, C. W. (2012). *Trending now: Using social media to predict and track disease outbreaks*. Retrieved May 15, 2013, from http://www.ncbi.nlm.nih.gov/pmc/articles/PMC3261963/

Schulz, R., & Beach, S. (1999). Caregiving as a risk factor for mortality: The caregiver health effect study. *Journal of the American Medical Association, 282*(23), 2215–2219. doi:10.1001/jama.282.23.2215 PMID:10605972

Schwarzer, R. (1999). Self-regulatory Processes in the Adoption and Maintenance of Health Behaviours. *J Health Psychol March, 4* (2), 115-127.

Segall, N., Saville, J. G., L'Engle, P., Carlson, B., Wright, M. C., Schulman, K., & Tcheng, J. E. (2011). Usability evaluation of a personal health record. In *Proceedings of AMIA Annual Symposium*. American Medical Informatics Association.

Selwyn, N. (2004). Reconsidering political and popular understandings of the digital divide. *New Media & Society, 6*(3), 341–362. doi:10.1177/1461444804042519

Senge, P. M. (1990). *The Fifth Discipline*. New York: Doubleday/Currency.

Shannon, C. E., & Weaver, W. (1949). *The mathematical theory of information*. Urbana, IL: University of Illinois Press.

Shaw, R. J., & Johnson, C. M. (2011). Health Information Seeking and Social Media Use on the Internet among People with Diabetes. *Online Journal of Public Health Informatics, 3*(1), 1–9. doi:10.5210/ojphi.v3i1.3561 PMID:23569602

Sherstyuk, A., Vincent, D., & Berg, B. (2008). *Creating Mixed Reality Manikins for Medical Education*. Paper presented at the Artificial Reality and Telexistance (ICAT, 2008). Yokohoma, Japan.

Shi, E., & Perrig, A. (2004). Designing secure sensor networks. *IEEE Wireless Communications, 11*(6), 38–43. doi:10.1109/MWC.2004.1368895

Shiffman, S., Stone, A. A., & Hufford, M. R. (2008). Ecological momentary assessment. *Annual Review of Clinical Psychology, 4*(1), 1–32. doi:10.1146/annurev.clinpsy.3.022806.091415 PMID:18509902

Shih, C. (2009). *The Facebook Era: Tapping Online Social Networks to Build Better Products and Sell More Stuff*. Hoboken, NJ: Prentice Hall.

Showell, C., & Turner, P. (2013). The PLU problem: are we designing personal ehealth for People Like Us? In *Proceedings of Information Technology and Communications in Health (ITCH) Conference*. IOS Press.

Siegenthaler, E., Wurtz, P., & Groner, R. (2010). Improving the usability of e-book readers. *Journal of Usability Studies, 6*(1), 25–38.

Siewiorek, D. Smailagic, Furukawa, A., Krause, A., Moraveji, N., Reiger, K., & Shaffer, J. (2003). Sensay: A context-aware mobile phone. In *Proceedings of the 7th IEEE International Symposium on Wearable Computers*. IEEE.

Siliquini, R., Ceruti, M., Lovato, E., Bert, F., Bruno, S., & De Vito, E. et al. (2011). Surfing the internet for health information: An Italian survey on use and population choice. *BMC Medical Informatics and Decision Making, 11*(1), 1–9. doi:10.1186/1472-6947-11-21 PMID:21211015

Simborg, D. (2010). Consumer empowerment versus consumer populism in healthcare IT. *Journal of the American Medical Informatics Association, 17*, 370–372. doi:10.1136/jamia.2010.003392 PMID:20595301

Sime Darby Healthcare. (2013). *Sime Darby Healthcare*. Retrieved May 15, 2013, from http://www.simedarby-healthcare.com/

Simon, S. K., & Seldon, H. L. (2012). Personal health records: Mobile biosensors and smartphones for developing countries. *Studies in Health Technology and Informatics, 182*, 125. PMID:23138087

Singh, R. I., Sumeeth, M., & Miller, J. (2011). Evaluating the Readability of Privacy Policies in Mobile Environments. *International Journal of Mobile Human Computer Interaction, 3*(1), 55–78. doi:10.4018/jmhci.2011010104

Sirajuddin, A. M., Osheroff, J. A., Sittig, D. F., Chuo, J., Velasco, F., & Collins, D. A. (2009). Implementation pearls from a new guidebook on improving medication use and outcomes with clinical decision support: Effective CDS is essential for addressing healthcare performance improvement imperatives. *Journal of Healthcare Information Management, 23*(4), 38–45. PMID:19894486

Sirianni, C. (2009). *Investing in democracy: Engaging citizens in collaborative governance*. Washington, DC: Brookings Press.

Sittig, D. F., Wright, A., Osheroff, J. A., Middleton, B., Teich, J. M., Ash, J. S., & Bates, D. W. (2008). Grand challenges in clinical decision support. *Journal of Biomedical Informatics, 41*(2), 387–392. doi:10.1016/j.jbi.2007.09.003 PMID:18029232

Skiba, D., & Barton, A. (2006). Adapting your Teaching to Accommodate the Net Generation of Learners. *The Online Journal of Issues in Nursing, 11*(2), Manuscript 4.

Skolasky, R. L., Green, A. F., Scharfstein, D., Boult, C., Reider, L., & Wegener, S. T. (2011). Psychometric properties of the patient activation measure among multimorbid older adults. *Health Services Research, 46*(2), 457–478. doi:10.1111/j.1475-6773.2010.01210.x PMID:21091470

Slagle, J. M., Gordon, J. S., Harris, C. E., Davison, C. L., Culpepper, D. K., Scott, P., & Johnson, K. B. (2010). MyMediHealth - Designing a next generation system for child-centered medication management. *Journal of Biomedical Informatics, 43*(5Suppl), S27–S31. doi:10.1016/j.jbi.2010.06.006 PMID:20937481

Smedley, A. (2005). The importance of informatics competencies in Nursing: An Australian Perspective. *Computers, Informatics, Nursing. CIN, 23*(2), 106–110. PMID:15772512

Smith, A. (2011, September 19). *Americans and text messaging*. Pew Internet & American Life Project: A Project of the Pew Research Center. Retrieved from http://www.pewinternet.org/~/media//Files/Reports/2011/Americans%20and%20Text%20Messaging.pdf

Smith, C. A., Hetzel, S., Dalrymple, P., & Keselman, A. (2011). Beyond readability: Investigating coherence of clinical text for consumers. *Journal of Medical Internet Research, 13*(4), e104. doi:10.2196/jmir.1842 PMID:22138127

Smith, C. E., Dauz, E. R., Clements, F., Puno, F. N., Cook, D., Doolittle, G., & Leeds, W. (2006). Telehealth services to improve nonadherence: A placebo-controlled study. *Telemedicine Journal and e-Health, 12*(3), 289–296. doi:10.1089/tmj.2006.12.289 PMID:16796496

Smith, J., Milberg, S., & Burke, S. (1996). Information Privacy: Measuring Individuals' Concerns about Organizational Practices. *Management Information Systems Quarterly, 20*(2), 167–196. doi:10.2307/249477

Solis, B., & Breakenridge, D. (2009). *Putting the public back in public relations*. Upper Saddle River, NJ: Pearson Education.

Solomon, M., Wagner, S. L., & Goes, J. (2012). Effects of a web-based intervention for adults with chronic conditions on patient activation: online randomized controlled trial. *Journal of Medical Internet Research, 14*(1), e32. doi:10.2196/jmir.1924 PMID:22353433

Sourceforge. (2013). *Android Screenshots and Screen Capture*. Retrieved November 8, 2013, from http://sourceforge.net/projects/ashot/

Spiegel, P. B. (2004). HIV/AIDS among conflict-affected and displaced populations: Dispelling myths and taking action. *Disasters, 28*(3), 322–339. doi:10.1111/j.0361-3666.2004.00261.x PMID:15344944

Spiekermann, S., & Lorrie, F. C. (2009). Engineering privacy. *IEEE Transactions on Software Engineering, 35*(1), 67–82. doi:10.1109/TSE.2008.88

Sposaro, F., & Tyson, G. (2009). iFall: An Android application for fall monitoring and response. In Proceedings of Engineering in Medicine and Biology Society, (pp. 6119-6122). IEEE.

Squirrels. (2013). Reflector. In *Products*. Retrieved November 8, 2013, from http://www.airsquirrels.com/reflector/

Staggers, N., Gassert, C., & Curran, C. (2002). A Delphi study to determine Informatics competencies for nurses at four levels of practice. *Nursing Research, 51*(6), 383–390. doi:10.1097/00006199-200211000-00006 PMID:12464758

Stajduhar, K., Funk, L., Toye, C., Grande, G., Aoun, S., & Todd, C. (2010). Part I: Home-based family caregiving at the end of life: A comprehensive review of quantitative research (1998-2008). *Palliative Medicine, 24*(6), 573–593. doi:10.1177/0269216310371412 PMID:20562171

Stanford, V. (2002). Pervasive Health Care Applications Face Tough Security Challenges. *IEEE Pervasive Computing / IEEE Computer Society [and] IEEE Communications Society, 1*(2), 8–12. doi:10.1109/MPRV.2002.1012332

Stergiou, N., Georgoulakis, G., Margari, N., Aninos, D., Stamataki, M., & Stergiou, E. et al. (2009). Using a web-based system for the continuous distance education in cytopathology. *International Journal of Medical Informatics, 78*(12), 827–838. doi:10.1016/j.ijmedinf.2009.08.007 PMID:19775933

Sterling, G. (2013). *Pew: 61 Percent in US Now Have Smartphones*. Retrieved September 30, 2013, from http://marketingland.com/pew-61-percent-in-us-now-have-smartphones-46966

Sterling, G. (2013, May 29). *Tablet Market Share iPad Remains Dominant, Samsung Shows Growth*. Retrieved from http://marketingland.com/tablet-market-share-ipad-remains-dominant-samsung-shows-growth-45974

Stewart, A. L., Hays, R. D., Wells, K. B., Rogers, W. H., Spritzer, K. L., & Greenfield, S. (1994). Long-term functioning and well-being outcomes associated with physical activity and exercise in patients with chronic conditions in the medical outcomes study. *Journal of Clinical Epidemiology, 47*(7), 719–730. doi:10.1016/0895-4356(94)90169-4 PMID:7722585

Stinson, J., Jibb, L., Nathan, P. C., Maloney, A. M., Dupuis, L. L., Gerstle, J. T., et al. (2012). *Development and Testing of a Multidimensional IPhone Pain Assessment Application for Adolescents with Cancer*. iPROCEEDINGS Medicine 2.0 Boston. Retrieved from http://www.medicine20congress.com/ocs/index.php/med/med2012/paper/view/910

Stojanovic, D. (2009). *Context-aware Mobile and Ubiquitous Computing for Enhanced Usability: Adaptive Technologies and Applications*. Hershey, PA: Information Science. doi:10.4018/978-1-60566-290-9

Strader, T. J., Ramaswarni, S. N., & Houle, P. (2007). Perceived Network Externalities and Communication Technology Acceptance. *European Journal of Information Systems, 16*(1), 54–65. doi:10.1057/palgrave.ejis.3000657

Struik, L. L., Bottorff, J. L., Jung, M., & Budgen, C. (2012). *Facebook Me: The Use of Social Networking Sites for Gender-Sensitive Tobacco Control Messaging*. iPROCEEDINGS Medicine 2.0 Boston. Retrieved from http://www.medicine20congress.com/ocs/index.php/med/med2012/paper/view/785

Sunwoo, J., Yuen, W., Lutteroth, C., & Wünsche, B. (2010). Mobile games for elderly healthcare. In *Proceedings of the 11th International Conference of the NZ Chapter of the ACM Special Interest Group on Human-Computer Interaction* (pp. 73-76). ACM.

Sutirtha, C., Suranjan, C., Saonee, S., Suprateek, S., & Lau, F. (2009). Examining Success Factors For Mobile Work In Healthcare: A Deductive Study. *Decision Support Systems, 46*(3), 620–633. doi:10.1016/j.dss.2008.11.003

Swan, M. (2009). Emerging patient-driven health care models: An examination of health social networks, consumer personalized medicine and quantified self-tracking. *International Journal of Environmental Research and Public Health, 6*(2), 492–525. doi:10.3390/ijerph6020492 PMID:19440396

Syed-Abdul, S., Fernandez-Luque, L., Jian, W.-S., Li, Y.-C., Crain, S., & Hsu, M. et al. (2013). Misleading Health-Related Information Promoted Through Video-Based Social Media: Anorexia on YouTube. *Journal of Medical Internet Research, 15*(2), e30. doi:10.2196/jmir.2237 PMID:23406655

Tang, P. C., Ash, J. S., Bates, D. W., Overhage, J. M., & Sands, D. Z. (2006). Personal health records: Definitions, benefits, and strategies for overcoming barriers to adoption. *Journal of the American Medical Informatics Association, 13*(2), 121–126. doi:10.1197/jamia.M2025 PMID:16357345

Tarasenko, E. (2012). *Facebook Me: Russian Social Media for Patients and Physicians: Problems and Perspectives*. iPROCEEDINGS Medicine 2.0 Boston. Retrieved from http://www.medicine20congress.com/ocs/index.php/med/med2012/paper/view/1025

Taylor, C. (2013). *250,000 social media users in U.S. said they got the flu*. Retrieved May 18, 2013, from http://mashable.com/2013/01/16/facebook-twitter-flu/

Teves, J., Chaparro, B., Chan, R., Copic, N., Riss, R., & Simmons, J. (2013). *Exploring iPad Usage by Healthcare Professionals in a Pediatric Hospital*. Retrieved from http://usabilitynews.org/exploring-ipad-usage-by-healthcare-professionals-in-a-pediatric-hospital/

Thackeray, R., Neiger, B. L., Hanson, C. L., & McKenzie, J. F. (2008). Enhancing promotional strategies within social marketing programs: Use of web 2.0 social media. *Health Promotion Practice*, 9(4), 338–343. doi:10.1177/1524839908325335 PMID:18936268

Thesaurus, C. R. I. S. P. (2006). Environmental Health Ontology. *BioPortal*. Retrieved June 11, 2011, from http://bioportal.bioontology.org/search

Thielst, C. B. (2011). Social Media: Ubiquitous Community and Patient Engagement. *Frontiers of Health Services Management*, 28(2), 3–14. PMID:22256506

Thompson, P. D., Buchner, D., Piña, I. L., Balady, G. J., Williams, M. A., & Marcus, B. H. et al. (2003). Exercise and physical activity in the prevention and treatment of atherosclerotic cardiovascular disease a statement from the Council on Clinical Cardiology (Subcommittee on Exercise, Rehabilitation, and Prevention) and the Council on Nutrition, Physical Activity, and Metabolism (Subcommittee on Physical Activity). *Circulation*, 107(24), 3109–3116. doi:10.1161/01.CIR.0000075572.40158.77 PMID:12821592

Thune, I., & Furberg, A.-S. (2001). Physical activity and cancer risk: dose-response and cancer, all sites and site-specific. *Medicine and Science in Sports and Exercise*, 33(6 Suppl), S530–50, discussion S609–10.

Tidd, J., & Bessant, J. (2009). *Managing innovation: Integrating technological, market and organizational change*. Academic Press.

Tong, R. (2007). Gender-based disparities east/west: Rethinking the burden of care in the United States and Taiwan. *Bioethics*, 21(9), 488–499. doi:10.1111/j.1467-8519.2007.00594.x PMID:17927625

Torning, K., & Oinas-Kukkonen, H. (2009). Persuasive system design: State of the art and future directions. In *Proceedings of the 4th International Conference on Persuasive Technology*. New York: ACM.

Trappenburg, J., Jonkman, N., Jaarsma, T., van Os-Medendorp, H., Kort, H., & de Wit, N. et al. (2013). Self-management: one size does not fit all. *Patient Education and Counseling*, 92(1), 134–137. doi:10.1016/j.pec.2013.02.009 PMID:23499381

Traxler, J. (2007). Defining, discussing and evaluating mobile learning: The moving Finger writes and having writ. *International Review of Research in Open and Distance Learning*, 8(2), 67–75.

Tremblay, D.-G. (2007). Communities of Practice (CoP), implementation challenges of e-working. *The Journal of E-Working*, 1, 69–82.

Treuer, P., & Jenson, J. (2003). Electronic Portfolios Need Standards to Thrive: The proliferation of e-portfolio applications requires compatible software and design standards to support lifelong learning. *EDUCAUSE Quarterly*, 2, 34–42.

Tseng, F.-C., & Kuo, F.-Y. (2014). A study of social participation and knowledge sharing in the teachers' online professional community of practice. *Computers & Education*, 72, 37–47. doi:10.1016/j.compedu.2013.10.005

Twitter. (2013). *Twitter Inc*. Retrieved May 18, 2013, from https://twitter.com/

Twomey, A. (2004). Web-based teaching in nursing: Lessons from the literature. *Nurse Education Today*, 24(6), 452–458. doi:10.1016/j.nedt.2004.04.010 PMID:15312954

U.S. Census Bureau. (2010, May). *The next four decades, the older population in the United States: 2010 to 2050*. Retrieved July 24, 2013 from http://www.census.gov/prod/2010pubs/p25-1138.pdf

U.S. Census Bureau. (2012). *The 2012 statistical abstract, the national databook*. Retrieved July 29, 2013 from http://www.census.gov/compendia/statab/cats/health_nutrition.html

U.S. Department of Health & Human Services (HHS). (2011). *We Can't Wait: Obama Administration takes new steps to encourage doctors and hospitals to use health information technology to lower costs, improve quality, create jobs*. Retrieved November 4, 2013, from http://www.hhs.gov/news/press/2011pres/11/20111130a.html

U.S. Department of Health and Human Services. (2010). *Health literacy online: A guide to writing and designing easy-to-use health Web sites.* Retrieved July 4, 2013, from http://www.health.gov/healthliteracyonline/

United Nations Fund for Population Activities (UNFPA). (n.d.). *Young people: The greatest hope for turning the tide.* Retrieved July 22, 2012, from http://www.unfpa.org/hiv/people.htm

University of Tasmania. (2010). *Social Media Guidelines.* Retrieved 15 January 2013, from http://www.utas.edu.au/__data/assets/pdf_file/0007/82843/Social-Media-Guidelines.pdf

UPMC. (2013). *HealthTrak: Your health online – and on your schedule.* Retrieved November 2, 2013, from https://myupmc.upmc.com/

Urbach, N., Smolnik, S., & Riempp, G. (2010). An empirical investigation of employee portal success. *The Journal of Strategic Information Systems*, *19*(3), 184–206. doi:10.1016/j.jsis.2010.06.002

Utterback, J. M. (1994). *Mastering the Dynamics of Innovation.* Harvard Business School Press.

Utterback, J. M., & Acee, H. J. (2005). Disruptive Technologies: An Expanded View. *International Journal of Innovation Management*, *9*(1), 1–17. doi:10.1142/S1363919605001162

Van De Belt, T. H., Engelen, L. J., Berben, S. A., & Schoonhoven, L. (2010). Definition of health 2.0 and medicine 2.0: A systematic review. *Journal of Medical Internet Research*, *12*(2), e18. doi:10.2196/jmir.1350 PMID:20542857

Van der Rijt, R., & Hoffman, S. (2013). Ethical considerations of clinical photography in an area of emerging technology and smartphones. *Journal of Medical Ethics.* PMID:23800451

van Gemert-Pijnen, J. E., Nijland, N., van Limburg, M., Ossebaard, H. C., Kelders, S. M., Eysenbach, G., & Seydel, E. R. (2011). A holistic framework to improve the uptake and impact of eHealth technologies. *Journal of Medical Internet Research*, *13*(4), e111. doi:10.2196/jmir.1672 PMID:22155738

van Mierlo, T., Voci, S., Lee, S., Fournier, R., & Selby, P. (2012). Superusers in Social Networks for Smoking Cessation: Analysis of Demographic Characteristics and Posting Behavior from the Canadian Cancer Society's Smokers' Helpline Online and StopSmokingCenter.net. *Journal of Medical Internet Research*, *14*(3), e66. doi:10.2196/jmir.1854 PMID:22732103

Van, S. C., Ilie, V., Lou, H., & Stafford, T. (2007). Perceived critical mass and the adoption of a communication technology. *European Journal of Information Systems.* doi: doi:10.1057/palgrave.ejis.3000680

Vargas, P. A., Robles, E., Harris, J., & Radford, P. (2010). Using information technology to reduce asthma disparities in underserved populations: A pilot study. *The Journal of Asthma: Official Journal of the Association for the Care of Asthma*, *47*(8), 889–894. doi:10.3109/02770903.2010.497887 PMID:20846082

Vavasseur, C. B., & MacGregor, S. K. (2008). Extending Content-Focused Professional Development through Online Communities of Practice. *Journal of Research on Technology in Education*, *40*(4), 517–536. doi:10.1080/15391523.2008.10782519

Venkatesh, V., Morris, M., & Davis, F. D. (2003). User acceptance of information technology: Toward a unified view. *Management Information Systems Quarterly*, *27*(3), 425.

Vestal, C. (2012). *Medicaid: a year of excruciating decisions.* Retrieved May 17, 2012, from www.stateline.org/live/prntable/story?contentId=624072

Vicente, K. J. (2004). *The human factor: Revolutionizing the way people live with technology.* New York: Routledge.

Vidrine, D. J., Arduino, R. C., & Gritz, E. R. (2006a). Impact of a cell phone intervention on mediating mechanisms of smoking cessation in individuals living with HIV/AIDS. *Nicotine & Tobacco Research: Official Journal of the Society for Research on Nicotine and Tobacco*, *8*(1), S103–S108. doi:10.1080/14622200601039451 PMID:17491177

Vidrine, D. J., Arduino, R. C., Lazev, A. B., & Gritz, E. R. (2006b). A randomized trial of a proactive cellular telephone intervention for smokers living with HIV/AIDS. *AIDS (London, England), 20*(2), 253–260. doi:10.1097/01. aids.0000198094.23691.58 PMID:16511419

Vilkoniene, M. (2009). Influence of augmented reality technology upon pupils' knowledge about human digestive system: The results of the experiment. *US-China Education Review, 6*(1), 36–43.

Vital Wave Consulting. (2009). *mHealth for Development: The Opportunity of Mobile Technology for Healthcare in the Developing World.* United Nations Foundation, Vodafone Foundation.

Vodafone. (2012). *Disease outbreak.* Retrieved May 22, 2013, from http://mhealth.vodafone.com/solutions/access_to_medicine/disease_outbreaks/

Wade, A., Abrami, P., & Sclater, J. (2005). An Electronic Portfolio to Support Learning. *Canadian Journal of Learning and Technology, 31*(3).

Wagner, E. H., Austin, B. T., Davis, C., Hindmarsh, M., Schaefer, J., & Bonomi, A. (2001). Improving chronic illness care: translating evidence into action. *Health Affairs, 20*(6), 64–78. doi:10.1377/hlthaff.20.6.64 PMID:11816692

Wagner, E. H., Austin, B. T., & Von Korff, M. (1996). Improving outcomes in chronic illness. *Managed Care Quarterly, 4*(2), 12–25. PMID:10157259

Walsh, B. (2013). *mHealth market poised for explosive growth.* Retrieved 25 July, from http://www.clinical-innovation.com/topics/mobile-telehealth/mhealth-market-poised-explosive-growth

Walters, B. H. (2012). *Telling Tales: Treatment Stories on an Eating Disorder Support Website.* iPROCEEDINGS Medicine 2.0 Boston. Retrieved from http://www.medicine20congress.com/ocs/index.php/med/med2012/paper/view/924

Wang, D., Kogashiwa, M., Ohta, S., & Kira, S. (2002). Validity and reliability of a dietary assessment method: The application of a digital camera with a mobile phone card attachment. *Journal of Nutritional Science and Vitaminology, 48*(6), 498–504. doi:10.3177/jnsv.48.498 PMID:12775117

Wang, H., Chung, J. E., Park, N., McLaughlin, M. L., & Fulk, J. (2012). Understanding Online Community Participation: A Technology Acceptance Perspective. *Communication Research, 39*(6), 781–801. doi:10.1177/0093650211408593

Wasko, M. M. L., & Faraj, S. (2005). Why should I share? Examining social capital and knowledge contribution in electronic networks of practice. *Management Information Systems Quarterly, 29*(1), 35–57.

Wasko, M. M. L., Teigland, R., & Faraj, S. (2009). The provision of online public goods: Examining social structure in an electronic network of practice. *Decision Support Systems, 47*(3), 254–265. doi:10.1016/j.dss.2009.02.012

Wavecrest Computing. (2009). *Social networking or social not-working?* Retrieved August 3, 2011, from http://www.wavecrest.net/editorial/include/SocialNetworking_SocialNotworking.pdf

WDREC. (2013). *Understanding Dementia Free online course.* Retrieved 23 July 2013, from http://www.utas.edu.au/wicking/wca/mooc

Webb, T. L., Joseph, J., Yardley, L., & Michie, S. (2010). Using the Internet to promote Health Behaviour Change: A systematic review and meta analysis of the impact of theoretical basis, use of behaviour change techniques, and mode of delivery on efficacy. *Journal of Medical Internet Research, 12*(1). doi:10.2196/jmir.1376 PMID:20164043

Wee, C. C., Davis, R. B., & Phillips, R. S. (2005). Stage of readiness to control weight and adopt weight control behaviors in primary care. *Journal of General Internal Medicine, 20*(5), 410–415. doi:10.1111/j.1525-1497.2005.0074.x PMID:15963162

Weinger, M. B., Gardner-Bonneau, D., & Wiklund, M. E. (2011). *Handbook of human factors in medical device design.* Boca Raton, FL: CRC Press.

Weitzel, M., Smith, A., Lee, D., de Deugd, S., & Helal, S. (2009). Participatory Medicine: Leveraging Social Networks in Telehealth Solutions. In *Ambient Assistive Health and Wellness Management in the Heart of the City (LNCS)* (Vol. 5597, pp. 40–47). Berlin: Springer. doi:10.1007/978-3-642-02868-7_6

Wenger, E. (1998). *Communities of practice: Learning, meaning, and identity*. Cambridge Univ Pr. doi:10.1017/CBO9780511803932

Wenger, E. (2004). Knowledge management as a doughnut: Shaping your knowledge strategy through communities of practice. *Ivey Business Journal, 68*(3), 1–8.

Wenger, E., McDermott, R., & Snyder, W. M. (2002). *Cultivating communities of practice: A guide to managing knowledge*. Cambridge, MA: Harvard University Press.

West, D., & Miller, E. (2006). The digital divide in public e-health: Barriers to accessibility and privacy in state health department web sites. *Journal of Health Care for the Poor and Underserved, 17*(3), 652–667. doi:10.1353/hpu.2006.0115 PMID:16960328

While, A., & Dewsberry, G. (2011). Nursing and information and communication technology (ICT), A discussion of trends and future directions. *International Journal of Nursing Studies, 48*(10), 1302–1310. doi:10.1016/j.ijnurstu.2011.02.020 PMID:21474135

Whitaker, J. (2008). *Health Privacy: What Consumers Want*. Retrieved 17 December 2012, from http://www.privacy.org.au/Papers/HealthInfoPrivacy-081110.pdf

White, G. (2008). *Digital learning: An Australian research agenda*. Retrieved 24 July 2013, from www.acer.edu.au/documents/TLL_DigitalLearningResearch.doc

White, R. W., & Horvitz, E. (2009). Cybercondria: Studies of the escalation of the medical concerns in web search. *ACM Transactions on Information Systems, 27*(4), 1–37. doi:10.1145/1629096.1629101

WHO. (1948). *Preamble to the constitution of the World Health Organization as adopted by the International Health Conference, New York, 19-22 June, 1946, signed on 22 July 1946 by the representatives of 61 states (official records of the World Health Organization, no. 2, p. 100) and entered into force on 7 April 1948*. WHO.

WHO. (2011). *mHealth: New Horizons for health through mobile technologies: Second survey on ehealth*. Retrieved 23 July 2013, from http://www.who.int/goe/publications/goe_mhealth_web.pdf

Wicklund, R. (2013). When mhealth and telehealth become just healthcare. *Government Health IT*. Retrieved 26 July 2013, from http://www.govhealthit.com/news/when-mhealth-and-telehealth-become-just-healthcare

Wicks, P., Massagli, M., Frost, J., Brownstein, C., Okun, S., & Vaughan, T. et al. (2010). Sharing Health Data for Better Outcomes on PatientsLikeMe. *Journal of Medical Internet Research, 12*(2), e19. doi:10.2196/jmir.1549 PMID:20542858

Wiklund, M. E., & Wilcox, S. B. (2005). *Designing usability into medical products*. Boca Raton, FL: Taylor & Francis/CRC Press. doi:10.1201/9781420038088

Wilkins, C., Casswell, S., Barnes, H. M., & Pledger, M. (2003). A pilot study of a computer assisted cell phone interview (CACI) methodology to survey respondents in households without telephones about alcohol use. *Drug and Alcohol Review, 22*(2), 221–225. doi:10.1080/09595230100100651 PMID:12850908

Windham, C. (2005). The Student's Perspective. *Educating the Net Generation, Educause*. Retrieved 14 February 2010, from www.educause.edu/educatingthenetgen

Wisconsin Department of Health Services. (2011). *Wisconsin Environmental Public Health Tracking*. Retrieved June 8, 2011, from http://www.dhs.wisconsin.gov/epht/DataInfo.htm

Wolf, J. A., Moreau, J. F., Akilov, O., Patton, T., English, J. C. III, Ho, J., & Ferris, L. K. (2013). Diagnostic inaccuracy of smartphone applications for melanoma detection. *JAMA Dermatology, 149*(4), 422–426. doi:10.1001/jamadermatol.2013.2382 PMID:23325302

Wong, D. H., Gallegos, Y., Weinger, M. B., Clack, S., Slagle, J., & Anderson, C. T. (2003). Changes in intensive care unit nurse task activity after installation of a third-generation intensive care unit information system. *Critical Care Medicine, 31*(10), 2488–2494. doi:10.1097/01.CCM.0000089637.53301.EF PMID:14530756

Woodfin, G. (2011). *How to find your twitter RSS Feed & Profile ID Number*. Retrieved August 25, 2011, from http://www.glenwoodfin.com/rss/how-to-find-your-twitter-rss-feed-in-2011/

Woods, D. D., & Hollnagel, E. (2006). *Joint cognitive systems: Patterns in cognitive systems engineering.* Boca Raton, FL: CRC/Taylor & Francis. doi:10.1201/9781420005684

Woodward, H., & Nanlohy, P. (2004). Digital portfolios: Fact or fashion? *Assessment & Evaluation in Higher Education, 29*(2), 228–238. doi:10.1080/0260293042000188492

World Bank. (2012). *Information and Communications for Development 2012: Maximizing Mobile.* Washington, DC: World Bank.

World Fact Book, C. I. A. (2012). The World Factbook Environment: Current issues. *Central Intelligence Agency.* Retrieved June 7 2011, from https://www.cia.gov/library/publications/the-world-factbook/fields/2032.html

World Health Organization. (2005). Malaysia Environmental Health Country Profile. *World Health Organization.* Retrieved June 8, 2011, from http://www.environment-health.asia/fileupload/malaysia_ehcp_07Oct2004.pdf

World Health Organization. (2008). *Foodborne disease outbreaks: Guidelines for investigation and control.* Retrieved August 29, 2011, from http://www.who.int/foodsafety/publications/foodborne_disease/outbreak_guidelines.pdf

World Health Organization. (2011). *Mhealth: New Horizons for Health Through Mobile Technologies.* Retrieved from http://www.himss.org/content/files/Code%20491%20-%20mHealth-New%20horizons%20for%20health%20through%20mobile%20technologies_WHO_2011.pdf

Wu, L., Forbes, A., Griffiths, P., Milligan, P., & While, A. A. (2010). Telephone follow-up to improve glycaemic control in patients with type 2 diabetes: Systematic review and meta-analysis of controlled trials. *Diabetic Medicine, 27*(11), 1217–1225. doi:10.1111/j.1464-5491.2010.03113.x PMID:20950378

Wu, X., Gu, Z., & Wei, Z. (2008). The construction of innovation networks and the development of technological capabilities of industrial clusters in China. *International Journal of Innovation and Technology Management, 5*(2), 179–199. doi:10.1142/S0219877008001321

Yambem, L., Yapici, M. K., & Zou, J. (2008). A new wireless sensor system for smart diapers. *IEEE Sensors Journal, 8*(3), 238–239. doi:10.1109/JSEN.2008.917122

Yamout, S. Z., Glick, Z. A., Lind, D. S., Monson, R. A. Z., & Glick, P. L. (2011). Using Social Media to enhance surgeon and patient education and communication. *Bulletin of the American College of Surgeons, 96*(7), 7–15. PMID:22315896

Yardley, L., Morrison, L. G., Andreou, P., Joseph, J., & Little, P. (2010). Understanding reactions to an Internet delivered healthcare intervention: Accommodating user preferences for information provision. *BMC Medical Informatics and Decision Making,* (1): 52. doi:10.1186/1472-6947-10-52 PMID:20849599

Year of the Big EHR Switch Confirms Physicians Favor iPad and Mobile Applications . (2013, May 30). Retrieved from http://www.prweb.com/releases/2013/5/prweb10553455.htm?PID=6150547

Yu, T. K., Lu, L. C., & Liu, T. F. (2010). Exploring factors that influence knowledge sharing behavior via weblogs. *Computers in Human Behavior, 26*(1), 32–41. doi:10.1016/j.chb.2009.08.002

Zayas-Caban, T., & Dixon, B. E. (2010). Considerations for the design of safe and effective consumer health IT applications in the home. *Quality & Safety in Health Care, 19*(Suppl 3), i61–i67. doi:10.1136/qshc.2010.041897 PMID:20959321

Zhang, J., Shi, H., & Zhang, Y. (2009). Self-organizing map methodology and Google maps services for geographical epidemiology mapping. In *Proceedings of Digital Image Computing: Technique and Application 2009* (DICTA '09) (pp. 229-235). DICTA. doi:10.1109/DICTA.2009.4610.1109/DICTA.2009.46

Zhang, T., Wang, J., Liu, P., & Hou, J. (2006). Fall detection by embedding an accelerometer in cellphone and using KFD algorithm. *International Journal of Computer Science and Network Security, 6*(10), 277–284.

Zhang, W., & Watts, S. (2003). Knowledge adoption in online communities of practice.[ICIS.]. *Proceedings of ICIS, 2003,* 96–109.

Zhang, Y., Fang, Y., Wei, K.-K., & Chen, H. (2010). Exploring the role of psychological safety in promoting the intention to continue sharing knowledge in virtual communities. *International Journal of Information Management*, *30*(5), 425–436. doi:10.1016/j.ijinfomgt.2010.02.003

Zickuhr, K., & Madden, M. (2012). *Older adults and Internet use*. Pew Internet & American Life Project. Retrieved from http://pewinternet.org/Reports/2012/Older-Adults-and-Internet-Use.aspx

Zvarova, K., Ursiny, M., Giebink, T., Liang, K., Blaivas, J. G., & Zvara, P. (2011). Recording urinary flow and lower urinary tract symptoms using sonouroflowmetry. *The Canadian Journal of Urology*, *18*(3), 5689–5694. PMID:21703041

Zviran, M., & Erlich, Z. (2003). Measuring IS User Satisfaction: Review and Implications. *Communications of the Association for Information Systems*, *12*(5), 81–104.

About the Contributors

Mowafa Househ is an Assistant Professor and former Research Director at the College of Public Health and Health Informatics, King Saud bin Abdulaziz University for Health Sciences, National Guard Health Affairs, Riyadh, Kingdom of Saudi Arabia. Dr. Househ is also an adjunct professor at the University Of Victoria, School of Health Information Science, BC, Canada and is the editor-in-chief of the *Journal of Health Informatics in Developing Countries*. Dr. Househ's primary research interests are on the use of information and communication technologies to empower patients and clinicians. His doctoral work focused on the empowerment of pharmacists, physicians, and academics in the use of collaborative technologies to facilitate knowledge translation research. His current work revolves on empowering patients through the use of social media, mobile health, and personal health records. Dr. Househ is a respected and published author within health informatics community. He has published in leading health informatics journals such as the *International Journal of Medical Informatics, The Yearbook of Medical Informatics*, and *Applied Clinical Informatics*.

Elizabeth Borycki, RN, PhD, is an Associate Professor in the School of Health Information Science and an Adjunct in Nursing at the University of Victoria. Elizabeth is a health informatics expert who conducts research in the areas of clinical informatics, patient safety, quality improvement, and organizational behaviour and change management involving Health Information Technology (HIT). Elizabeth employs qualitative, quantitative, and mixed methods approaches in her study of the effects of HIT upon patients, caregivers, and clinicians (e.g. physicians, nurses). She has represented Canada (as academic representative) and North America (member of the board of directors) to the International Medical Informatics Association, and her work is known internationally.

Andre Kushniruk is a Professor at the School of Health Information Science at the University of Victoria in Canada. Dr. Kushniruk conducts research in a number of areas including evaluation of the effects of technology, human-computer interaction in healthcare and other domains, as well as cognitive science. His work is known internationally, and he has published widely in the area of health informatics. Dr. Kushniruk has held academic positions at a number of Canadian universities and worked with major hospitals in both Canada, the United States, and internationally. He holds undergraduate degrees in Psychology and Biology, as well as a MSc in Computer Science from McMaster University and a PhD in Cognitive Psychology from McGill University.

* * *

Haitham Alali is a chief knowledge officer in Balqa Health Directorate at Ministry of Health/ Hashemite Kingdom of Jordan. He received his Doctorate in MIS from the Universiti Kebangsaan Malaysia (UKM), Department of Systems Science and Management, Faculty of Information Science and Technology, and holds an MMIS from the University of Banking and Financial Sciences. Prior to getting his doctorate, he had worked in healthcare services and management for nine years. His research interests include knowledge management in healthcare sector, development of virtual communities of practice, strategic human resource management of healthcare professionals, medical informatics, and collaborative systems.

Urs-Vito Albrecht is Deputy Director of the Peter L. Reichertz Institute for Medical Informatics of Braunschweig Technical University and Hannover Medical School in Hannover and Principal Investigator for mHealth at this facility. He leads the multidisciplinary research group PLRI MedAppLab that is focused on research questions on ethical, legal, and technical aspects of using smart devices and apps in the medical field. Urs is a physician by profession who gained his work experience in several medical disciplines ranging from Emergency Medicine to Forensic Medicine. He holds a doctorate in Medicine and a degree in Public Health with focus on Public Health Ethics and Epidemiology. Urs is Secretray of the Institutional Review Board at Hannover Medical School and a coeditor of several medical informatics journals with the scope encompassing mHealth.

Shilo Anders, PhD, has conducted research and specialized training in human factors engineering and health services research and applied these principles to medical and military contexts. Her research has explored the needs, adaptations, and interactions in systems as the environment and tools evolve, specifically medical informatics. She conducted research in user interface design and evaluation, patient safety, coordination, and decision making during her academic career and has continued this line of research in the private sector. Dr. Anders is a human factors engineer at Applied Research Associates. Prior to her current position, she was a National Library of Medicine postdoctoral fellow and assistant professor in Vanderbilt University's Departments of Biomedical Informatics and Anesthesiology and part of the Center for Research and Innovation in Systems Safety (CRISS).

Sharazade (Shari) Balouchi is an undergraduate student at Sewanee: The University of the South in Tennessee, where she pursues an International and Global Studies degree with minors in Economics and in Physics/Astronomy. Shari has worked with InfoClin as an undergraduate intern for 2 years, during which time she has created an e-marketing campaign, developed software architecture, and managed data for the company. She also designed an electronic poster entitled *Creating Infrastructure and Evaluating the Market for Patient eTools in Healthcare* for the eHealth 2013 Conference on Accelerating Change. As a student of international studies, she is passionate about communicating global issues such as health, energy, and promoting crosscultural understanding. She recently studied in Africa focusing on alternative energy physics and taking up another language. In her spare moments, Shari is an enthusiastic science writer and served as an editorial intern in 2013 for the astronomical magazine *Sky & Telescope*.

Tridib Bandyopadhyay is an Associate Professor and Program Director of Information Systems at Coles College of Business in Kennesaw State University. He is also a continuing Faculty Research Associate of The KSU Center for Information Security Education. He earned his PhD in MIS from

The University of Texas at Dallas. He teaches both undergrad and grad course in Systems Analysis and Design, Information Security, Emerging Technologies and Innovations in the BSIS, BSISA, and MSIS programs of Kennesaw State University. Dr. Bandyopadhyay's research interests include Information Security and Assurance, Cyber Insurance, Cyber Terrorism, and ICT in Development including health issues. Dr. Bandy welcomes collaborative research and has worked with professors and students from universities in US and Africa. His research works have been published in peer-reviewed journals like ISF, CACM, ITM, IJICTE, and also in the proceedings of national and international conferences. Before coming to academics, he worked as a Manager (Planning and Systems) in the Energy Sector.

Jeff Barnett joined the BC Cancer Agency in 1982. Initially, he was a clinical pharmacist and Director of Pharmacy at the Vancouver Island Cancer Centre. In 2007, he completed a Master's of Science in Health Informatics at the University of Victoria and became the Director of Clinical Informatics for the BC Cancer Agency. He was involved in a number of informatics projects and worked on a variety of clinical systems. Jeff recently retired from the BC Cancer Agency but continues to be active in research and teaching in clinical informatics. He is an adjunct assistant professor in the School of Health Information Science at the University of Victoria and an instructor in the Masters of Health Administration, School of Population and Public Health at the University of British Columbia.

Tshepo Batane is a Senior Lecturer in the Department of Educational Technology at the University of Botswana. She received her PhD in Curriculum and Instruction with specialization in Instructional Technology from Ohio University in the United States in June 2002. Dr. Batane is currently Head of the Department of Educational Technology and teaches courses in technology application to learning. Her research interests are centered around exploring innovative ways of utilizing technology to improve different aspects of life. This has included integration of technology into the curriculum, preparing teachers to use technology in their classrooms, and utilization of technology to improve healthcare. Currently, Dr. Batane is working on research that explores the applicability of Activity Theory frameworks to improve technology adoption in various contexts.

Lau Tiu Chung completed his Master of Science by research at Swinburne University of Technology in 2013. Prior to his Master degree, he completed a Bachelor degree in Business Information System from the same University in 2009. His research interest includes environmental health data mining and knowledge discovery and develops applications to improve the public health. He has published various articles in peer-reviewed journals, book chapters, and conference papers.

Elisabetta Cioni (PhD) is full professor of Sociology of Culture and Communication at the Department of Political Sciences, Communication Sciences and Information Engineering (University of Sassari, Italy). She teaches "Strategy of Public Communication," "Public Communication," and "Communication and Organization." Among her research interests are public communication, health communication, sociology of family, and new forms of participation enabled by digital technologies. Her research approach prefers mixed-methods, by integrating qualitative instruments, in particular in-depth interview and participant observation, with the secondary analysis of quantitative data.

Elizabeth Cummings, RN, RM, BA, BIS(Hons), PhD, is currently a Senior Lecturer and Graduate Research Coordinator in the School of Health Sciences (Nursing), and coordinator of the University of Tasmania eHealth Research Centre, at the University of Tasmania. She is a registered Nurse and Midwife with 35 years experience in the health sector including acute and primary care, administration, and education. She has significant experience in ehealth implementation and evaluation and has worked in the area of health informatics for over 12 years. She has significant experience in a diverse range of research relating to ICTs in health and ageing, patient-centred chronic disease self-management, and the use of qualitative methods for evaluation of health information systems. She has been involved in a European Commission-funded project on ICT and ageing.

Kerstin Denecke is scientific director of the Digital Patient Modeling group at ICCAS at the Medical Faculty of the University of Leipzig. Dr. Denecke holds a Diploma in Computer Science and was awarded a Doctoral degree in Computer Science by the Technical University of Braunschweig. Before she joined the University of Leipzig, she worked as a researcher at L3S research center and as a software architect at an IT company providing software for hospitals. She coordinated several research projects, among others the EU-funded project M-Eco: Medical Ecosystem on event-driven surveillance of infectious diseases and was involved in the EU Projects Terence and LivingKnowledge. Her main research interests are natural language processing and text and data mining. The specific areas she has been working on include medical language processing, information extraction, sentiment analysis, and text classification. She has published a number of research papers in several international conferences and journals.

Judith W. Dexheimer, PhD, is a Research Assistant Professor in the divisions of Emergency Medicine and Biomedical Informatics at Cincinnati Children's Medical Center. Judith is an informatics expert who conducts research in clinical decision support, computerized applications for emergency medicine, and evidence-based medicine. She has a background in developing and implementing clinical informatics applications including organizational and workflow aspects of integration and development, emergency medicine, guideline integration and implementation, and evidence-based medicine.

Leonie Ellis, B Com, BComp(Hons), PhD, is currently a Senior Lecturer and Graduate Research Coordinator in the School of Engineering and ICT at the University of Tasmania. She is a qualitative researcher and is a member of the eHealth Research Methods Group within the school with a special interest in Social Media and eHealth. She has experience in a diverse range of research relating to eHealth, Social Media, and ICT in Education. Her PhD investigated the implementation of technology in a paramilitary organisation.

Ute von Jan received her computer science diploma in 1997 from the University of Hildesheim and started working at the Medical Computing Center of Hannover Medical School. In 2000, she transferred to the Institute of Medical Informatics, which later merged with the Institute of Medical Informatics at the University of Braunschweig under the name of "Peter L. Reichertz Institute for Medical Informatics." Until a few years ago, she specialized in medical image processing, and in 2007, she finished her doctoral thesis in this area. Currently, she is a member of the PLRI MedAppLab research group that concentrates on ethical, legal, and technical issues of using mobile smartdevices in the medical field.

Karim Keshavjee is a family physician with a part-time practice in Ontario Canada. Karim has over 20 years of experience with designing, developing, researching, and implementing electronic medical records. He has consulted with many organizations and has presented on EMRs at national and international conferences. Karim has designed and implemented several clinical decision support tools in primary care and is particularly interested in how technology can better support the patient-physician interaction. Karim is an Associate Member of the Centre for Evaluation of Medicines at McMaster University and an Adjunct Assistant Professor at the University of Victoria.

Alessandro Lovari (Ph.D) is an assistant professor of Sociology of Culture and Communication at the University of Sassari's Department of Political Sciences, Sciences of Communication, and Information Engineering, where he teaches Corporate Communication and Social Media for Public Administrations. He has been a visiting scholar at the Department of Communication at Purdue University (USA). His main research interests are public communication, public relations, and the relationships between institutions, media, and citizens. He also studies the characteristics of Web 2.0 and social media and their impact on healthcare organizations, and on citizens' behaviors.

Carey Mather, RN, BSc, PGrad Dip Hlth Prom, GradCert ULT, GradCert Creative Media Tech, MPH, is a lecturer and PhD candidate in the School of Health Sciences (Nursing) at the University of Tasmania. Carey has worked in the health sector for 28 years in various capacities and settings including the acute, palliative, health promotion, and community environments. During 2010, as part of her role as the Teaching Fellow, Emerging Technologies, she investigated innovative technologies including e-portfolios to facilitate the learning and teaching of undergraduate students. Recently, she has been involved with facilitating high quality work integrated learning experiences for students. Part of this work has focused on the needs of clinical supervisors and the development of salient mobile learning strategies to support them in their role.

Ramona McNeal is an associate professor in the Department of Political Science at the University of Northern Iowa. Her chief research interest is the impact of technology on participation, including its relationship to voting, elections, and public opinion. She also studies e-government, campaign finance reform, telehealth and telecommunication policy. She has published work in a number of journals including the *Journal of Information Technology & Politics*, *Social Science Quarterly*, *Political Research Quarterly*, *Government Information Quarterly,* and *Telemedicine and E-Health.* She is a co-author of *Digital Citizenship: The Internet, Society and Participation* (MIT Press, 2007) with Karen Mossberger and Caroline Tolbert.

Helen Monkman is a PhD Candidate at the School of Health Information Science at the University of Victoria in Canada. She earned her BSc and MA in Psychology from Carleton University. Helen has a passion for research in consumer health informatics. She is an advocate for the importance of design in lowering demands on health literacy and optimizing usability in systems for laypeople. Helen has collaborated on a wide range of projects with various Canadian health organizations. These projects have included research on and evaluation of public health information systems, personal health records, electronic medication reconciliation, and human aspects of system interoperability.

Chris Paton is a researcher at the University of Oxford and is the founder of New Media Medicine Ltd., a digital health company that develops Massive Open Online Courses (MOOCs), e-learning, mHealth, and social media projects for the healthcare industry. He trained as a medical doctor in the UK and has worked for the NHS, Cambridge University, and Oxford University in clinical and academic roles. He has also spent several years in New Zealand working as a Senior Research Fellow for the National Institute for Health Innovation at the University of Auckland where he earned his Executive MBA.

Oliver Pramann is an attorney at law specialized in medical law, namely in pharmaceutical law and law concerning medical devices within the context of clinical trial regulation. Since 2008, Oliver Pramann has been working in this field as a fully qualified lawyer. He earned his doctorate in 2006 with a legal dissertation about publication policies in clinical study agreements. Before then, he was educated at the Georg August University in Göttingen and worked at the local Centre for Medical Law. As a consultant of the PLRI MedAppLab research group that concentrates on ethical, legal, and technical issues of using mobile smart devices in the medical field, he associates his interests in law concerning medical informatics and his experiences as a lawyer in the fields he is specialized in.

Shaina Reid is a passionate healthcare information technology Professional and Project Manager with over 10 years of experience in clinical informatics. Currently, Shaina represents IMITS as the Senior Manager of Clinical and Systems Transformation Project, aiming to transform care delivery and clinical information systems across Provincial Health Services Authority, Vancouver Coastal Health Authority, and Providence Health Care in BC. Additionally, she is responsible for oversight on various other related clinical information system projects across PHSA. Specializing in project planning, workflow analysis, requirements gathering, system design, clinician engagement, and change management, Shaina has successfully led and managed large-scale clinical information systems and technology projects across British Columbia, Canada, and the United States.

Juhana Salim is a professor at the Faculty of Information Science and Technology, PhD (Infomration Science – Universiti Kebangsaan Malaysia), Masters of Science in Librarianship (Western Michigan University, Kalamazoo), Bachelor of Arts (Western Michigan University, Kalamazoo). Her research interests include strategic information system, knowledge technology, and information science.

Mary Schmeida, PhD, has served as a researcher for several organizations in the United States and is also affiliated with Kent State University, USA. She holds a doctoral degree in Political Science, Public Policy. Her research areas of expertise are information technology and mobile health, telehealth, social and welfare policy in the U.S., healthcare reform policy, mental health policy, and rural health disparities. Her research has been published in scholarly books and journals and presented to national and international professional audiences.

Lee Seldon currently teaches near the Straits of Malacca in West Malaysia. Before that, he worked in Sarawak on the northwest edge of Borneo. Before that, he was a Senior Lecturer (for Health Informatics) at Monash University's Frankston campus in Australia. Before that, he worked as a telemedicine consultant for a company in Melbourne. Before that, he was a Senior Research Fellow associated with the

Australian Bionic Ear Institute. Before that, he was an ENT resident at University Hospital in Cologne, Germany. Before that, he was a student of medicine, a postgrad student of biology, an undergraduate student of physics in, respectively, Cologne, West Berlin, and Cambridge, Massachusetts.

Lau Bee Theng completed her PhD in 2006. Presently, she is a senior lecturer and ICT program coordinator at Faculty of Engineering, Computing, and Science, Swinburne University of Technology, Sarawak Campus. Her research interest is mainly on assistive technologies utilizing ICT for the special people. She has published more than 60 articles in peer-reviewed journals, book chapters, and conference papers. She has successfully supervised postgraduate students to completion and coordinated a few research projects on assistive technologies for special children, injury recognition and activity monitoring using multi depth sensors, wireless, and Bluetooth devices, and brain interfaced human-computer interaction.

Eh Eh Tin is a student at the University of Tasmania, Australia. He studied Information Systems and received his BA (Hons) from University of Tasmania. His special interests include systems analysis, business analysis, data management, information security, health informatics, and consulting business professionals on how to design and implement information systems. His previous research was on transforming paper tools into electronic in aged care policy setting. Mr. Tin moved to Australia with his wife and son as refugees in 2008. He was born in a small village called Kawh Pawn in Myanmar, and he spent many years fleeing from civil war. His education was interrupted as he often had to hide in the jungles during Myanmar's civil war. When was asked how he feels to be in Australia, he said, "God blessed me so much by bringing me to Australia, which I consider a paradise." He is an IT consultant for a small legal firm in Tasmania and also teaches computer basics to refugees from Myanmar.

Jastinder Toor has over eight years of Project Management experience through a variety of jobs in multiple sectors. She has a Bachelor of Technology from Ryerson University and a Diploma in Health Informatics from Centennial College. She is currently looking to make her mark in the health informatics field. She is passionate about improving quality of care and empowering patients to take charge of their own health.

Paul Turner, PhD, MSc, BA(Hons), MACS, is currently A/Professor and Research Coordinator (ICT Disciplines) in the School of Engineering and ICT at the University of Tasmania. He is Director, eHealth Services Research group and eLogistics Research group at the University of Tasmania. He has published more than 175 peer-reviewed papers, obtained more than $7.5m research funding, and supervised to graduation 15 PhDs in the last 10 years. In the domain of eHealth, he has a focus on human-centred systems, quality and safety systems, and the development, implementation, and evaluation of health information systems across primary and acute care.

Karim Vassanji is an experienced health professional with a special interest in process design and clinical architecture. His clinical background as a dentist both in the United Kingdom and Portugal has provided him with the necessary skills to understand information requirements in healthcare settings, and the ability to integrate information technologies for the betterment of the care provided. Karim holds a post-graduate diploma in Health Services Management and is currently pursuing a Masters in eHealth from McMaster University in Canada. Karim is especially interested in mobile technology that can assist a variety of healthcare providers and patients simultaneously, as means to empower patients and caregivers as well as foster relationships, reducing perceived boundaries. Karim believes that technology can only be as good as our understanding of human behavior.

John Waldron is a health informatics professional with broad experience in both public and private-sector healthcare organizations. John's focus has been on clinical system requirements, design, development, and integration, most recently as the Director of Enterprise Architecture and Security for a large health service provider. John strives to bridge the gap between the business of healthcare and the technologies needed to deliver on those objectives.

Jonn Wu joined the BC Cancer Agency in 1999 and is a radiation oncologist at the Vancouver Cancer Centre. His research interests include developing a provincial platform to support population-based oncology outcomes research (OaSIS), as well as developing novel computerized radiotherapy planning and delivery systems. He is the Provincial H&N Tumour Group Chair and the Chief Medical Information Officer for the BC Cancer Agency.

Bahman E. Zadeh is a Graduate Research Assistant in the Department of Information Systems at Kennesaw State University. In 2009, he earned his Bachelor of Science Degree in Computer Science with minor in Information Systems from Kennesaw State University. He also was awarded a Master of Science in Information Systems from Kennesaw State University in 2012. He currently is working as a software developer focusing on distributed computer systems in Atlanta area. Mr. Zadeh's main research interest lies with the design and implementation of image processing in healthcare and adoption of mobile technology for healthcare delivery. As a result of his existing research work, he was petitioned by Well Star Health Group for a research project, which he is currently working on.

Ahmad M Zbib MD, CPHIMS-CA, is a non-practicing physician and entrepreneur, passionate about putting technology to meaningful use in healthcare. Ahmad is a digital health strategist leading Canada's longest running consumer ehealth program within a non-profit organization. He currently is responsible for a suite of evidence-informed online health behaviour change tools and disease management portals. Ahmad's expertise is unique, combining a medical education with professional certification in healthcare information management. He is considered one of Canada's thought leaders in digital health matters including mobile health solutions.

Index